TIBIAL PLATEAU FRACTURES

TIBIAL PLATEAU FRACTURES

John T. Riehl, MD

Orthopaedic Surgery
Texas Bone and Joint
Coastal Orthopaedic Trauma
Dallas, Texas, USA

ELSEVIER

Elsevier
1600 John F. Kennedy Blvd.
Ste 1800
Philadelphia, PA 19103-2899

Tibial Plateau Fractures, FIRST EDITION
ISBN: 978-0-323-82568-9

ISBN: 978-0-323-82568-9

Content Strategist: Belinda Kuhn
Content Development Specialist: Ranjana Sharma
Publishing Services Manager: Shereen Jameel
Project Manager: Nadhiya Sekar
Design Direction: Ryan Cook

Printed in India

Last digit is the print number: 9 8 7 6 5 4 3 2 1

LIST OF CONTRIBUTORS

J.D. Adams, MD
Assistant Professor
Department of Orthopedic Surgery
Prisma Health
Greenville
SC
USA

Jesse Jay Caballero, MD
Resident
Orthopaedics
Indiana University School of Medicine
Indianapolis
IN
USA

James Gainer, MD
University of Louisville

Brandi Hartley, MD
Program Director, Assistant Professor
Orthopaedic Surgery
University of Louisville
Louisville
KY
USA

Yohan Jang, DO, FAAOS
Assistant Professor
Orthopaedic Surgery
Indiana University, School of Medicine
Indianapolis
IN
USA

Daniel Oscar Johansen, MD
Orthopaedic Surgery
Department of Orthopaedic Surgery
UCLA
Los Angeles
CA
USA

Adam D. Kessler, D.O.
Orthopedic Traumatologist
Deptarment of Orthopedics
Freeman Hospital-West
Joplin
MO
USA

Christopher Lee, MD
Assistant Professor
Orthopaedic Surgery
UCLA
Los Angeles
CA
USA

Travis Parkulo, MD, MS
MD
Orthopaedic Surgery
University of Louisville
Louisville
KY
USA

Cassandra Anne Ricketts, BS, MD
Orthopaedic Surgery Resident
Orthopaedic Surgery
Geisinger
Danville
PA
USA

John T. Riehl, MD
Orthopaedic Surgeon and CEO
Orthopaedic Surgery
Coastal Orthopaedic Trauma
Dallas
TX
USA

Adam A. Sassoon, MD, MS
Associate Professor
Orthopaedic Surgery
UCLA
Santa Monica
CA
USA

Abhijit Seetharam, MD
Resident Physician
Orthopaedic Surgery
Indiana University School of Medicine
Indianapolis
IN
USA

David Seligson, MD
Professor
Orthopedics
University of Louisville
Louisville
KY
USA

Brendan Shi, MD
Resident Physician
Orthopaedic Surgery
UCLA Medical Center
Los Angeles
CA
USA

Jan Szatkowski, MD, MBA
Assistant Professor, Chief of Foot and Ankle
Orthopedic Surgery
Indiana University
Indianapolis
USA

James Widmaier Jr., MD
Physician
Orthopaedic Trauma
Geisinger Medical Center
Danville
PA
USA

PREFACE

Tibial plateau fractures present a challenging and diverse array of clinical problems to the treating surgeon. The approach, reduction strategy, and fixation can vary widely from fracture to fracture and from patient to patient. When you add to that the recent advances in precontoured plating for the tibial plateau coupled with advances in soft tissue management around the knee, tibial plateau fractures constitute a complex injury worthy of an entire textbook devoted to the evaluation, initial management, definitive management, and aftercare.

Tibial Plateau Fractures has been written to provide a single text that covers every aspect of treatment of these complex fractures with a focus on practical clinical knowledge. Modern treatment strategies have been clearly defined based on recent literature and cutting-edge fixation techniques. Case examples and high yield points are highlighted at the end of every chapter in order to help the reader come away with the most crucial aspects of care as determined by the surgeon experts who have authored each chapter. Reduction techniques for percutaneous and open surgical treatment of these fractures has been emphasized. Additionally, an entire chapter has been devoted to soft tissue injuries that occur in conjunction with tibial plateau fractures. This is an important distinction from other books, chapters, and journal articles, on the subject, as soft tissue injuries are often overlooked in prior works with a focus on the bony injury only. Untreated soft tissue injuries can be a source of long-term disability and poor outcomes in these multifaceted injuries. This book intends to help the reader identify all aspects of care in the treatment of tibial plateau fractures and help the surgeon to achieve the best possible outcome.

I am greatly indebted to the contributors for all of their hard work in putting together each chapter. The time, effort, dedication, and expertise involved is tremendous, and their commitment to education and advancement in the field of orthopaedics is acknowledged and appreciated. Additional thanks are due to the publisher Elsevier and the personnel who have worked to produce a final product that is now available as a clear and concise text to help the reader in treating their patients. Finally, I would like to thank my friends, mentors, colleagues, operating room and clinic staff, and loved ones for their support and encouragement they have given me throughout my career.

I hope you enjoy *Tibial Plateau Fractures* and I wish you great success in the treatment of all your patients.

John Riehl, M.D.
www.johnriehl.com

"The price of success is hard work, dedication to the job at hand, and the determination that whether we win or lose, we have applied the best of ourselves to the task at hand." -Vince Lombardi

CONTENTS

1

Anatomy and Surgical Approaches

John T. Riehl, MD

INTRODUCTION

The anatomy of the proximal tibia involves a complex interaction between bone, ligaments and their attachment sites, cartilage, and muscles. The knee is an intricate hinge joint consisting of the tibia, femur, and patella. Ligamentous and muscular attachment sites also include the proximal fibula. Rather than being a purely rotational motion around a fixed axis, the tibiofemoral articulation involves posterior translation of the femoral condyles in relation to the tibia during flexion. This phenomenon is often termed "posterior rollback" and permits higher degrees of knee flexion by preventing impingement between the posterior tibial plateau and posterior distal femur. Additionally, when going into full knee extension, the distal femur articular surface internally rotates in relation to the tibial plateau. This is termed the "screw-home mechanism" and helps provide stability to the knee in full extension.[1,2] This occurs partly as a result of the bony anatomy in the knee, with the lateral femoral condyle being larger than the medial condyle from anterior to posterior, and the medial condyle extending further distally than the lateral condyle.

The undersurface of the patella articulates with the femur and provides additional torque for knee extension. Normal patella height is such that on a lateral x-ray with the knee in 30 degrees of flexion, the distal pole of the patella should rest at or slightly proximal to the tibiofemoral joint line. Forces transmitted across the patellofemoral joint can reach magnitudes of 3 times body weight during normal activities of daily living and can approach up to 20 times body weight during sporting activities.[3,4]

RELEVANT SURGICAL ANATOMY

The tibia is a long bone that is somewhat triangular in shape when viewed in an axial plane. The proximal tibia widens significantly when going proximally from the diaphysis to the metaphysis and articular surface. The articular surface ranges in width from approximately 75 to 90 mm at its maximum, and these will be common screw lengths used in fixation of tibial plateau fractures. The articular surface width of the proximal tibia closely matches or is slightly wider than the articular width of the distal femur.[5,6] The medial and lateral tibial plateau are asymmetric with the lateral plateau being slightly proximal and concave compared to the medial surface. Although it can vary among individuals, the posterior slope of the tibial articular surface in the sagittal plane is approximately 10°. Separating the medial and lateral articular surfaces of the proximal tibia are the medial and lateral tibial spines (also referred to as the intercondylar eminence). The tibial spines are two surface projections in the midline of the plateau that are points of attachment for the menisci, anteriorly as the attachment point for the anterior cruciate ligament (ACL) and posteriorly as the attachment site for the posterior cruciate ligament (PCL). The intercondylar eminence does not come into contact with the distal femur under normal loading conditions and as such is void of hyaline cartilage.

The articular surface is covered by two C-shaped rings, the medial and lateral menisci. The menisci contain attachments to the periphery of the tibial plateau through coronary (or meniscotibial) ligaments. The lateral meniscus is larger and more mobile than the medial meniscus. The menisci increase articular congruency in the knee and help to transmit load across the knee. They are made up primarily of type I collagen and have a blood supply that is greater in the periphery than in the interior of the ring. Blood supply for the menisci comes from the middle and inferior genicular arteries and from diffusion.

The proximal tibial metaphysis serves as an attachment site for several important structures (Figs. 1.1–1.3). The tibial tubercle is located anteriorly in the midline of the proximal tibial metaphysis and serves as the insertion of the patellar tendon. Gerdy's tubercle sits slightly lateral and proximal to the tibial tubercle and serves as the insertion of the iliotibial (IT) band. Halfway between Gerdy's tubercle and the fibular head and just beyond the lateral articular margin is the attachment point of the anterolateral ligament (ALL). Avulsion fracture of this insertion is termed a "Segond fracture" and is often associated with ACL tears. The proximal medial tibial metaphysis serves as the insertion point of the pes anserinus which is the confluence of tendons of (from anterior to posterior and superficial to deep) the sartorius, gracilis, and semitendinosus. Beneath this tendon structure is the anserine bursa which can become inflamed and therefore a source of pain over the medial tibial plateau. The medial collateral ligament contains superficial and deep portions with a broad insertion from the medial meniscus and medial edge of the plateau (deep medial collateral ligament [MCL]) to the medial tibial metaphysis (superficial MCL) approximately 6 cm distal to the joint line.[7]

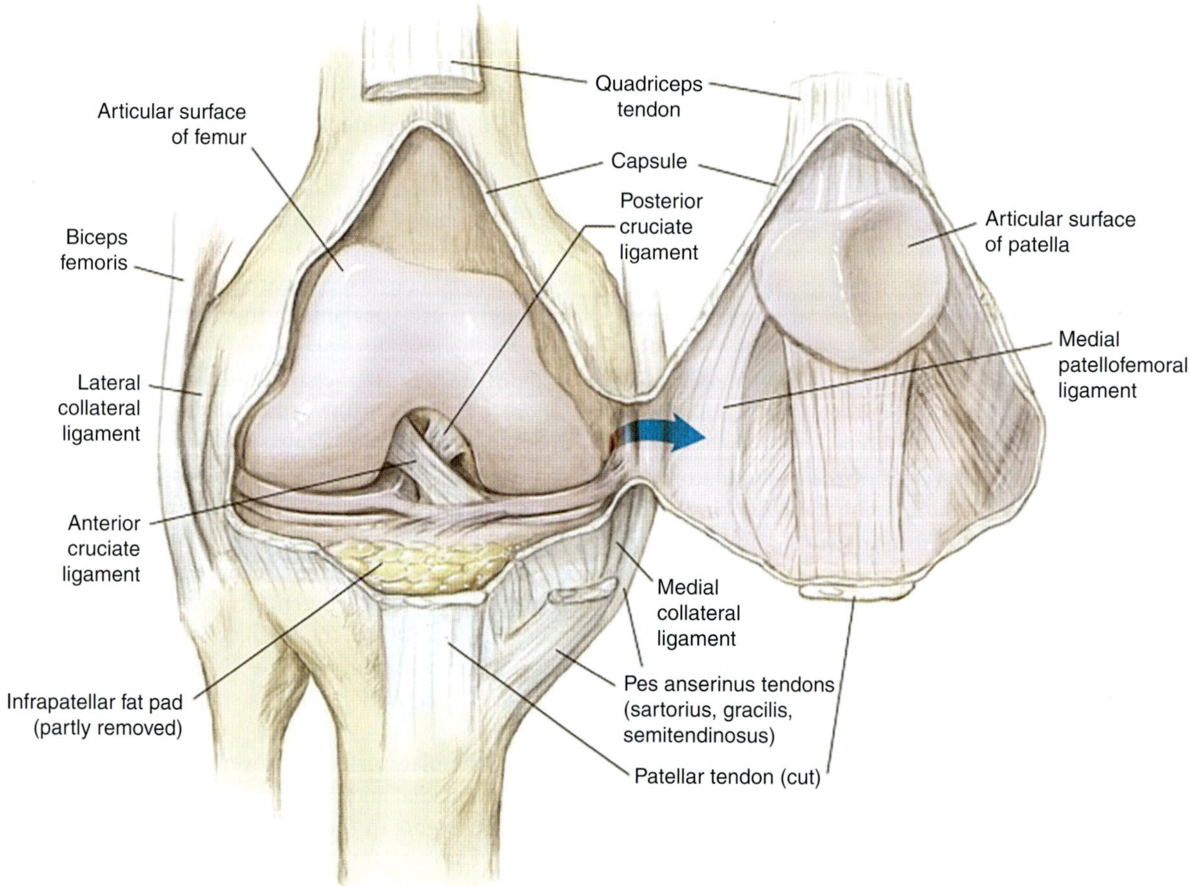

Fig. 1.1 Knee anatomy. (From Miller M, Chhabra A, Park J, Shen F, Weiss D, Browne J. *Orthopaedic Surgical Approaches*. 2nd ed. Philadelphia, PA: Elsevier; 2014. Fig. 7-4.)

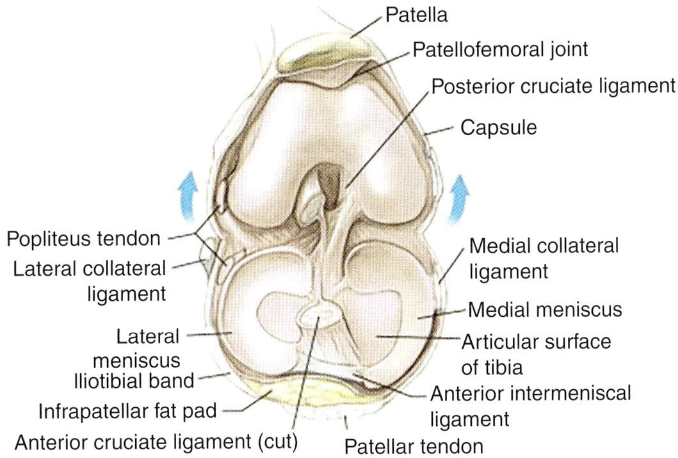

Fig. 1.2 Knee joint (hinged open). (From Miller M, Chhabra A, Park J, Shen F, Weiss D, Browne J. *Orthopaedic Surgical Approaches*. 2nd ed. Philadelphia, PA: Elsevier; 2014. Fig. 7-5.)

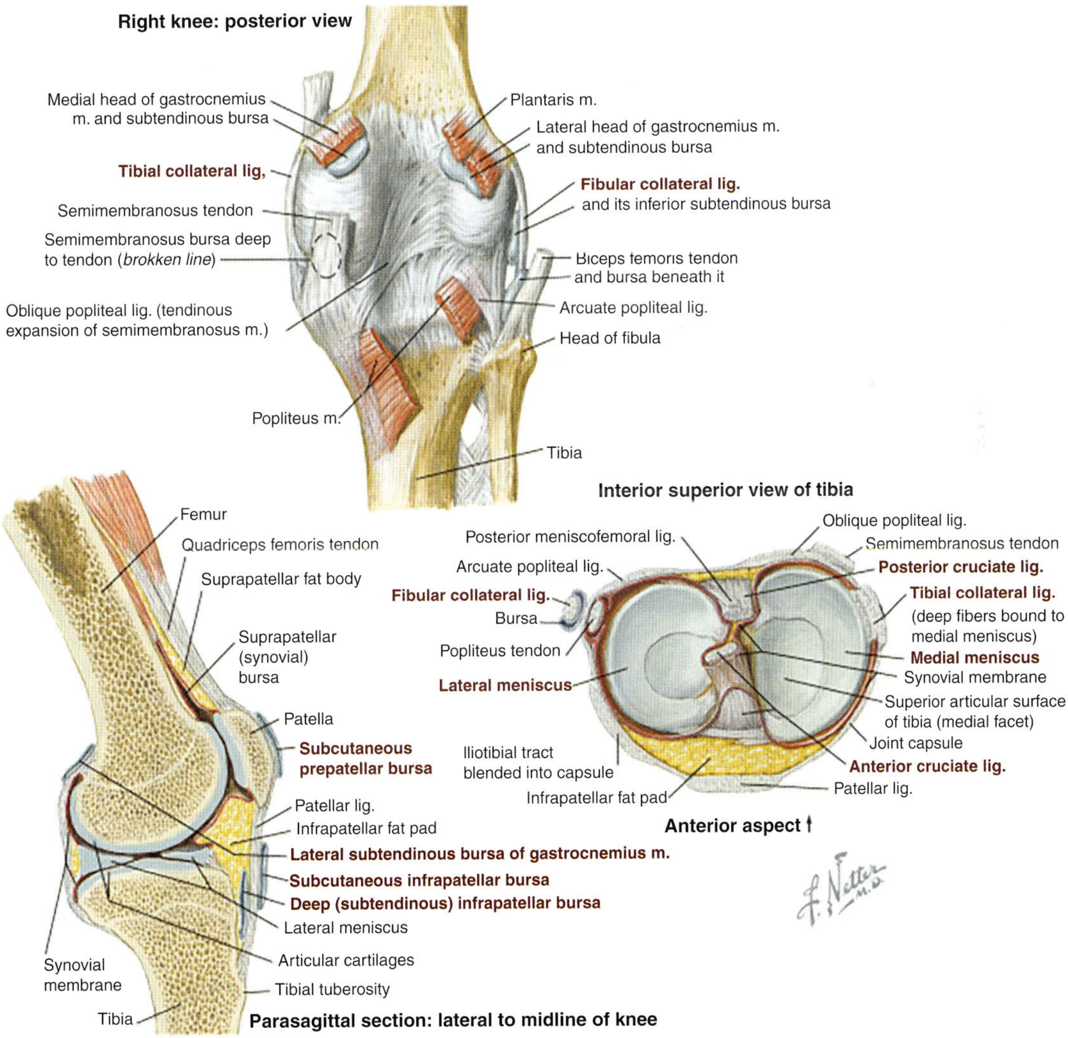

Fig. 1.3 Knee joint ligaments, tendons, and bursae. (From Hansen JT, Netter FH, Machado CAG. *Netter's Clinical Anatomy*. 4th ed. Philadelphia, PA: Elsevier; 2009. Fig. 6-19.)

The fibula is located posterolaterally and articulates with the tibia through the proximal tibiofibular joint. This is an arthrodial joint (allows only gliding motion) at the level of the tibial metaphyseal flare. The anterior and posterior fibular head ligaments constrain this joint with the anterior ligament being broader and stronger than the posterior ligament. Also inserting on the head of the fibula are the biceps femoris tendon and lateral collateral ligament (LCL). The peroneal nerve wraps from posterior to anterior around the lateral fibular neck before dividing into superficial and deep branches.

The cruciate ligaments (ACL and PCL) prevent anterior and posterior translation of the tibia in relation to the femur. The ACL originates on the lateral femoral condyle posterior to the intercondylar ridge of the femur. It inserts into the tibial intercondylar eminence just posterior to the transverse meniscal ligament and has a variable broad insertion that can measure approximately 1.1 ×1.5 cm from medial to lateral and anteroposterior. The shape of the tibial insertion has been described in many different ways including oval, triangular, C-shaped, and "duck foot–like".[8] The PCL originates on the medial femoral condyle and travels between the posterior meniscofemoral ligaments (Humphrey—anterior to PCL; Wrisberg—posterior to PCL) and inserts posteriorly into the intercondylar eminence and extends distally below the articular surface.[9] The PCL is slightly longer and larger in diameter than the ACL. Fractures involving the intercondylar eminence can be functionally equivalent to cruciate ligament tears and may require fixation.

As noted earlier, the MCL has a broad insertion on the medial tibia. It possesses an intimate relationship with the medial meniscus through direct attachments. The MCL attaches to the posterior half of the tibia when viewed in the sagittal plane. The MCL, its position, and its attachments can somewhat limit the exposure to the articular surface with medial approaches to the tibial plateau. The MCL resists valgus forces across the knee. The posterior oblique ligament (POL) contains obliquely oriented fibers that originate posterior to the MCL on the femur and fan out posteriorly inserting on the posteromedial tibia, meniscus, joint capsule, and semimembranosus tendon[7] (Fig. 1.4).

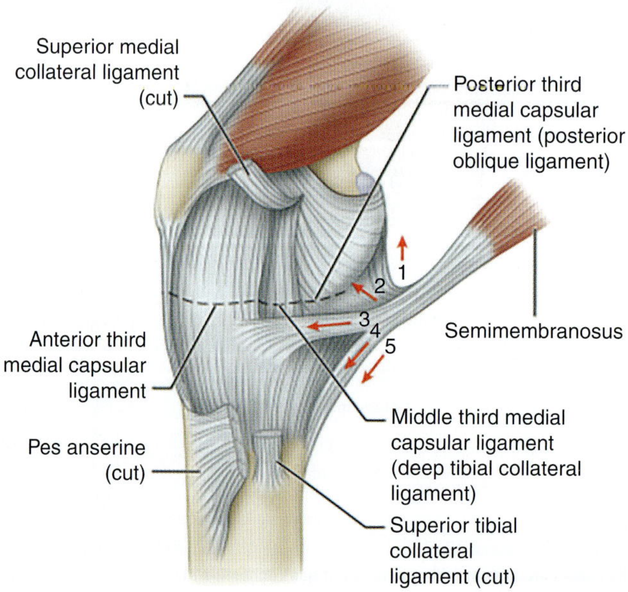

Fig. 1.4 Medial knee structures. *1*, Oblique popliteal ligament; *2*, posterior capsule and posterior horn of medial meniscus; *3*, anterior or medial tendon of semimembranosus; *4*, direct head of semimembranosus; and *5*, distal portion of semimembranosus tendon. (From Campbell WC, Canale ST, Beaty JH. *Campbell's Operative Orthopaedics*. 11th ed. Philadelphia, PA: Elsevier; 2008. Fig. 45.3.)

Laterally, the LCL resists varus stress at the knee. It originates roughly at or just posterior to the lateral epicondyle in a small bony depression and inserts into a small depression on the lateral fibular head 8 mm posterior to the fibular head anterior margin and 28 mm distal to the tip of the fibula.[10] The popliteus tendon (PLT) originates approximately 18.5 mm anterior and distal to the LCL origin just posterior to the femoral articular margin. The PLT travels posterior and inferior and has a broad insertion along the posterior medial tibia. The biceps femoris also contributes to the lateral structures of the knee with attachment sites primarily on the fibular head (Fig. 1.5)

The anterolateral tibial plateau is covered by the anterior compartment musculature of the lower leg. These muscles are elevated in order to gain access to the proximal tibia for reduction and placement of plate fixation. Posteriorly, the gastrocnemius muscle originates from the medial and lateral femoral condyles. Deep to the gastrocnemius and arising from the posterior tibia and posterior fibular head is the soleus muscle. From medial to lateral, the popliteal artery, vein, and tibial nerve travel through the popliteal space and dive deep to the soleus arch before giving off additional branches. Geniculate arteries branch off of the popliteal artery prior to entering the soleus arch and provide blood supply to the knee. The saphenous vein and nerve travel subcutaneously along the medial side of the knee and can be injured during medial approaches (Fig. 1.6).

APPROACHES

The following approaches can be performed with or without a tourniquet placed high on the thigh. It is the author's preference to apply a tourniquet in all cases but to leave the tourniquet deflated during exposure in most cases, inflating only if necessary to visualize joint reduction. With prone approaches, it is helpful to apply the tourniquet with the patient supine prior to flipping prone. In all approaches, padding of bony prominences is advised. In supine approaches, where hip internal rotation is desired, a bump is placed under the ipsilateral hip and the ipsilateral arm is often brought over the chest and secured

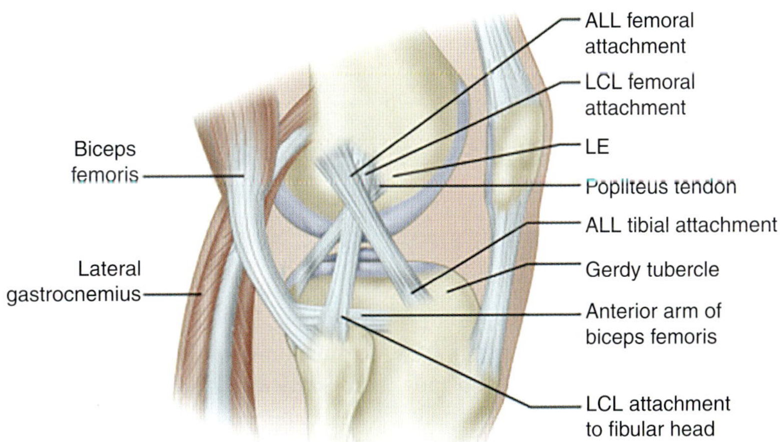

Fig. 1.5 Knee joint, lateral view. Osseous landmarks and attachment sites of the main structures of the lateral knee (IT band and nonanterolateral ligament–related capsule removed). The femoral attachment of the ALL is located posterior and proximal to the lateral collateral ligament; it courses anterodistally to its anterolateral tibial attachment approximately midway between the center of Gerdy's tubercle and the anterior margin of the fibular head. *ALL*, Anterolateral ligament; *LCL*, lateral collateral ligament; *LE*, lateral epicondyle. (From Campbell WC, Canale ST, Beaty JH. *Campbell's Operative Orthopaedics*. 11th ed. Philadelphia, PA: Elsevier; 2008. Fig. 45.24.)

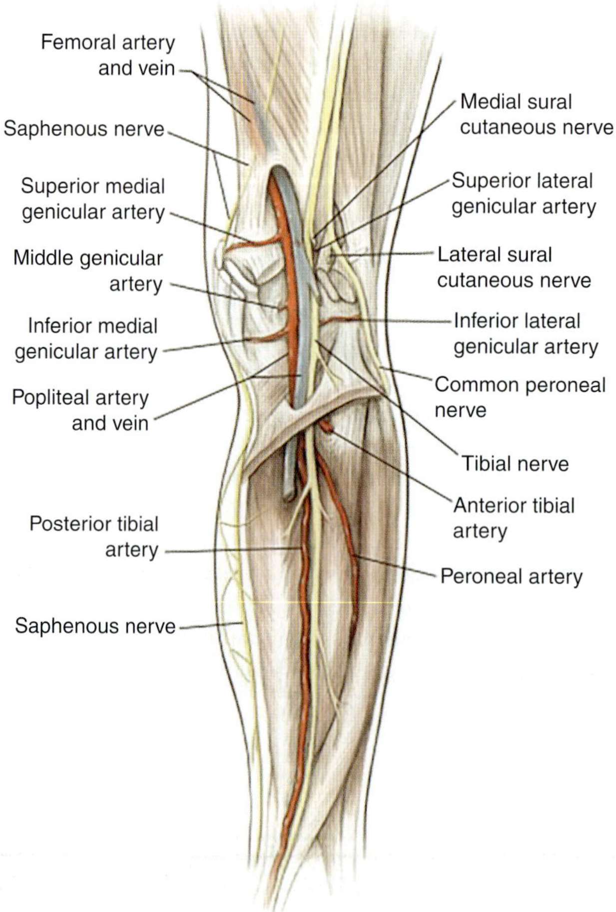

Fig. 1.6 Posterior structures surrounding the knee. (From Miller M, Chhabra A, Park J, Shen F, Weiss D, Browne J. *Orthopaedic Surgical Approaches.* 2nd ed. Philadelphia, PA: Elsevier; 2014. Fig. 7.16.)

rather than being placed abducted on an armboard. It is the author's preference to prewash the entire extremity with a scrub brush followed by alcohol, then to prep and drape the leg from the tourniquet to the toes, and to apply a second prep after draping. The vast majority of tibial plateau fractures can be exposed and treated with the use of one or both of the first two approaches described here, anterolateral and posteromedial.

Anterolateral Approach

The anterolateral approach is the most common open approach used in fixing tibial plateau fractures. This approach provides access to the lateral tibial plateau and, in conjunction with a transverse submeniscal arthrotomy, will often allow visualization from the lateral articular margin to the lateral tibial spine. A varus force applied at the knee will improve visualization by opening up the space in the lateral tibiofemoral compartment. A steady and constant force can be applied easily and quickly with the use of a femoral distractor or a simple external fixator (Fig. 1.7). The primary indication for use of the anterolateral approach is for displaced fractures involving the lateral condyle that require open reduction. Fixation can then be achieved with independent lag screws, buttress plating, or a combination thereof.

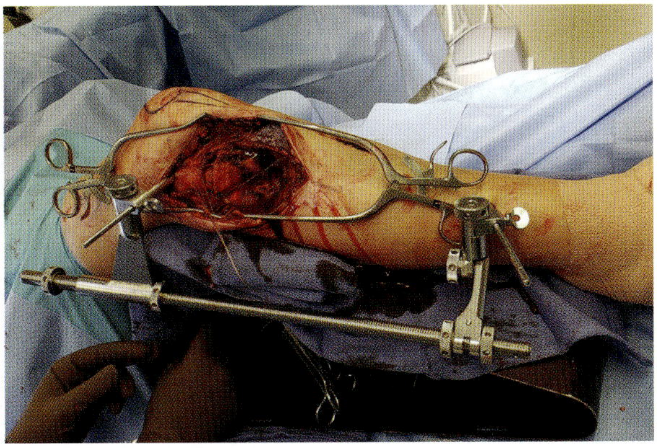

Fig. 1.7 Anterolateral approach with femoral distractor applying distraction and varus to the knee joint. Note the position of the femoral distractor rod posterior to the leg, which will avoid interference with x-ray and instrumentation. Additional information regarding intraoperative distraction can be found in Chapter 5, Internal Fixation.

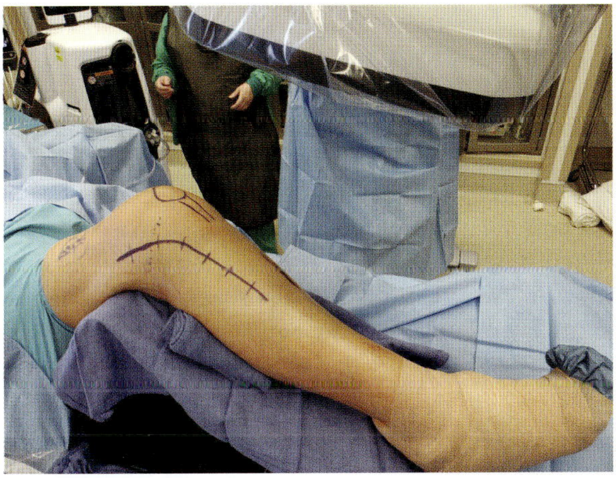

Fig. 1.8 Anterolateral approach with knee flexed over a radiolucent triangle. Note rolled towels placed under the leg. Despite a bump placed beneath the hip, the leg may still externally rotate. Rolled towels placed on the lateral side of the leg or triangle will allow the leg to internally rotate as desired for exposure.

Patient positioning is supine with a bump under the ipsilateral hip to prevent hip external rotation. Nonsterile positioning bumps can then be placed under the leg prior to prepping and draping to create a flat platform for the lower leg with the hip and knee each flexed approximately 20 degrees to elevate the operative knee from the table. Alternatively, a radiolucent triangle can be used to flex the knee after prepping and draping (Fig. 1.8).

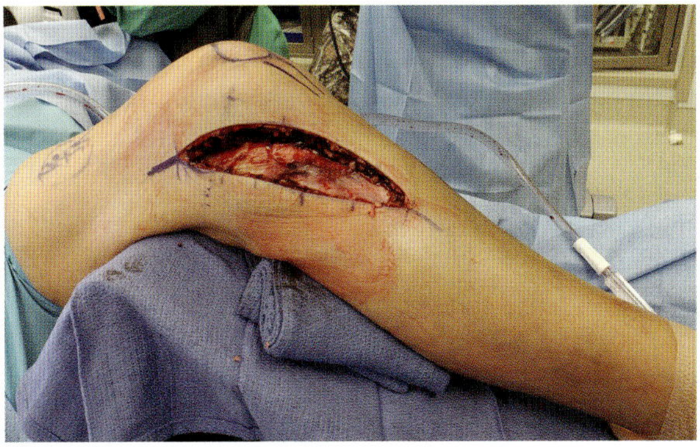

Fig. 1.9 Anterolateral approach with incision made through skin and subcutaneous tissue.

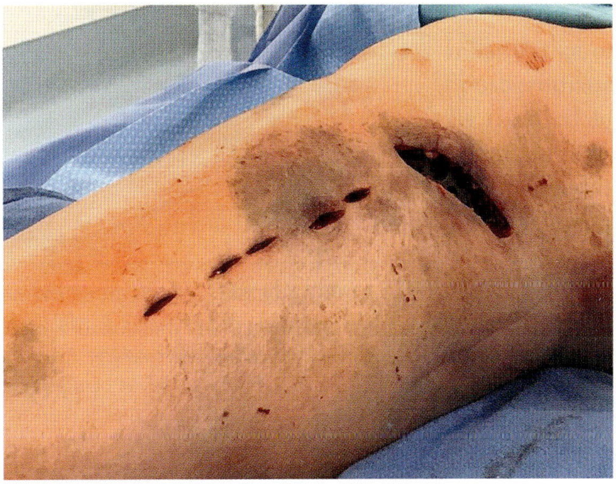

Fig. 1.10 Straight incision made proximally for percutaneous plate insertion.

The incision can be performed in several different ways. The incision can be performed as a lazy S-shaped incision with the transverse limb centered over the tibial articular surface, the anterior limb over the lateral compartment distally, and the posterior limb extending up to the lateral femoral condyle. When the knee is flexed, this incision will no longer appear S shaped and will have the appearance of a smooth arc (Fig. 1.9). Alternatively, the incision may be made in a "hockey stick" shape or in a straight line from approximately the level of the lateral femoral condyle traveling over the Gerdy's tubercle and the lateral tibial plateau toward the tibial crest. This straight incision is particularly useful when using an anterolateral approach for lateral joint reduction and percutaneous plate fixation (Fig. 1.10).

Sharp dissection is performed through subcutaneous tissues down to fascia, exposing the lateral knee retinaculum and anterior compartment musculature. Anterior muscle fascia is then incised approximately 1 cm lateral from the tibial crest. Fascia is incised and the IT band is proximally cut in line with its fibers through the retinaculum of the knee without incising through the synovial layer. Fascia and the IT band are reflected anteriorly up to the level of the tibial tubercle. Both the IT band and the ALL are released and preserved for repair at the completion of the case. A knife or electrocautery is then used to elevate the lateral musculature from the lateral tibial metaphysis. With the knife held straight up and down and deep to the posterior fascial flap and the tibialis anterior origin, the blade is brought flat against the lateral plateau and taken proximally between the retinacular layer and synovial layer to divide the two layers posteriorly as far as the fibular head (Fig. 1.11). Holding the knife straight up and down (anterior to posterior) and parallel to the lateral tibial cortex allows the surgeon to more easily stay within the plane between the retinaculum and synovium.

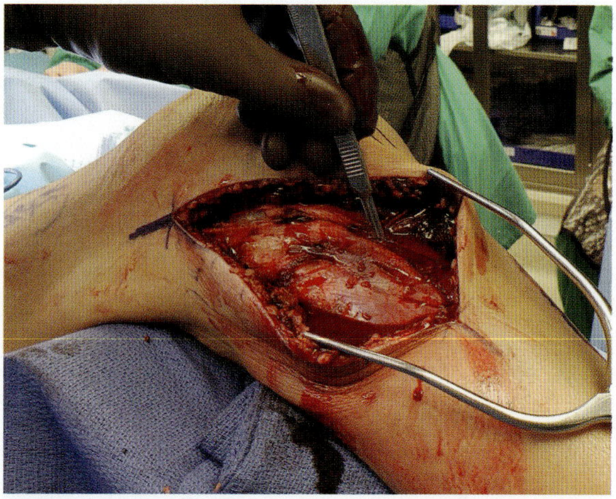

Fig. 1.11 Elevation of anterior compartment musculature along its origin at the lateral plateau continued proximally to the division of the retinacular layer from the synovial layer of the knee capsule. By keeping the blade flat against the lateral plateau, the knife will remain between the retinacular and synovial layers and allow consistently for separation of the two layers without violating the synovium.

The tibialis anterior muscle is then elevated from the lateral face of the tibia as far distally as needed for plate placement. This can be done with sharp dissection or the use of a Cobb elevator (Fig. 1.12).

A transverse submeniscal arthrotomy can then be performed in order to gain direct visualization into the joint. A 15-blade scalpel is used to incise the lateral knee capsule and coronary ligaments between the lateral articular surface and the lateral meniscus. This capsular incision can begin beneath the anterior horn of the lateral meniscus and continue lateral and then posterior to the posterolateral condyle. With the knee in a 60-degree flexed position, the LCL and common peroneal nerve move more posterior and allow exposure along the entire lateral tibial plateau. Sutures can then be placed

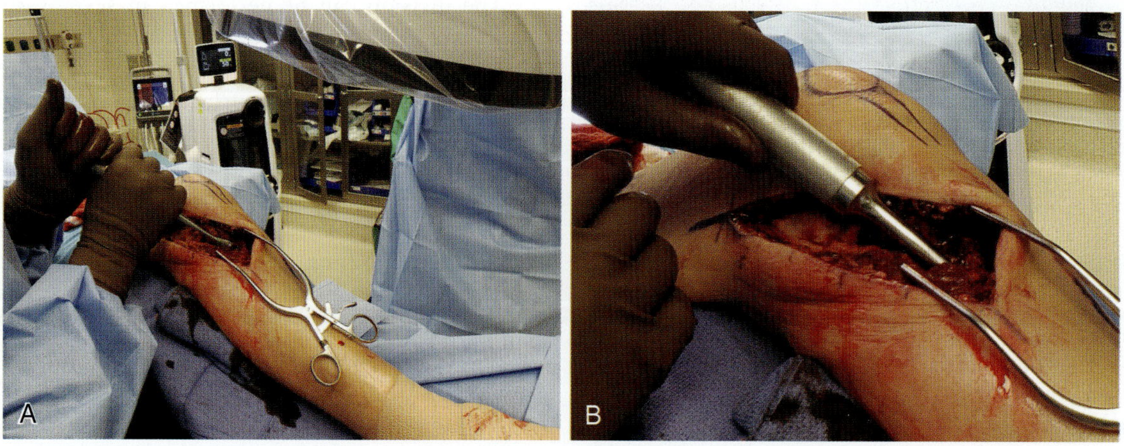

Fig. 1.12 (A and B) Cobb elevator being used to elevate the tibialis anterior muscle from the lateral tibial cortex.

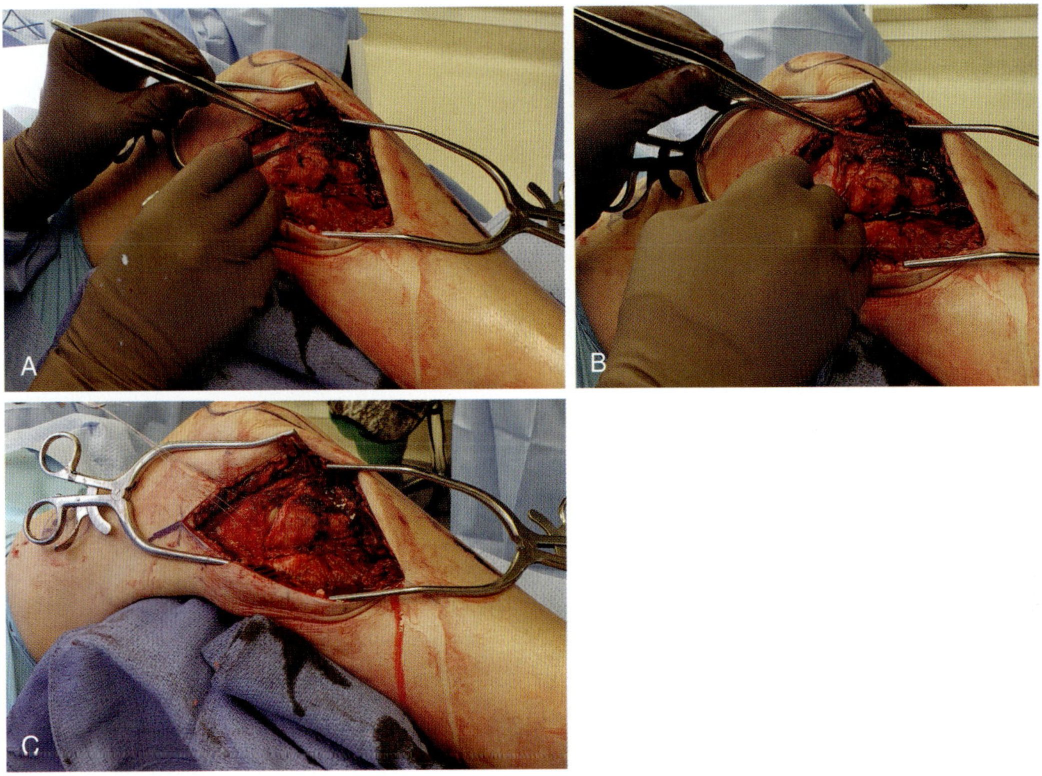

Fig. 1.13 Transverse submeniscal arthrotomy performed through the anterolateral approach to the tibial plateau. Arthrotomy is begun anteriorly with knife held parallel to the articular surface (A) and continues posteriorly to expose the joint surface (B). Sutures can then be placed in the periphery of the meniscus and capsule for retraction and can be used for repair at the completion of the case (C).

in the lateral portion of the lateral meniscus and capsule and can be used to retract the meniscus and facilitate repair at the end of the case (Fig. 1.13).

Further exposure of depressed articular surface fragments can be achieved by working through the anterior fracture line. A Cobb elevator or osteotome can be placed within the main sagittal fracture fragment on the lateral tibial plateau and can be used to "hinge" or "book" open the fracture site, exposing comminuted fracture fragments existing centrally and posteriorly (Fig. 1.14). This fracture site can then be held open with a lamina spreader or a Gelpi retractor, while fracture reduction takes place (Fig. 1.15). If no anterior fracture line exists, an osteotomy can be made anteriorly just lateral to the patellar tendon and tibial tubercle in the sagittal plane with a corresponding transverse cut in the

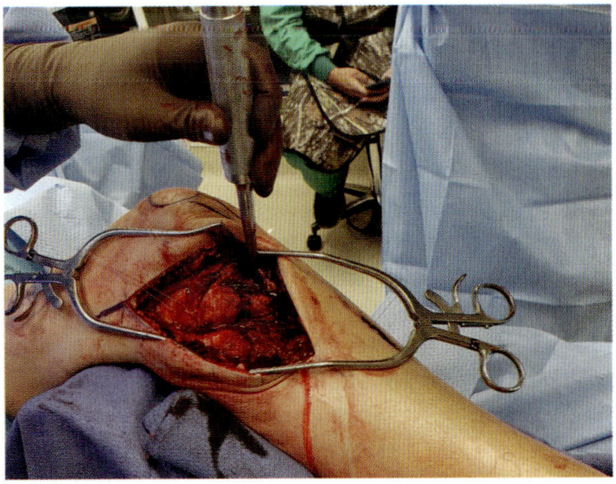

Fig. 1.14 Cobb elevator is being used to develop and "book" open sagittal plane fracture line in this lateral tibial plateau fracture.

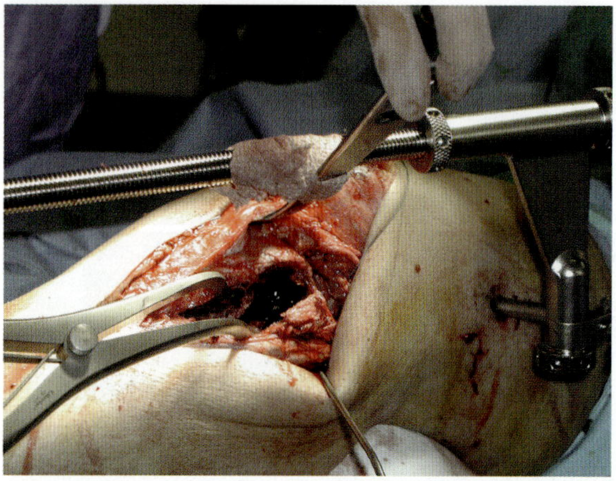

Fig. 1.15 A lamina spreader is being used to hold the lateral plateau in a booked open position. Note the use of Coban (3M, Saint Paul, MN) and femoral distractor to aid in holding the Hohmann retractor in place. (Picture and retraction technique courtesy of James Widmaier, MD.)

anterolateral metaphysis. This osteotomized fragment can then be booked open to provide access to centrally and posteriorly depressed fragments. Alternatively, a cortical window can be made in the metaphysis of the lateral plateau with an osteotome or large drill bit, and a curved tamp can then be used to elevate depressed articular fragments (Fig. 1.16). Once exposure is obtained, a helpful tip for retraction is to utilize a heavy nylon suture as a radiolucent retractor of the skin edges (Fig. 1.17). When this retraction stitch is used there is no need for the assistant to hold a retractor and no barrier to x-ray visualization.

When exposure of the posterolateral tibial plateau is needed, this can often be achieved through the anterolateral approach.[11–13] With the knee flexed, the posterior IT band (which has previously been split) is retracted posteriorly and peeled off all the way back to the lateral fibular head. Dissection can be performed along the rim of the lateral tibial plateau posteriorly deep to the biceps femoris, and a retractor can be placed behind the posterolateral corner. With the knee flexed to 60 degrees, the LCL and popliteal tendon are mobilized and retracted posteriorly (protecting the peroneal nerve). The knee can then be extended and tibia internally rotated to view the posterolateral aspect of the plateau, providing access for reduction and pinning. Plating can then be performed by flexing the knee again to allow retraction of the LCL.

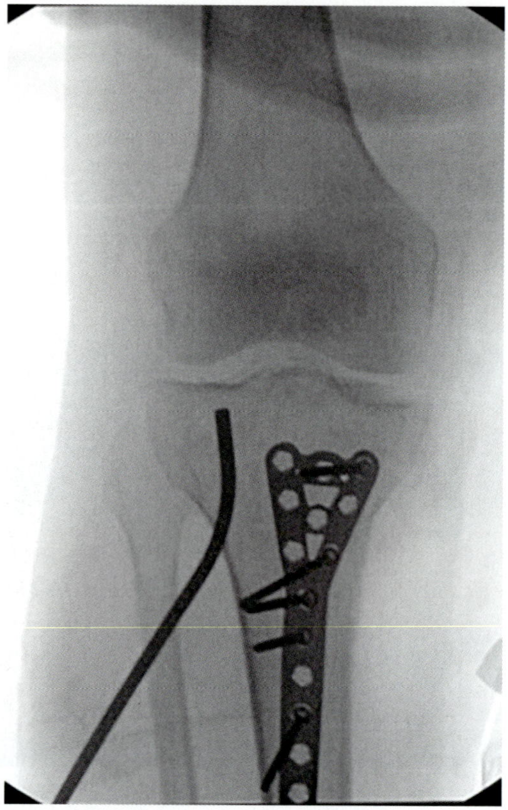

Fig. 1.16 Following open treatment of a displaced posteromedial tibial plateau fracture fragment, lateral joint depression was addressed through a cortical window made with a 4.5-mm drill bit. A tamp was inserted to elevate the depressed articular fragment as shown here.

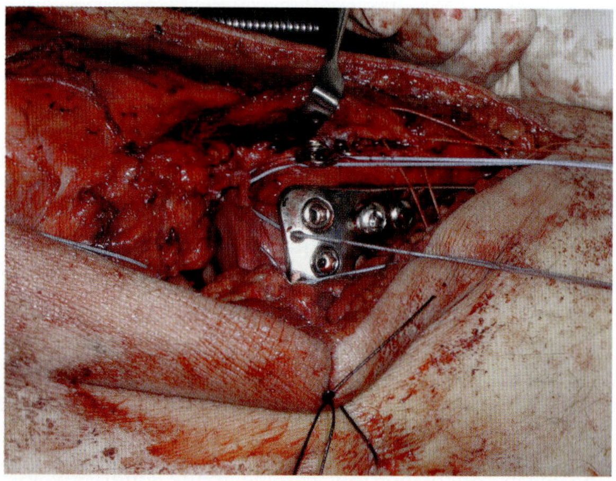

Fig. 1.17 Nylon suture (2-0) used as a "radiolucent retractor" with a no-hands technique to retract the posterior skin flap with anterolateral exposure of the tibial plateau. (Picture and retraction technique courtesy of James Widmaier, MD.)

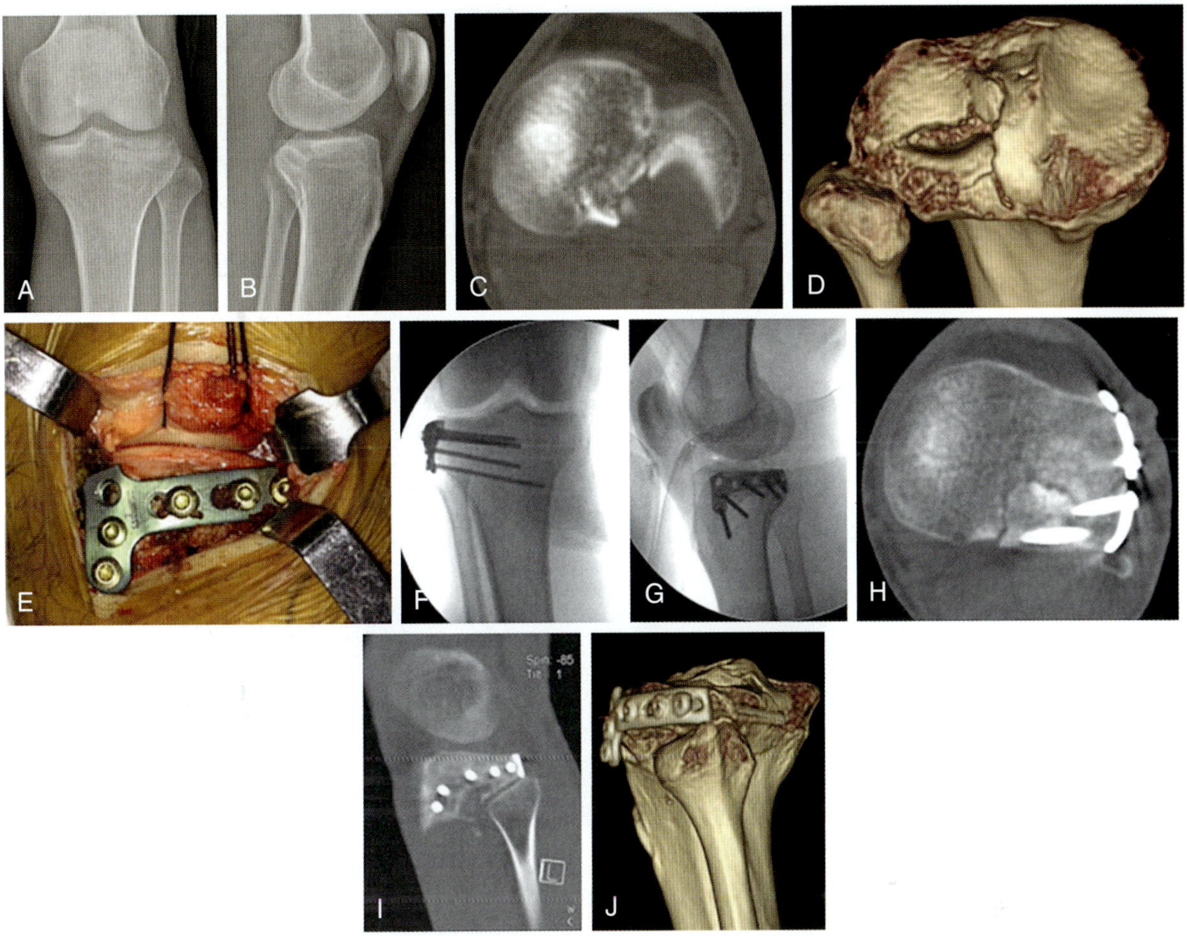

Fig. 1.18 Extended anterolateral approach with exposure of the posterolateral tibial plateau. Anteroposterior [AP] (A) and lateral (B) view preoperatively showing a posterolateral tibial plateau fracture; (C and D) CT scan images before the operation showed that the fragment was on the posterolateral quadrant of the tibial plateau. Intraoperative photograph (E) showed that the fracture was reduced and fixed with a mini-fragment plate. (F and G) AP and lateral intraoperative fluoroscopy images showed that the fracture was anatomically reduced. (H–J) Images of CT scan and reconstruction after operation. The fragment was elevated and fixed by a horizontal belt plate. *CT*, Computed tomography. (From Hu SJ, Chang SM, Zhang YQ, Ma Z, Du SC, Zhang K. The anterolateral supra-fibular-head approach for plating posterolateral tibial plateau fractures: a novel surgical technique. *Injury*. 2016;47:502-507. Fig. 5.)

A cadaver study with an accompanying clinical cohort of patients was performed to assess the anatomic considerations and clinical outcomes of patients with posterolateral tibial plateau fractures treated through an extensile anterolateral approach as described previously.[12] The fibular head was found to be on average 12.2 mm from the tibial articular surface in a superior to inferior direction. The LCL was found to be 6.7 and 21.1 mm with the knee extended and flexed to 60 degrees, respectively, in a transverse measurement from the lateral plateau articular surface to the LCL. Knee flexion of 60 degrees relaxes the LCL and allows greater access to the posterolateral tibial plateau. Depending on fracture comminution, plating of the posterolateral tibia can be performed through this incision with the use of standard tibial plateau plates placed more posteriorly than normal or with rim plates (Fig. 1.18). Plates designed with extensions to reach around the plateau proximally can be used here as well. Patients achieved good clinical outcomes of radiographic alignment on x-ray and

CASE 1.1

A 61-year-old male slipped on wet leaves and fell from a standing height. He developed immediate pain and inability to bear weight through the right knee. He was found to have a Schatzker type II tibial plateau fracture (Fig. 1.19).

An extensile anterolateral approach was chosen to expose the entire lateral plateau including the posterolateral fracture fragment. The patient was positioned on a foam ramp with a bump under the hip and a curved incision made over the joint (Fig. 1.20). Fascia was released posteriorly to the posterolateral tibia and submeniscal arthrotomy was performed (Fig. 1.21). After reducing and fixing the articular portion with a rim plate, a lateral tibial plateau plate was placed using minimally invasive techniques (Fig. 1.22). A meniscal tear was debrided through the arthrotomy. Final fixation construct can be seen in Fig. 1.23.

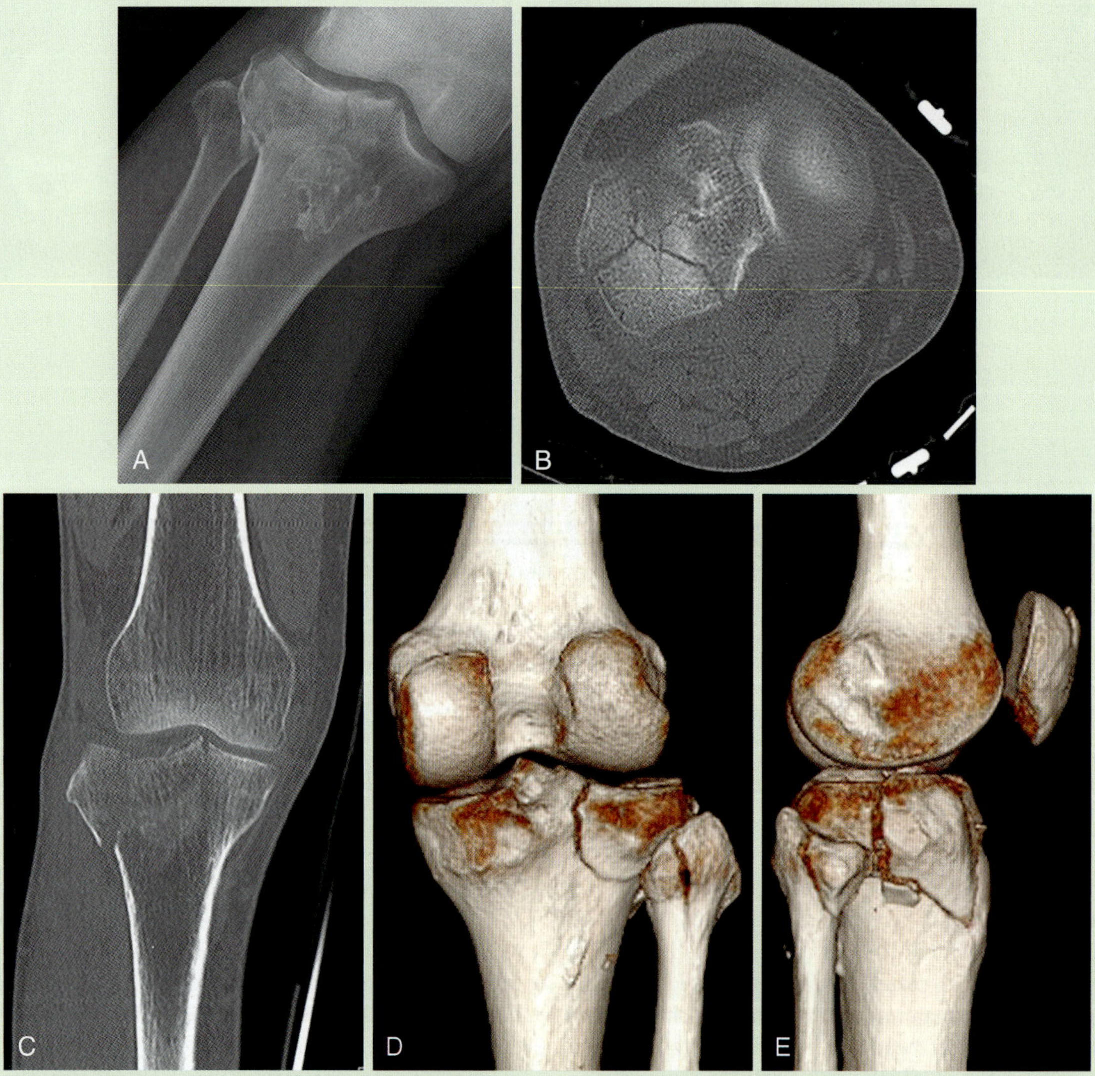

Fig. 1.19 AP x-ray (A) and CT scan (B–E) showing fracture of the lateral tibial plateau with displacement and plateau widening. Incidental finding of bone infarct is seen as well. *CT*, Computed tomography.

CASE 1.1—CONT'D

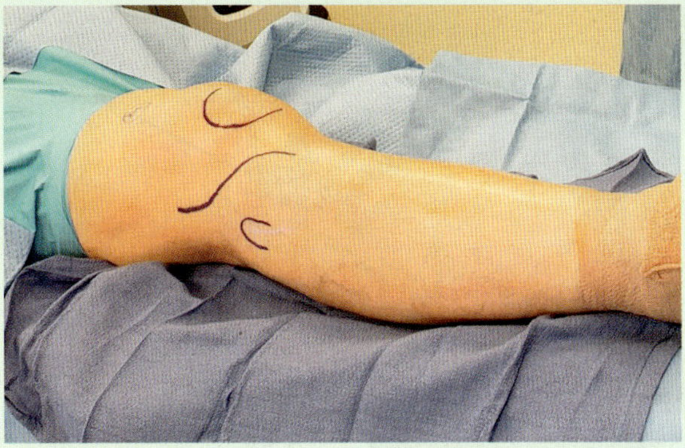

Fig. 1.20 Positioning and incision for extended anterolateral exposure to the tibial plateau.

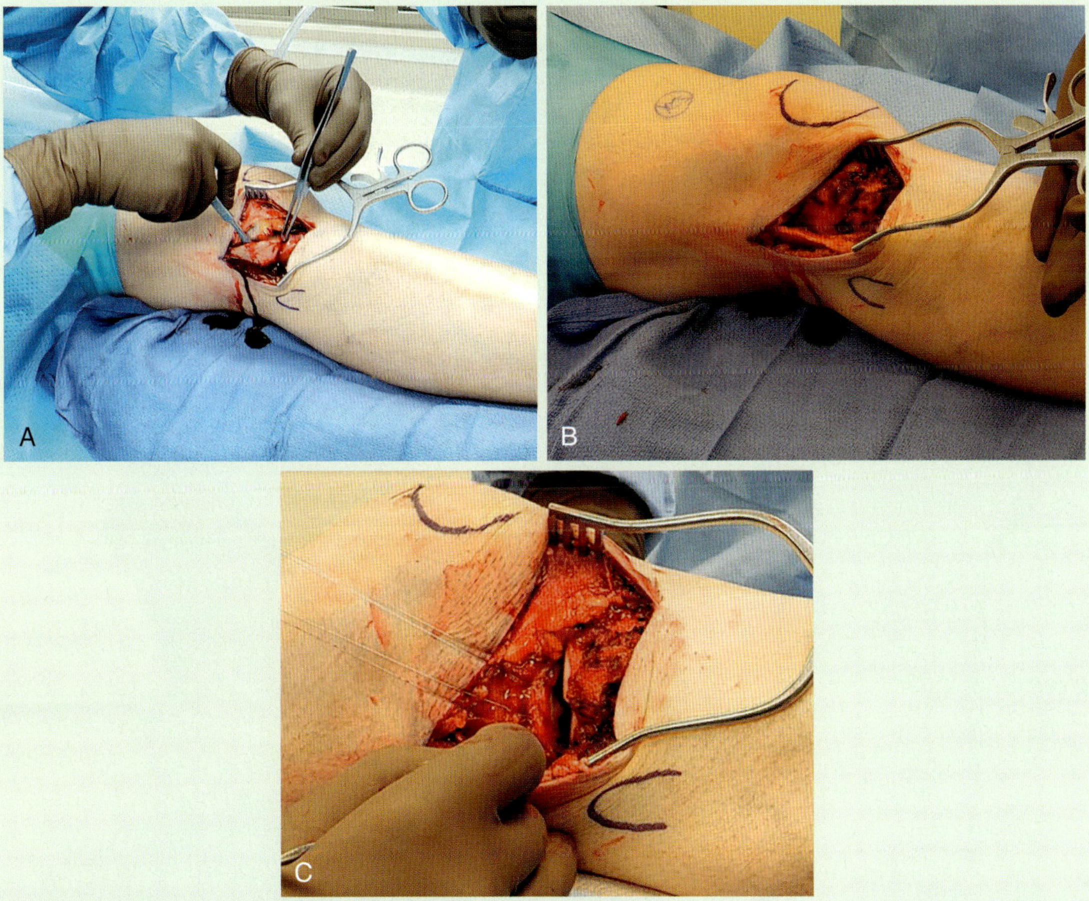

Fig. 1.21 Extended anterolateral exposure of the tibial plateau exposing posterolateral fracture fragment. Fascial incision made with knife brought up against the lateral plateau and metaphysis to peel fascia off lateral plateau (A). As knife is carried proximally in the same plane knee synovium is exposed (B). Transverse submeniscal arthrotomy is then performed (C).

Continued

CASE 1.1—CONT'D

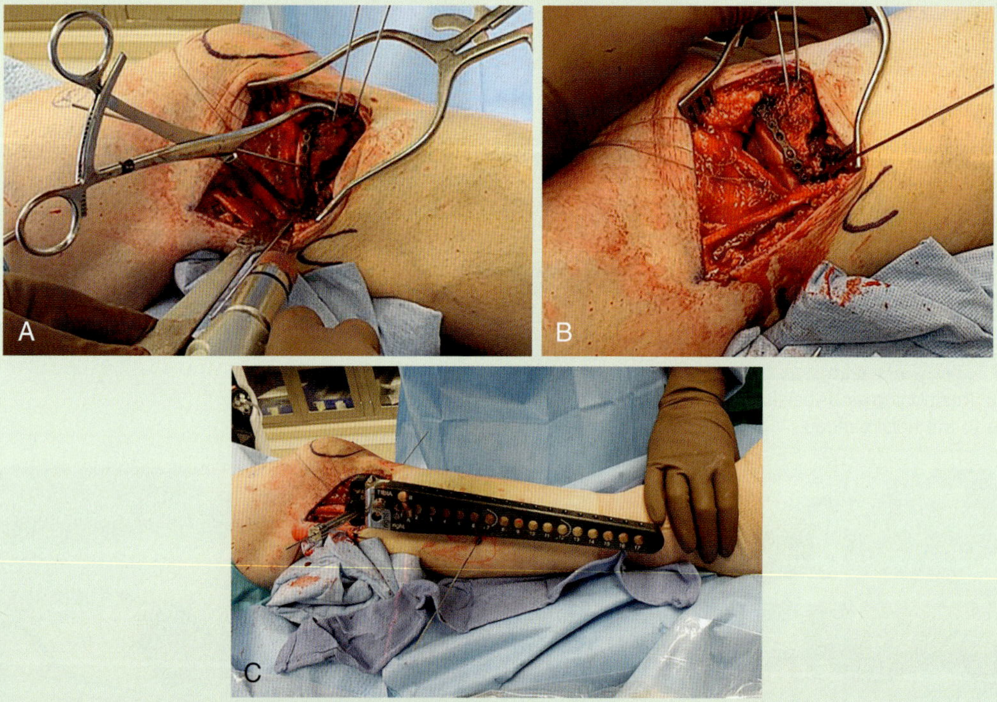

Fig. 1.22 With the entire lateral plateau exposed, reduction is then performed, clamps placed, and rim plate applied (A). With varus force applied at the knee, the entire lateral plateau can be seen to assess fracture reduction (B). A precontoured lateral plateau plate can then be placed using minimally invasive techniques (C).

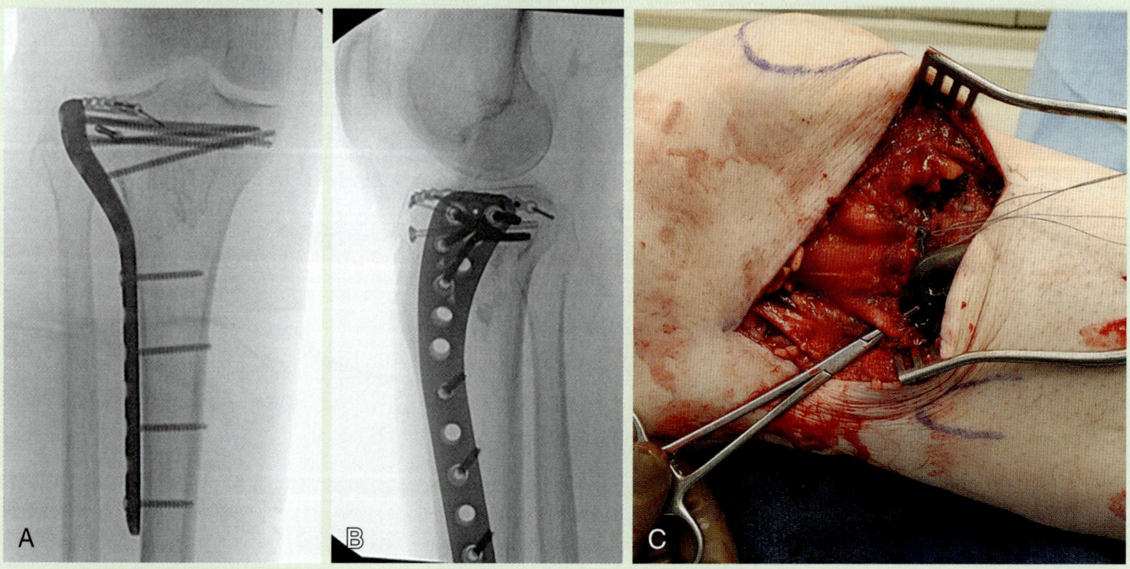

Fig. 1.23 X-rays showing final fixation construct in Case 1.1 (A and B). Capsule was repaired back to the lateral plateau using sutures placed in the periphery of the meniscus (C). The LCL can be seen posteriorly in the wound (overlying the clamp). *LCL*, Lateral collateral ligament.

computerized tomography (CT) scans, healing, range of motion, and Hospital for Special Surgery (HSS) and Short Musculoskeletal Function Assessment (SMFA) scores in this study.

Posteromedial

Many bicondylar tibial plateau fractures require direct access to the medial condyle. The posteromedial approach provides access to the medial and posterior aspects of the medial tibial plateau. Indications for its use are displaced medial condyle fractures requiring reduction and isolated medial condyle and bicondylar plateau fractures requiring medial buttress fixation that cannot be adequately stabilized percutaneously or with lateral locked fixation. Posteromedial fracture lines, particularly, tend to be unstable fractures that when present often require a direct approach and fixation. In some instances, posterolateral fractures may be repaired through posteromedial approaches, and posterior plate designs with projections that wrap around posterolaterally can assist with repair of these fractures from a posteromedial approach.

One of the main advantages of the posteromedial approach is that it can be performed with the patient in the supine position while still providing access to the posteromedial and direct posterior (DP) aspects of the tibial plateau (Fig. 1.24). This allows for dual approaches anterolaterally and posteromedially during one single prep and can be used to treat most bicondylar tibial plateau fractures.

The patient is placed supine on a radiolucent table. The hip is allowed to externally rotate, and the surgeon stands or sits on the side of the bed opposite to the injured extremity. The leg can be placed on a towel bump with the knee flexed approximately 45 degrees. The length of the incision will depend on the fracture pattern and the degree of exposure needed. The more posterior and proximal access that is needed, the more proximal the incision should be carried up to the femoral condyles. The distal extent of the incision will depend on where the distal portion of any plate being applied will ultimately come to rest.

For wide exposure, the incision begins directly anterior to the semitendinosus at the proximal aspect

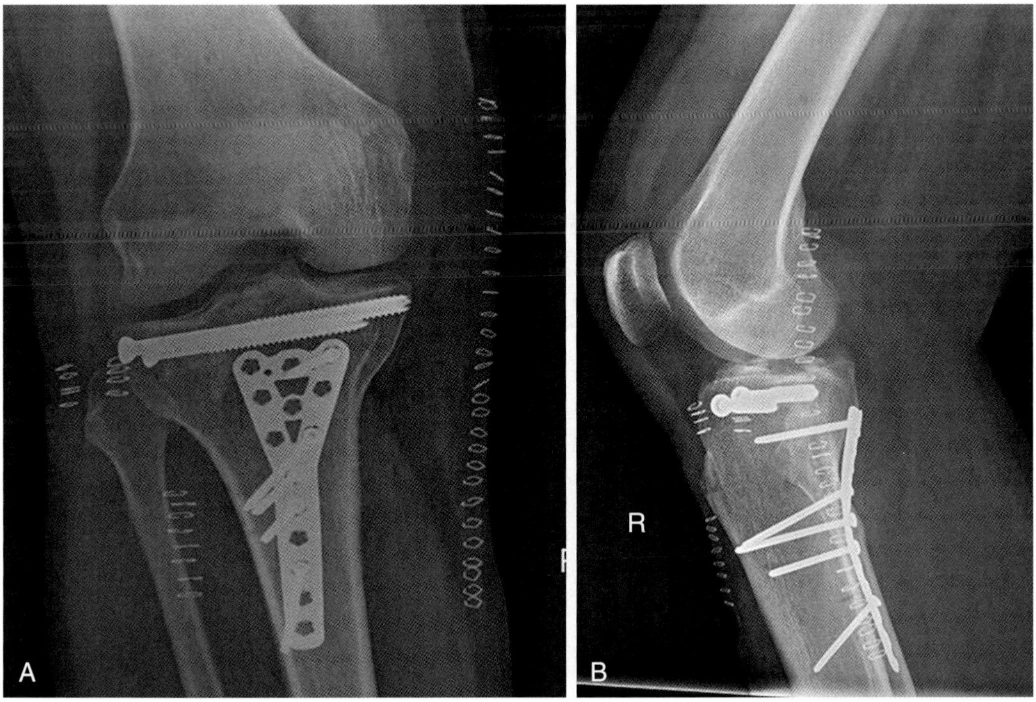

Fig. 1.24 AP and lateral x-ray of plate placed directly posterior on the tibial plateau through a posteromedial approach (A and B). Note staples posteromedially indicating the location of the incision.

of the medial femoral condyle. The incision continues across the posteromedial aspect of the knee joint in a curved fashion and continues 2 cm posterior to the palpable posteromedial edge of the tibia. With the knee fully extended, this incision will appear as a straight line and with the knee flexed the incision will be curved (Fig. 1.25). During dissection, care is taken to preserve the saphenous vein. Fascia is exposed and is incised proximally in line with the semitendinosus fibers between the hamstring and the medial head of the gastrocnemius, while distally it is incised along the anterior edge of the gastrocnemius. A Cobb elevator is used to elevate the gastrocnemius and the popliteus off of the posterior tibia and capsule (Fig. 1.26). Working between this interval of the semitendinosus and medial head of the gastrocnemius—and with flexion and external rotation of the tibia—access can be gained to the posterior tibia proximally (Fig. 1.27).

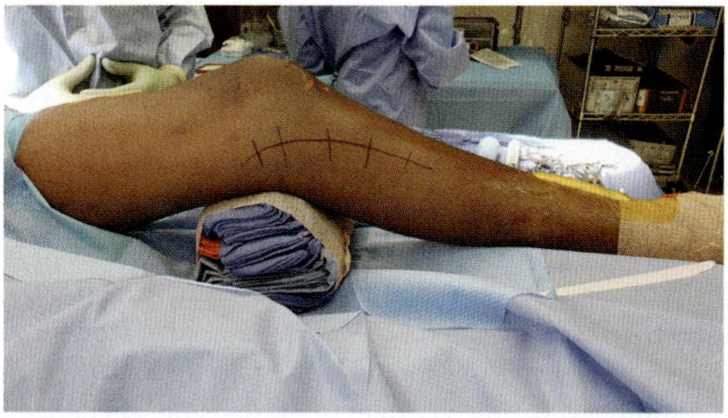

Fig. 1.25 Supine patient position with skin incision drawn for the posteromedial approach to the tibial plateau. Note that the incision is a straight line when the knee is extended and will appear curved when the knee is flexed.

Occasionally, a split in the pes tendons in line with the fibers or elevation of the tendons down to the insertion can facilitate sliding a plate into a posteromedial position and is needed when more superior exposure is necessary (Fig. 1.28). If needed, the pes tendons can also be released from their insertion, leaving a cuff of tissue, and repaired at the end of the case. Working proximally along the anterior border of the medial hamstring also allows direct access to

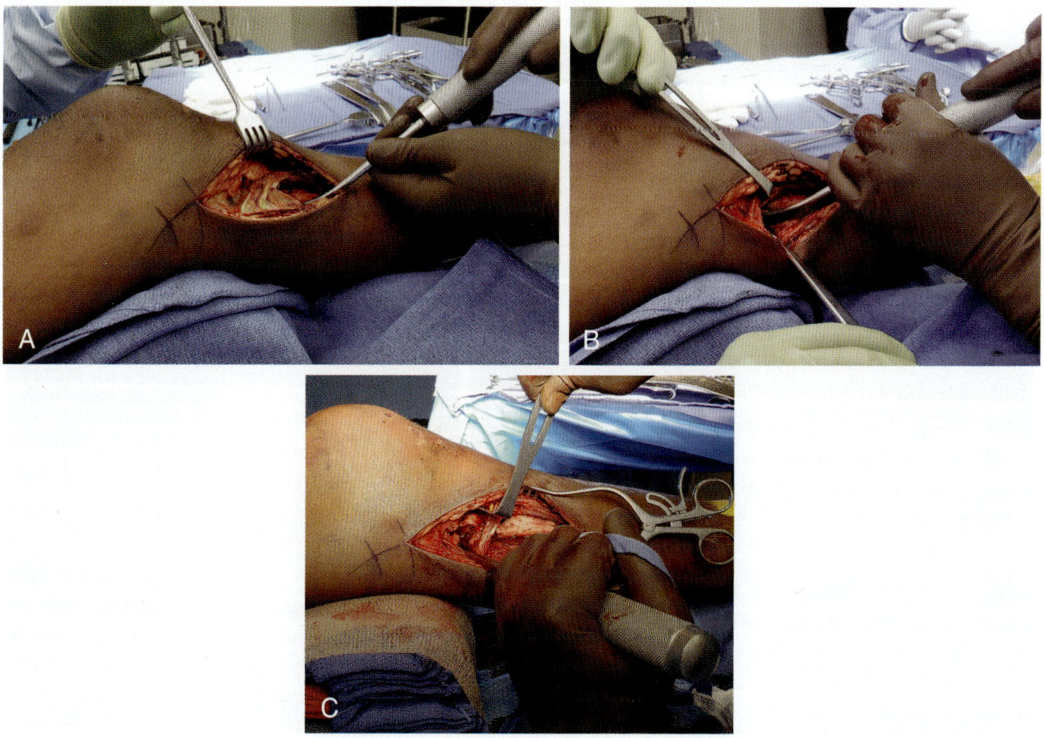

Fig. 1.26 Cobb elevator used to elevate gastrocnemius/soleus from the posterior surface of the tibia (A) and elevation of the popliteus proximally (B and C).

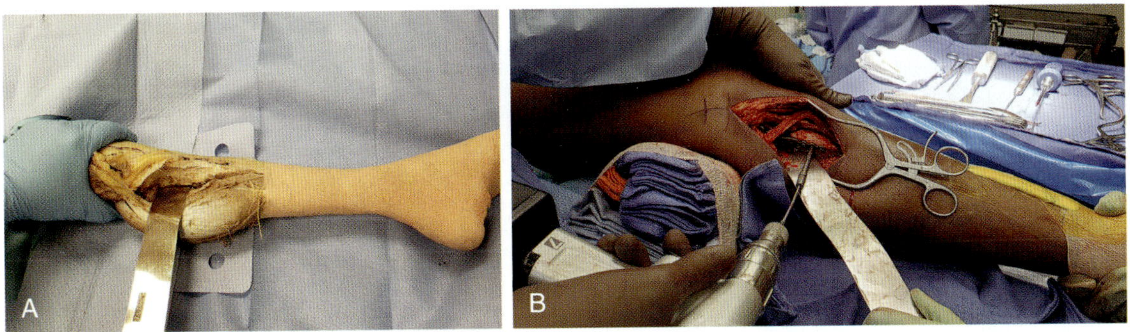

Fig. 1.27 Posterior exposure of the proximal tibia through posteromedial exposure. Malleable retractor is placed around the posterolateral cortex of the tibia and retracting posterior structures. Knee flexion and external rotation of the tibia allow for greater posterior access. A, cadaveric specimen demonstrating exposure. B, intraoperative photograph demonstrating drilling from direct posterior to anterior using the posteromedial approach with flexion and external rotation at the knee.

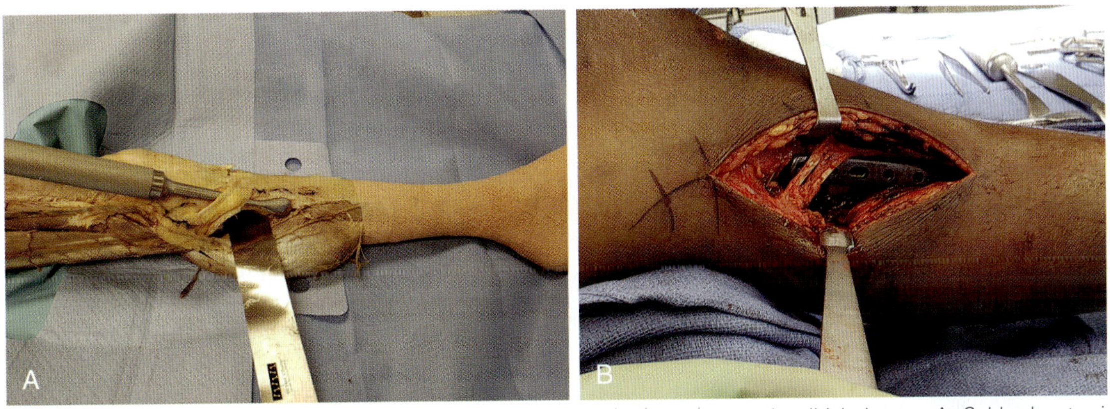

Fig. 1.28 Posteromedial exposure with pes tendon elevated out to its insertion on the tibial plateau. A, Cobb elevator is slid beneath the tendon simulating a plate placed underneath the tendon from superior to the tendon. B, Intraoperative photograph demonstrating plate placement beneath the pes tendon. The tendon can be retracted superiorly and inferiorly, as needed, to place screws.

the medial gastrocnemius origin. This can also be divided to reflect the medial gastrocnemius further and allow greater dissection toward the posterolateral tibial plateau. Large Hohmann and malleable retractors are helpful in retracting the gastrocnemius out of the way for reduction and plate placement, and as noted previously, further knee flexion (60–90 degrees) and external rotation of the tibia increase access and allow for proper hand positioning in instrumentation (Fig. 1.29).

A sometimes helpful and useful tip when performing a posteromedial approach is to use a radiolucent triangle to provide knee flexion and as a retractor holder. With the approach made and the knee flexed on a radiolucent triangle, a malleable retractor can be slightly contoured and hooked around the lateral tibial cortex. The retractor can then be placed into one of the slots on the triangle to hold it in place and free up extra hands for reduction and fixation (Fig. 1.30).

One recent description of this approach that can provide access to the posterior column uses the analogy of the posterior tibial plateau approach being like the flexor carpi radialis (FCR) approach to the distal radius.[14] In this description, the incision is placed medially over the medial head of the gastrocnemius (analogous to FCR) in a straight line. Gastrocnemius fascia is incised; the medial head is retracted laterally and semimembranosus is retracted medially. The popliteus (analogous to pronator quadratus) is then elevated from medial to lateral to expose the posterior plateau. This description uses the

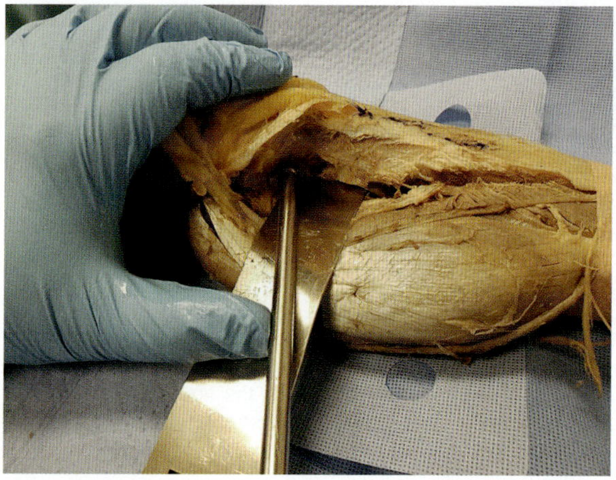

Fig. 1.29 Posteromedial exposure with ball spike placed at the posterolateral tibial plateau. Note with retraction and tibial external rotation, instrumentation can come at an angle almost directly posteriorly.

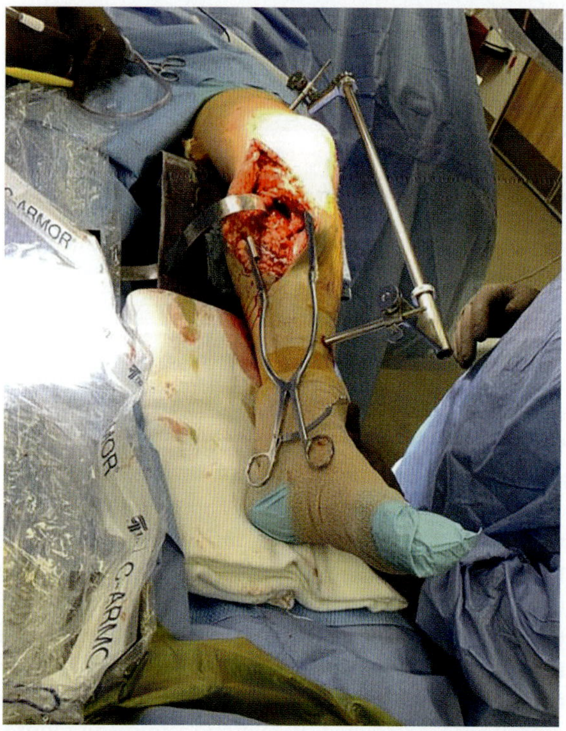

Fig. 1.30 Radiolucent triangle used as a retractor holder. Malleable retractor is placed through a slot in the triangle. (Picture and technique courtesy of James Widmaier, MD.)

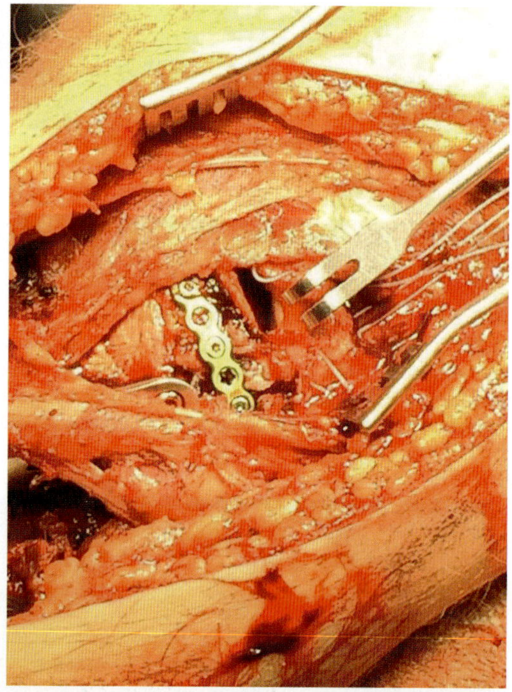

Fig. 1.31 Posteromedial approach to the tibial plateau. The pes tendons are shown here crossing over the buttress plate. A rim plate has been placed here as well. Arthrotomy was performed with a vertical split in the capsule posterior to the MCL. Note placement of sutures in order to repair medial meniscus back to capsule. *MCL*, Medial collateral ligament.

same interval and technique described earlier for posteromedial exposure with the exception that the authors of that study have described taking this approach in a prone position.

In the event that direct medial exposure is needed (as opposed to posteromedial), the incision can be made slightly anterior and the medial face of the tibia exposed, or a full-thickness anterior flap can be raised to gain access to more anterior aspects of the medial plateau. If making the incision more anterior, it is helpful to still keep this incision just posterior to where the final plate placement is planned. Due to its broad insertion, the pes anserinus will have to be elevated or split in direct medial plate applications. The superficial MCL insertion can be elevated and repaired at the end of the case as well. Because of the deep MCL, direct visualization of the joint surface is typically less than that achieved on the lateral plateau. The MCL can be

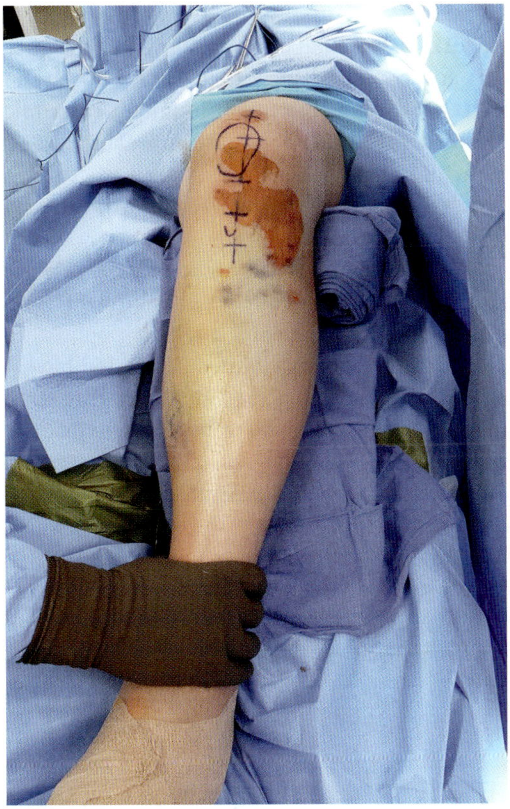

Fig. 1.32 Anterior midline incision used for direct anterior approach to the tibial plateau.

dissected along its anterior and posterior edges and the joint surface exposed leaving the deep MCL intact. When absolutely necessary, the deep MCL can be released from its tibial attachment along with a submeniscal arthrotomy (Fig. 1.31). Meticulous repair of the coronary ligaments and MCL insertion in addition to changes in postoperative care are necessary when this is done.

Direct Anterior

The direct anterior approach to the tibial plateau allows for direct visualization of nearly the entire articular surface and can be extremely helpful in cases of severe articular comminution. Additionally, in cases of fracture extension into the tibial shaft, the direct anterior approach provides simultaneous exposure for articular reduction and fixation, as well as access to the starting point for placement of tibial intramedullary fixation. In the event of the need for future total knee arthroplasty, the same midline incision may be used. When using a direct anterior approach, it is important that dissection along the tibial plateau proceeds in only one direction in order to prevent devascularization of the entire tibial plateau.

The patient is positioned supine with a bump under the hip. A radiolucent triangle is used to provide flexion at the knee. The incision is made anterior in the midline from two finger breadths above the patella down to the expected distal end of the plate (Fig. 1.32). The incision distally travels lateral to the tibial tubercle and remains just lateral to the tibial crest. The incision can be shortened distally in the case where minimally invasive plating techniques are used. In that instance, the incision can usually end inferiorly at the level of the tibial tubercle. This will allow enough access to the articular surface fracture site for reduction and plate placement laterally with percutaneous screw placement distally. Sharp dissection continues to the level of the knee retinaculum and anterior compartment of the lower leg, creating a full-thickness lateral skin flap (Fig. 1.33). It is important to avoid the creation of a large dead space and avoid raising large skin flaps in both directions (medial and lateral).

A lateral parapatellar arthrotomy is then performed. Care is taken at the level of the knee joint line to avoid cutting the anterior horn of the lateral meniscus. The knee capsule is retracted medially and laterally, and the lateral compartment musculature is elevated laterally from the tibial plateau, exposing the lateral fracture site and meniscus (Fig. 1.34).

A suture (2-0) can then be placed into the meniscus for retraction and later repair. If visualization of the tibial eminence and medial plateau is needed, excision of the infrapatellar fat pad can be performed. Rarely, in some isolated medial plateau fractures (where posteromedial plating is not necessary), a midline anterior incision can be similarly used with dissection proceeding medial with a medial parapatellar arthrotomy and elevation of capsule from the medial tibial condyle to complete exposure.

Direct Posterior

The DP approach is performed with the patient prone. It provides DP access to the proximal tibia and can be used to fix posterior plateau fracture fragments and

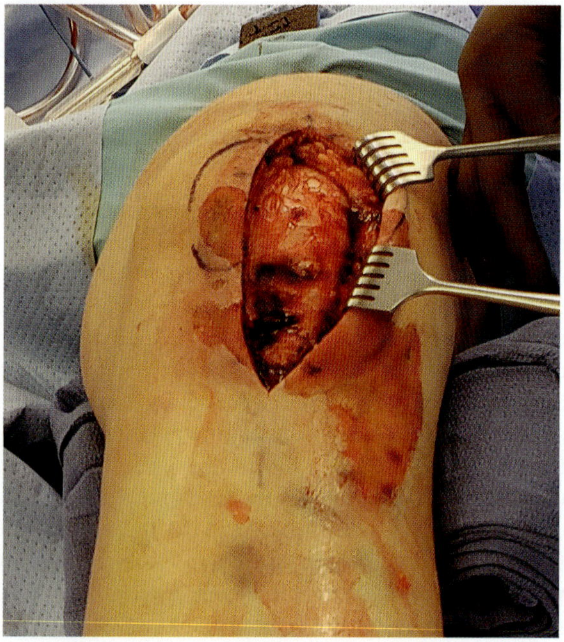

Fig. 1.33 Full-thickness skin and subcutaneous exposure made just prior to lateral parapatellar arthrotomy.

PCL avulsion fractures. With the access to the posteromedial plateau that can be achieved in the posteromedial approach and the access to the posterolateral plateau that can be obtained through an anteromedial or anterolateral approach, the DP approach is not often necessary for fixation of tibial plateau fractures. This approach also provides direct access to the posterior neurovascular structures around the knee and the posterior medial and lateral femoral condyles. A pillow or small bump can be positioned under the feet to provide slight flexion at the knee and relax the popliteal fascia and knee flexors. Many different incisions have been described for posterior exposure of the tibial plateau (Fig. 1.35). One such incision begins proximal lateral along the biceps femoris and curves obliquely into the knee flexion crease and continues distal medial in a lazy S fashion (Fig. 1.36). The saphenous vein and medial sural cutaneous nerve can be seen in the midline in this incision within the subcutaneous tissue and should be found and protected (Fig. 1.37). The medial sural cutaneous nerve can be followed back to the tibial nerve.

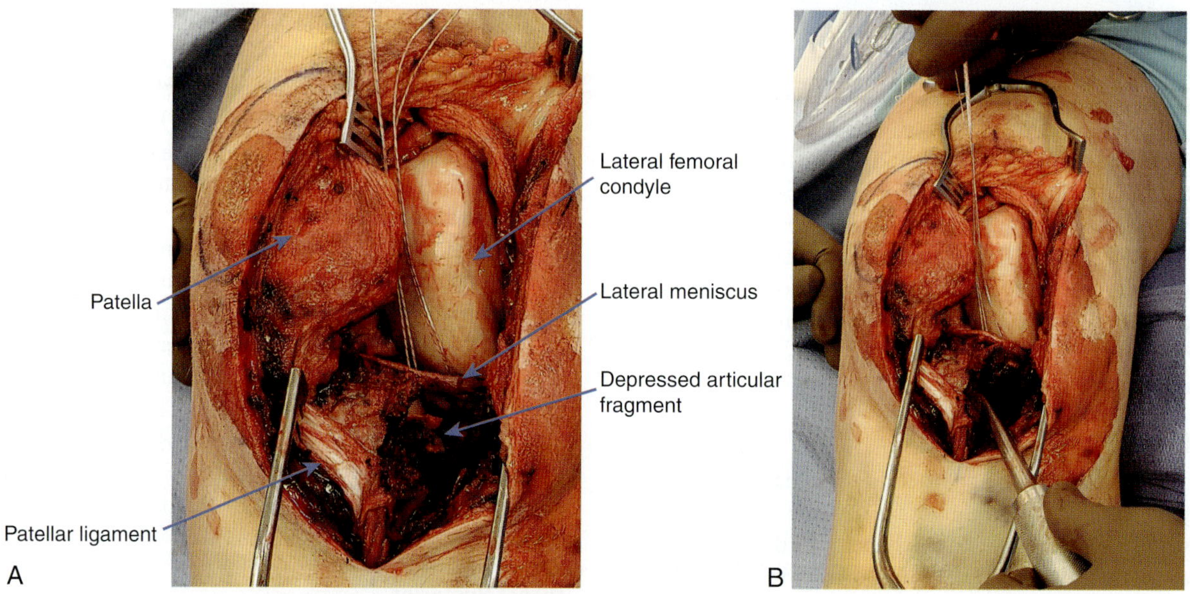

Fig. 1.34 Exposure of the lateral tibial plateau through a direct anterior approach. Note that the lateral cortex has been booked open and is being held with a self-retaining retractor. Depressed articular segment can be seen before (A) and after (B) elevation.

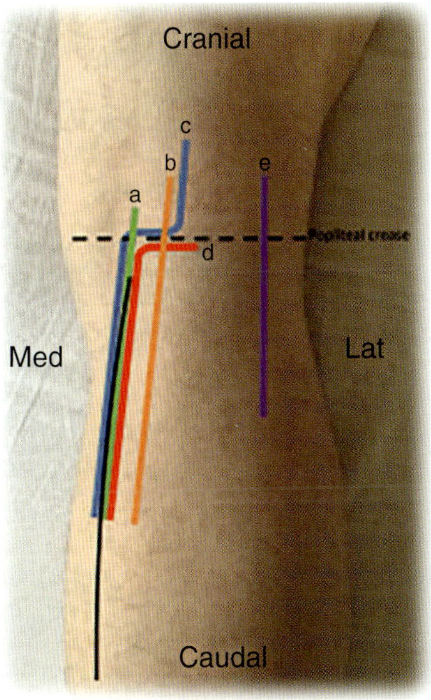

Fig. 1.35 Posterior approaches to the tibial plateau. *a,* Lobenhoffer or direct posteromedial approach *(green line)*; *b,* "FCR" or direct posterior approach *(orange line)*; *c,* S-shaped posteromedial approach *(blue line)*; *d,* posteromedial reversed L-shaped approach *(red line)*; *e,* posterolateral approach *(purple line)*. The medial border of the medial head of the gastrocnemius muscle is indicated by the *black line*. All described approaches with medial-based incisions dissect along the medial border of the gastrocnemius muscle, in order to retract it laterally. Some authors propose transection of the medial gastrocnemius tendon (leaving sufficient stump for reattachment) in order to gain further exposure. The popliteus muscle is longitudinally incised at the medial border and dissected off of the posterior tibia. Careful dissection below the popliteus muscle and its retraction will protect the popliteal neurovascular bundle. *FCR,* Flexor carpi radialis. (From Van den Berg JD, Quintens L, Zhan Y, Hoekstra H. Why address posterior tibial plateau fractures? *Injury.* 2020;51(12):2779-2785. Fig. 2.)

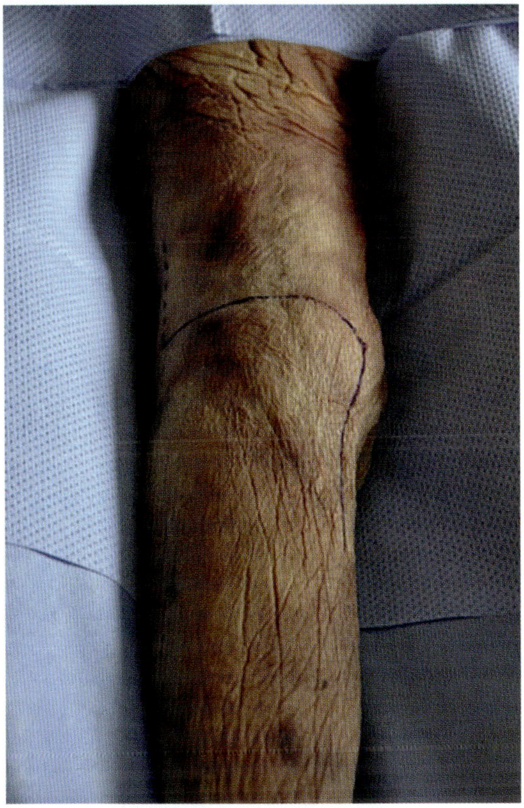

Fig. 1.36 Direct posterior curved incision. (From Berber R, Lewis CP, Copas D, Forward DP, Moran CG. Postero-medial approach for complex tibial plateau injuries with a postero-medial or postero-lateral shear fragment. *Injury.* 2014;45(4):757-765.)

Fascia is incised, and the boundaries of the popliteal fossa are identified (hamstring muscles and gastrocnemius). The common peroneal nerve lies just deep to the biceps femoris at the superolateral border of the popliteal fossa. Moving from lateral to medial lies the tibial nerve, popliteal vein, and popliteal artery (Fig. 1.38). These structures should not be individually dissected out, unless necessary for the operation, to avoid disruption in lymphatic flow of the lower extremity.

To visualize the posterior medial tibial plateau, the medial head of the gastrocnemius is identified and retracted laterally with medial retraction of the semimembranosus. For additional exposure, the medial gastrocnemius origin can be released and retracted inferolaterally with a cuff of tissue left for repair at the completion of the case. Incision and reflection of the posterior capsule will allow direct visualization of the PCL insertion (Fig. 1.39).

Lateral exposure can be obtained by retraction of the lateral head of the gastrocnemius. The common

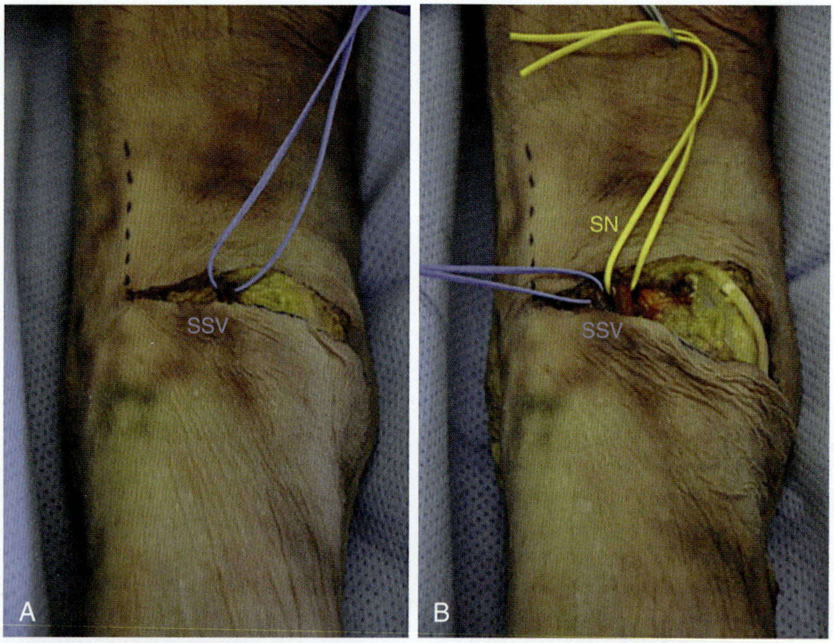

Fig. 1.37 SN and SSV seen in the posterior midline following incision during direct posterior approach. *SN*, Sural nerve; *SSV*, short saphenous vein. (From Berber R, Lewis CP, Copas D, Forward DP, Moran CG. Postero-medial approach for complex tibial plateau injuries with a postero-medial or postero-lateral shear fragment. *Injury*. 2014;45(4):757-765.)

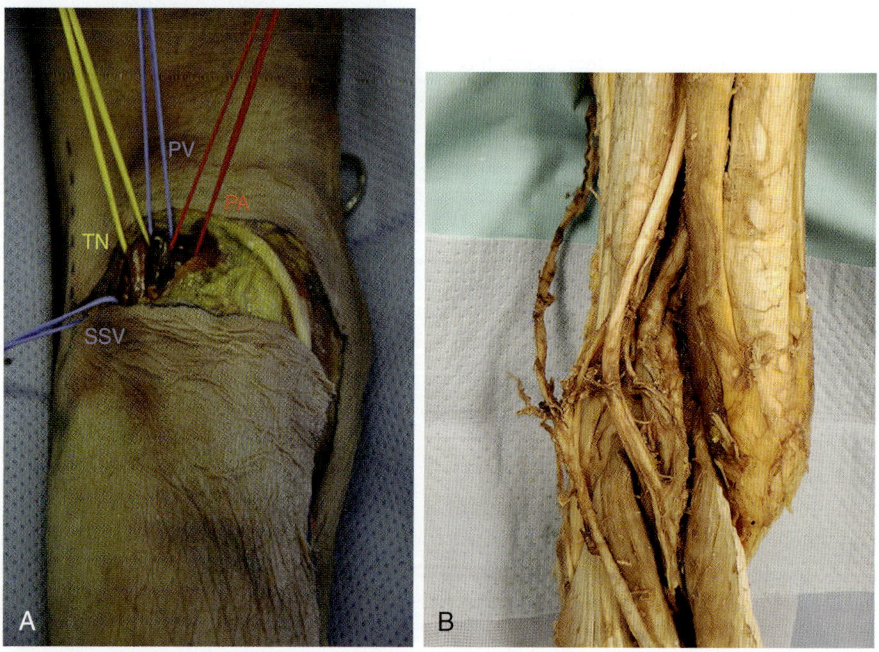

Fig. 1.38 Popliteal structures seen through a direct posterior approach in cadaveric specimens with (A) and without (B) skin. During a clinical approach, it is recommended to not individually dissect artery and nerve unless necessary. (From Berber R, Lewis CP, Copas D, Forward DP, Moran CG. Postero-medial approach for complex tibial plateau injuries with a postero-medial or postero-lateral shear fragment. *Injury*. 2014;45(4):757-765.)

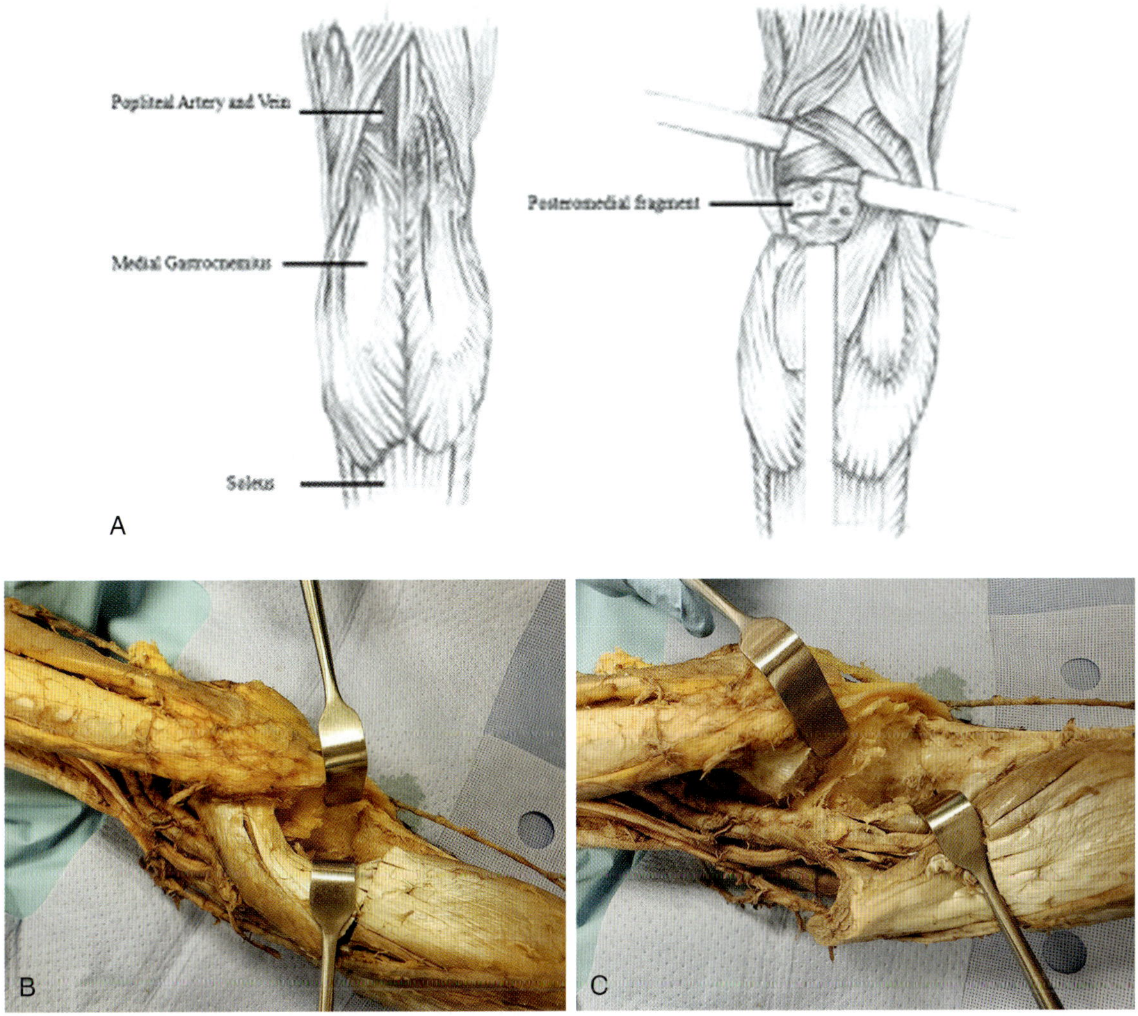

Fig. 1.39 Drawing (A) and cadaver specimen (B and C) showing exposure of the posteromedial corner of the tibial plateau through the direct posterior approach. In C, the origin of the medial head of the gastrocnemius has been divided with a cuff left for later repair. (A, From Lin KC, Tarng YW, Lin GY, Yang SW, Hsu CJ, Renn JH. Prone and direct posterior approach for management of posterior column tibial plateau fractures. *Orthop Traumatol Surg Res.* 2015;101(4):477-482.)

peroneal nerve should be exposed, mobilized, and protected. As with medial exposure, lateral exposure can be increased with the release of the origin of the lateral head of the gastrocnemius and distal reflection (Fig. 1.40).

As an alternative to the release of the gastrocnemius origins, additional exposure can be obtained by dividing the gastrocnemius in its midline.[15] The neurovascular bundle and lateral gastrocnemius are then retracted laterally, while the medial gastrocnemius is retracted medially, and the inferior medial genicular artery is seen overlying the popliteus muscle and ligated. The popliteus is then split and elevated off of the tibia (Fig 1.41). This approach provides wide exposure to the posterior plateau and has been described with a midline incision beginning

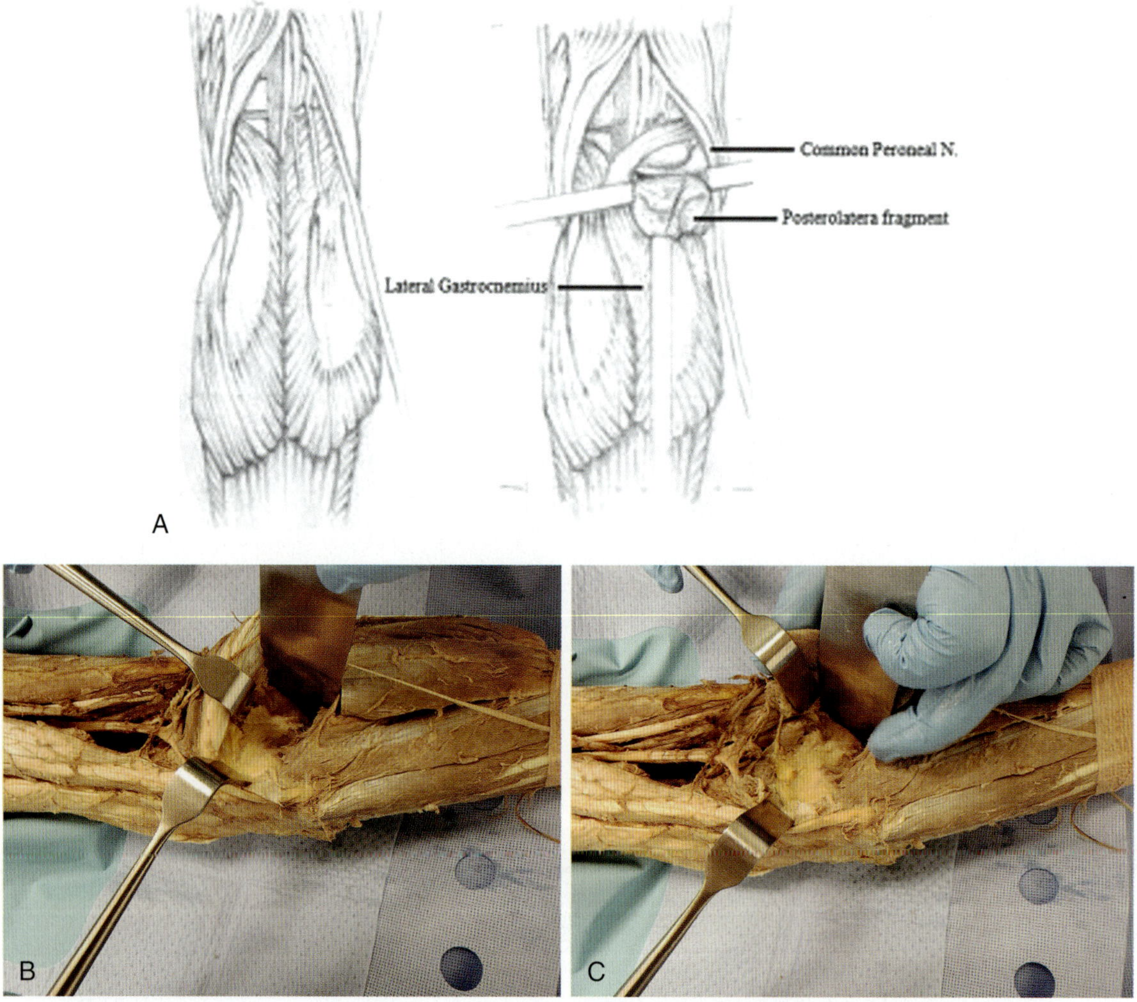

Fig. 1.40 Drawing (A) and cadaver specimen (B and C) showing exposure of the posterolateral corner of the tibial plateau through the direct posterior approach. In C, the origin of the lateral head of the gastrocnemius has been divided with a cuff left for later repair. (A, From Lin KC, Tarng YW, Lin GY, Yang SW, Hsu CJ, Renn JH. Prone and direct posterior approach for management of posterior column tibial plateau fractures. *Orthop Traumatol Surg Res*. 2015;101(4):477-482.)

just below the level of the knee flexion crease and can cross the knee joint in a zig-zag fashion to avoid scar contracture if needed.

Several additional variations of this approach have been described throughout the literature with curved, "L-shaped", and straight incisions (as depicted in Fig. 1.35), and some authors claim that these approaches provide excellent access to the posterior tibia with good clinical and radiographic results in small case series.[16–20]

Posterolateral

Although posterolateral exposure for fracture fixation can be achieved through DP and anterolateral approaches as described earlier, in some cases it may be preferable to perform a direct posterolateral exposure. This can be done with the patient prone or in a lateral position. Exposure can be performed through an L-shaped incision with the vertical limb overlying the posterolateral condyle of the tibia or with a slightly

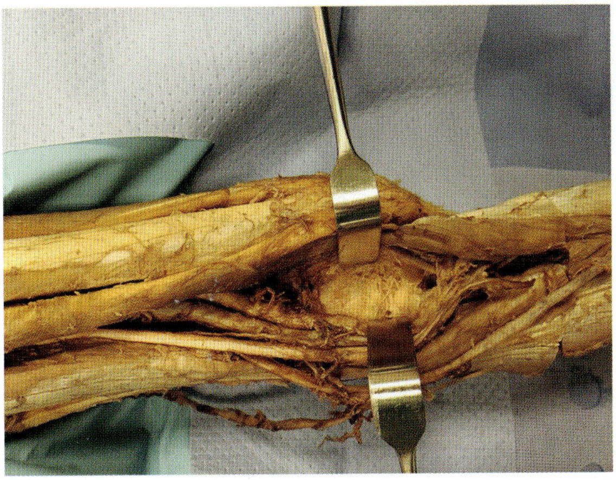

Fig. 1.41 Central exposure with lateral gastrocnemius and neurovascular bundle retracted laterally with medial gastrocnemius retracted medially.

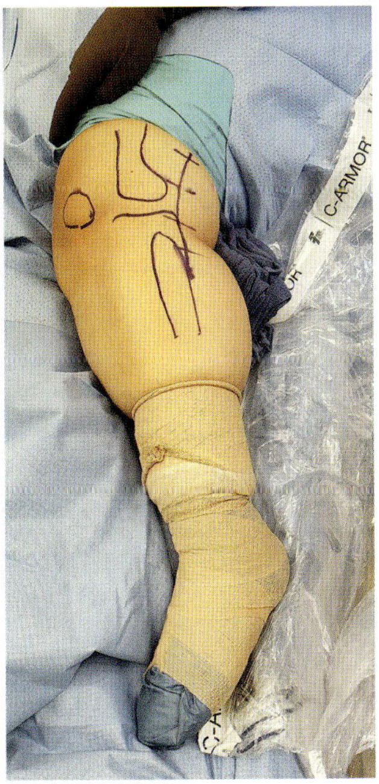

Fig. 1.42 Curved incision for posterolateral approach to the tibial plateau. The patient is in a lateral position.

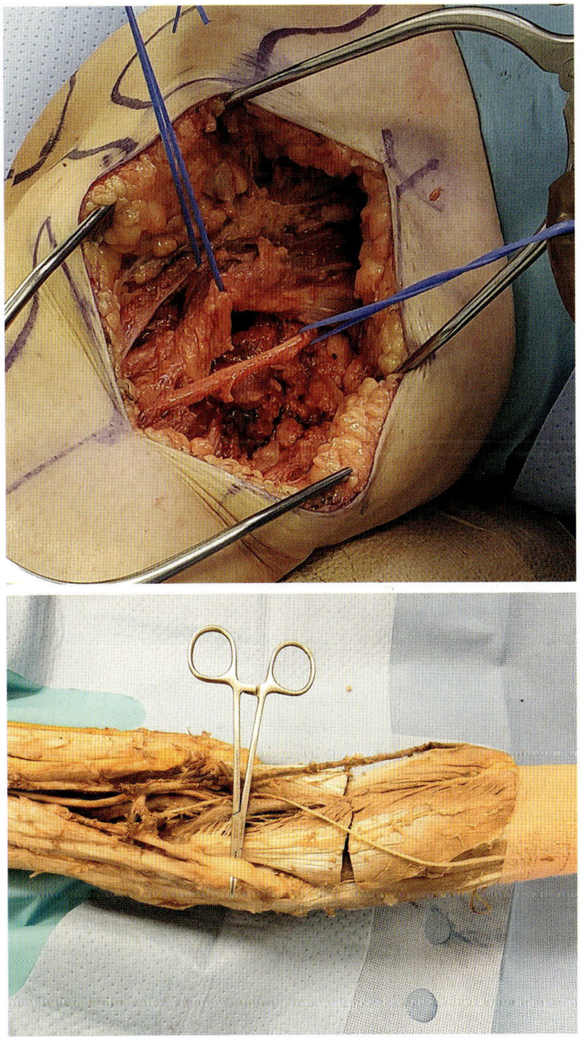

Fig. 1.43 Posterolateral approach. (A) The common peroneal nerve is seen lying posterior to the biceps femoris (both identified with vessel loops, peroneal nerve on the right in this picture, biceps femoris on the left). (B) Cadaveric specimen in prone position with clamp underneath and identifying the common peroneal nerve.

curved incision posterolaterally overlying the biceps femoris and continuing down posterior to the fibula (Fig. 1.42). The common peroneal nerve is identified deep to the biceps femoris (Fig. 1.43), mobilized along its course to the fibula, and protected. The nerve and biceps femoris can be retracted anterolateral and the lateral head of the gastrocnemius can be retracted posteromedial to expose the posterolateral tibia and capsule (Fig. 1.44). The soleus is elevated from the proximal tibia. The PLT will cross the surgical field and can be retracted superiorly. A submeniscal arthrotomy can then be performed if needed. This provides direct access posterolaterally for buttress plating and, if more anterior exposure is needed, the IT band can be incised in line with its fibers and retracted to provide access to the

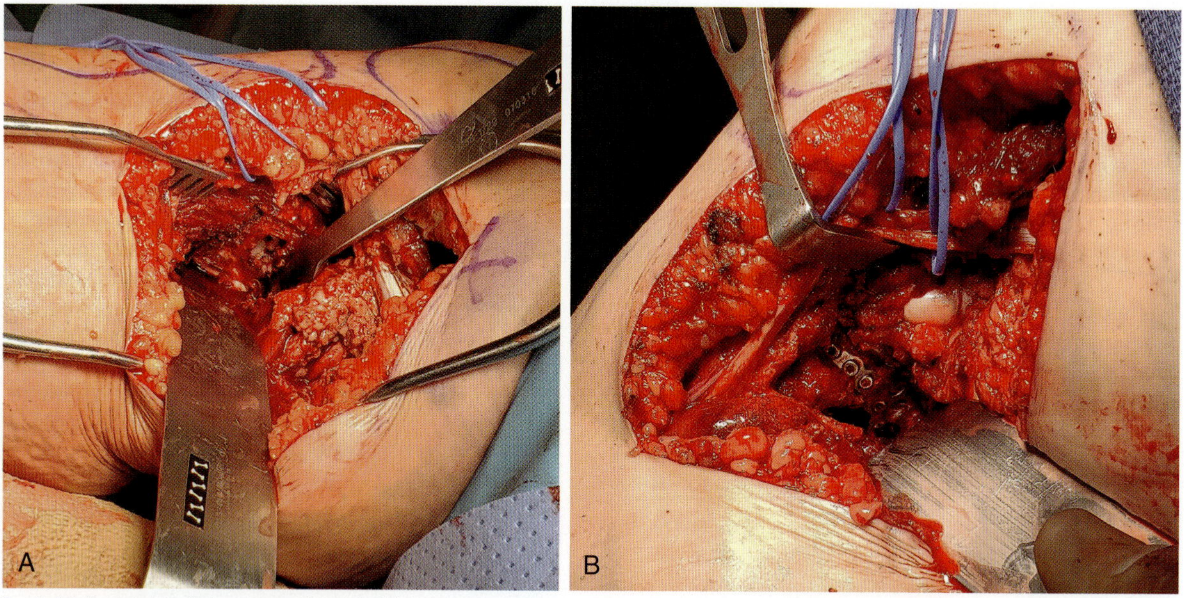

Fig. 1.44 Exposure of the posterolateral tibial plateau. (A) Posterolateral joint depression can be seen just anterior to the malleable retractor. Superficial peroneal nerve and biceps femoris are marked by vessel loops anteriorly. (B) The joint surface has been reduced and 2.7-mm plate applied.

lateral plateau as well. Several descriptions of approaches to the posterolateral tibia are present in the literature. Older approaches describe the use of a proximal fibula osteotomy, while more recent descriptions do not.[17,21–25]

Arthroscopic Approach

Standard anteromedial and anterolateral arthroscopic portals can be established with vertical or transverse incisions at the joint line on either side of the patellar tendon (Fig. 1.45). An inflow portal is sometimes necessary superolaterally as well to allow for high flow and flushing of hematoma from the joint. Gravity flow of fluid is used to prevent excess fluid extravasation into the leg, which could predispose the patient to the development of compartment syndrome. For this reason, dry scoping without fluid can also be used. A suction shaver is often needed to remove hematoma from within fracture lines. Arthroscopic visualization and probing of the articular surface can be performed through anterolateral and anteromedial parapatellar portals. Accessory incisions are then made for reduction and instrumentation as needed for the particular fracture pattern.

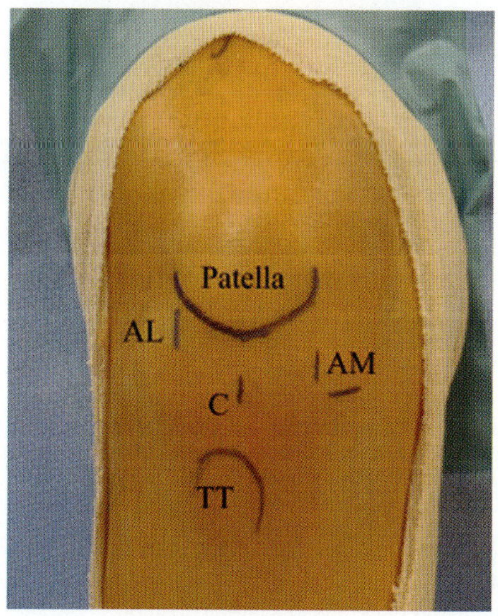

Fig. 1.45 Arthroscopic portal placement, right knee. *AL*, Anterolateral portal; *AM*, anteromedial portal; *TT*, tibial tubercle; *C*, central portal.)

Arthroscopic visualization can also be performed in conjunction with open approaches in order to better visualize articular surfaces not readily seen through the approach being performed. For example, a medial portal can provide direct visualization of the medial condyle during anterolateral exposure. Additionally, if medial or

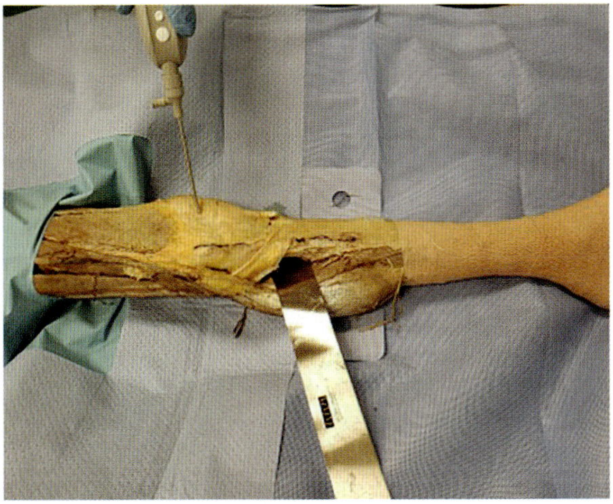

Fig. 1.46 Arthroscope placed and used without fluid for visualization of the joint with open approach. This can be performed through a standard anterior arthroscopic portal (as seen here) or used through a submeniscal arthrotomy to "see around and over" the edge of the tibial plateau for better visualization.

posterior visualization of the lateral plateau is suboptimal during anterolateral exposure, an arthroscope can be used without fluid to better view the plateau through a small medial portal or the submeniscal arthrotomy (Fig. 1.46).

RIEHL'S TIPS AND TRICKS

- A femoral distractor (or external fixator) can be used to provide increased visualization of the joint surface.
- The direct anterior approach provides good visualization of the joint surface and is especially useful in combined plating/nailing procedures.
- Do not hesitate to extend an incision proximally and/or distally if visualization of the fracture is suboptimal.
- Knee flexion and external rotation of the tibia allow for DP tibial access in the posteromedial approach.
- Repair of the ALL and IT band should be performed at the completion of the case with the anterolateral approach.[26]
- Dry scoping with scope inserted through standard portals or through arthrotomy can assist with greater visualization of the articular surface in tibial plateau fractures.

REFERENCES

1. Ishii Y, Terajima K, Terashima S, Koga Y. Three-dimensional kinematics of the human knee with intracortical pin fixation. *Clin Orthop Relat Res.* 1997;343:144–150.
2. Kim HY, Kim KJ, Yang DS, Jeung SW, Choi HG, Choy WS. Screw-home movement of the tibiofemoral joint during normal gait: three-dimensional analysis. *Clin Orthop Surg.* 2015;7(3):303–309.
3. Loudon JK. Biomechanics and pathomechanics of the patellofemoral joint. *Int J Sports Phys Ther.* 2016;11(6):820–830.
4. Schindler OS, Scott WN. Basic kinematics and biomechanics of the patella-femoral joint part 1: the native patella. *Acta Orthop Belg.* 2011;77(4):421–431.
5. Thamyongkit S, Fayad LM, Jones LC, Hasenboehler EA, Sirisreetreerux N, Shafiq B. The distal femur is a reliable guide for tibial plateau fracture reduction: a study of measurements on 3D CT scans in 84 healthy knees. *J Orthop Surg Res.* 2018;13(1):224.
6. Johannsen AM, Cook AM, Gardner MJ, Bishop JA. Defining the width of the normal tibial plateau relative to the distal femur: critical normative data for identifying pathologic widening in tibial plateau fractures. *Clin Anat.* 2018;31(5):688–692.
7. LaPrade RF, Engebretsen AH, Ly TV, Johansen S, Wentorf FA, Engebresten L. The anatomy of the medial part of the knee. *J Bone Joint Surg Am.* 2007;89(9):2000–2010.
8. Quiles C, Constantino JA, Ganan Y, Macias D, Quiles M. Stereophotogrammetric surface anatomy of the anterior cruciate ligament's tibial footprint: precise osseous structure and distances to arthroscopically-relevant landmarks. *Knee.* 2018;25(4):531–544.
9. Sheps DM, Otto D, Fernhout M. The anatomic characteristics of the tibial insertion of the posterior cruciate ligament. *Arthroscopy.* 2005;21(7):820–825.
10. James EW, LaPrade CM, LaPrade RF. Anatomy and biomechanics of the lateral side of the knee and surgical implications. *Sports Med Arthrosc Rev.* 2015;23(1):2–9.
11. Chen HW, Luo CF. Extended anterolateral approach for treatment of posterolateral tibial plateau fractures improves operative procedure and patient prognosis. *Int J Clin Exp Med.* 2015;8(8):13708–13715.
12. Hu SJ, Chang SM, Zhang YQ, Ma Z, Du SC, Zhang K. The anterolateral supra-fibular-head approach for plating posterolateral tibial plateau fractures: a novel surgical technique. *Injury.* 2016;47:502–507.
13. Cho JW, Smal P, Jeon YS, Oh CW, Oh JK. Rim plating of posterolateral fracture fragments (PLFs) through a modified anterolateral approach in tibial plateau fractures. *J Orthop Trauma.* 2016;30(11):e362–e368.

14. Berwin JT, Donovan RL, Riddick A, Kelly MB. The "FCR" approach to the knee for the management of posterior tibial plateau fractures. *J Orthop Trauma.* 2020;34(6):e221–e224.
15. Yin Z, Yang W, Gu Y, et al. A modified direct posterior midline approach for the treatment of posterior column tibial plateau fractures. *J Knee Surg.* 2020;33:646–654.
16. Luo CF, Sun H, Zhang B, Zeng BF. Three-column fixation for complex tibial plateau fractures. *J Orthop Trauma.* 2010;24(11):683–692.
17. Carlson DA. Posterior bicondylar tibial plateau fractures. *J Orthop Trauma.* 2005;19(2):73–78.
18. Lin KC, Tarng YW, Lin GY, Yang SW, Hsu CJ, Renn JH. Prone and direct posterior approach for management of posterior column tibial plateau fractures. *Orthop Traumatol Surg Res.* 2015;101(4):477–482.
19. Alpert JM, McCarty III LP, Bach BRJR. The direct posterior approach to the knee: surgical and anatomic approach. *J Knee Surg.* 2008;21(1):44–49.
20. Berber R, Lewis CP, Copas D, Forward DP, Moran CG. Postero-medial approach for complex tibial plateau injuries with a postero-medial or postero-lateral shear fragment. *Injury.* 2014;45(4):757–765.
21. Lobenhoffer P, Gerich T, Bertram T, Lattermann C, Pohlemann T, Tscheme H. [Particular posteromedial and posterolateral approaches for the treatment of tibial head fractures]. *Unfallchirurg.* 1997;100(12):957–967.
22. Garner MR, Warner SJ, Lorich DG. Surgical approaches to posterolateral tibial plateau fractures. *J Knee Surg.* 2016;29(1):12–20.
23. Frosch KH, Balcarek P, Walde T, Sturmer KM. A new posterolateral approach without fibula osteotomy for the treatment of tibial plateau fractures. *J Orthop Trauma.* 2010;24(8):515–520.
24. Chen C, Huang L, Zheng H, et al. Combined direct posterior split-gastrocnemius approach for the posterolateral tibial plateau involved fractures. *Ther Clin Risk Manag.* 2019;15:1461–1467.
25. Chang SM, Zheng HP, Li HF, et al. Treatment of isolated posterior coronal fracture of the lateral tibial plateau through posterolateral approach for direct exposure and buttress plate fixation. *Arch Orthop Trauma Surg.* 2009;129(7):955–962.
26. Wei X, Wang Z, Lu Y, Sun J, Riehl J. Surgical treatment for avulsion fractures of the anterolateral ligament associated with periarticular fractures of the knee. *J Knee Surg.* 2021. PMID 34507364. Online ahead of print.

2

Mechanism, Evaluation, and Temporary Fixation

Jesse Jay Caballero, MD, Jan Szatkowski, MD, MBA, Abhijit Seetharam, MD, and Yohan Jang DO, FAAOS

INTRODUCTION

Demographics

Fractures involving the tibial articular surface account for a little over 1% of all long bone fractures, 56.9% of all proximal tibia fractures/dislocations, and 8% of all fractures in the elderly.[1–4] These fractures have an annual incidence of 10.3 per 100,000.[5] The combined incidence of a patient having a tibial plateau fracture with associated polytrauma on admission has been estimated at 16% to 40%.[6–8] The age distribution is bimodal for both males and females, which is similar to what is seen in other periarticular injuries.[2] The majority of fractures occur in males (70%), with men aged 40 to 44 years being the most affected patient population overall.[4,5] Comminuted fractures are more common in males.[3] There is a shift of incidence between males and females that occurs after the age of 60, with females (61%) predominating.[4,9] With an increase in life expectancy and a large aging population in many developed countries, it is expected that the incidence of low-energy tibial plateau fractures will continue to increase. Medical comorbidities and certain medications can affect bone quality, increase the risk of postoperative infection, and inhibit wound healing.

Mechanism of Injury

The mechanism of tibial plateau fractures varies by the age of the patient. The majority of tibial plateau fractures in the elderly are due to low-energy falls. Osteopenia and osteoporosis play a large role in the fracture mechanisms and patterns observed. The forces acting on bone determine the resulting fracture patterns in conjunction with bone quality. Low bone density decreases the force necessary for injury. In the elderly, lateral fracture patterns are seen more commonly than medial ones. A higher incidence of compression fracture patterns tends to be seen in such cases with lower-energy injury mechanisms. In younger individuals, high-energy mechanisms predominate. The injury mechanism can involve motor vehicles, sports, and falls from height. The most common mechanism of injury overall is pedestrians being struck by motorized vehicles (30%), followed by low-energy falls (22%).[10]

The magnitude and direction of the injury force will often influence the fracture pattern. Angular, axial, and compression forces can all lead to failure of the condyles. Axial load is usually a predominant component of the injury mechanism and produces higher energy at failure than angular forces. In general, greater axial load results in more severe fractures with increased comminution, fragment displacement, and associated soft-tissue injury. In a cadaver study[11] that looked at mechanisms of injury, it was found that pure valgus forces resulted in the typical lateral split fractures, axial forces resulted in joint compression fractures, and a combination of axial and valgus forces resulted in split depression fractures. In isolated lateral plateau fractures, the medial collateral ligament can act as a pivot point causing the lateral femoral condyle to impact the lateral tibial plateau. The proximal tibia is more vulnerable to valgus force because of the 5 to 7 degrees of knee valgus in normal anatomic alignment. In addition, lateral side impacts tend to occur as a common injury mechanism in these fractures.

CLINICAL EVALUATION

Initial Emergency Department Evaluation

Evaluation and management of tibial plateau fractures in the emergency department will set the stage for successful patient outcomes. One should suspect a tibial plateau fracture in a patient who presents with pain and tenderness around the knee following an injury. The pain may be localized to the proximal tibia at the fracture site. The patient may present with a visible knee hemarthrosis secondary to an intraarticular fracture. The patient may also report deep pain secondary to a ligamentous or meniscal injury. Evaluation of a suspected tibial plateau fracture begins with a history and physical examination, as described later. The reported mechanism of injury is important to determine, as it helps predict the severity of the injury, the fracture pattern, and the associated injuries. For example, a fall from standing is a low-energy mechanism, and the risk of associated soft tissue, neurovascular injury, or compartment syndrome (CS) is low. However, if the mechanism is of high energy (as seen with motor vehicle accidents, a pedestrian struck, or a fall from height), then a higher degree of vigilance is necessary to detect associated injuries that may require urgent or emergent management. A thorough physical examination results in the diagnosis of associated injuries and helps establish future surgical timing and treatment.

Examination of the soft-tissue envelope will reveal the presence or absence of significant swelling, abrasions, blisters, and open injury. Open fractures require immediate antibiotics as the delay in the initial dose of antibiotic administration markedly increases the risk of infection.[12] Antibiotic coverage is guided by the severity of injury and contamination and typically includes coverage for gram-positive bacteria. If the open fracture injury appears to be of higher severity, prophylaxis against gram-negative organisms is recommended, and in the case of soil contamination, penicillin may be added as well.[13,14] As previously discussed, a thorough neurovascular examination should be performed. Any neurological deficits should be documented, whether complete or partial. There is a higher incidence of peroneal stretch injuries with medial plateau and higher-energy mechanisms.[15] If there are abnormalities of the distal leg pulses, further evaluation should ensue, including ankle-brachial index (ABI) measurement and possibly additional evaluation with a computed tomography arteriogram (CTA) or vascular consultation. Furthermore, the importance of assessment of the leg compartments cannot be overemphasized. If CS is evident, based either on classic signs and symptoms or on measured compartment pressures, plans should be set in place for urgent fasciotomies. Patients who present with injury following high-energy mechanisms should be strongly considered for close observation for the development of CS.

Radiographs ultimately guide treatment decisions and determine the risks of associated injuries. A CT scan is often necessary to optimally characterize a tibial plateau fracture; however, it should not always be ordered during the emergency department evaluation. When temporary external fixation is planned and fracture comminution and shortening are present, CT scans will provide a better picture of the fracture fragments after the application of an external fixator.

History

It is important to obtain a thorough history in all tibial plateau fractures. One should attempt to determine the mechanism of injury, its severity, and whether there is a need for emergent management. Low-energy falls or twisting injuries are less likely to cause neurovascular injury or CS, whereas falls from height, motor vehicle accidents, and pedestrians being struck by a vehicle may necessitate more urgent management. The fracture pattern is important in determining the treatment approach and risk of complications. The location and severity of pain, the timing of the injury, the associated injuries, and any treatments administered are helpful pieces of information. One should also assess tobacco use, prior knee problems, ambulatory status prior to the injury, and medical comorbidities such as pulmonary disease, diabetes, vascular disease, cancers, renal disease, nutritional deficiencies, previous poor dual-energy X-ray absorptiometry (DEXA) scan results, as well as the use of immunosuppressive medicines. Medical comorbidities and certain medications can affect bone quality, increase the risk for postoperative infection, and inhibit wound healing. The patient's activity level, social support, mental condition, and employment status should be known in order to make an appropriate treatment plan and manage postoperative expectations.

Physical Examination

As a part of the initial assessment of tibial plateau fractures, one should attempt to rule out soft-tissue compromise, open fractures, CS, and neurovascular injury. The injured limb should be circumferentially assessed, paying special attention to the overlying skin and the neurovascular baseline status. Circumferential skin and soft-tissue inspection and palpation should be done to assess for open injury and severity of soft-tissue injury. The severity of soft-tissue injury may be further described by the size, character, and location of swelling, contusions, and fracture blisters. Soft-tissue assessment is key to determining surgical approaches and timing.

A noncompressible, firm extremity, paresthesias, and pain with passive stretching suggest CS. Because it can develop even days after injury, CS should be monitored for throughout the patient's stay. Consideration should be given to measuring compartment pressures in those with high-energy fracture patterns or in unresponsive patients, and this may need to be repeated based on clinical assessment. Whether diagnosed by elevated compartment pressures or by physical examination alone, CS is treated by urgent fasciotomy. More details on CS are given later.

For high-energy injuries, especially fracture-dislocations and metaphyseal-diaphyseal dissociation patterns, it is imperative to obtain a thorough neurovascular assessment. Vascular injury is rare overall, but delays in diagnosis and surgical intervention by more than 8 hours can result in lower extremity amputation rates as high as 86%.[16–18] Neurovascular assessment should include testing for sensation patterns in the distribution of the tibial, superficial peroneal, saphenous, and sural nerves, and motor function of the tibial and peroneal nerves. Likewise, it should include extremity color assessment, capillary refill, and palpation of the distal pulses, including the posterior tibial and dorsalis pedis arteries. Findings should be compared with the contralateral side. Any differences in pulses or sensation can be further investigated with an ABI measurement. For some high-energy fractures, one might obtain an ABI regardless. An ABI >0.8 has a remarkably high negative predictive value, approaching 100%. With ABI <0.9, further vascular assessment with a CTA and/or a vascular surgery consultation should be obtained.[16]

If instability is suspected but not clear on radiographic assessment, varus and valgus stress testing may be required. Valgus instability is a potential indication for surgical management, especially in lateral tibial plateau fractures. Instability may not resolve without surgical fracture reduction and fixation.[19,20]

IMAGING AND EVALUATION

Imaging is a critical part of the initial evaluation. Imaging modalities range from plain radiographs to CT with three-dimensional reconstruction and magnetic resonance imaging (MRI). Imaging is necessary to evaluate the injury and determine what type of treatment may be necessary.

Plain Radiographs

Plain radiographs are usually the first imaging study to evaluate suspected tibial plateau fractures (Fig. 2.1). For some simple fractures, this may be the only imaging modality necessary. Typically, one orders anteroposterior (AP) and lateral view plain radiographs of the knee. An additional view, the caudal view (also known as the "tibial plateau view"), is shot 10 to 15 degrees caudally from a typical 90-degree AP view. This is done to account for the 15-degree posteroinferior slope of the plateau surface. The caudal view plain radiograph provides a view in line with the plane of the plateau. In this view, the proximal articular surface can be viewed as a single radiodense line that allows better assessment than lateral and AP views of articular depression.[21] One should also obtain radiographs of the entire tibia. Oblique views were once used to assess the fracture lines and degree of displacement; however, CT scans have largely replaced them. Notably, it has been shown that plain radiographs alone can miss insufficiency fractures in osteopenic patients.[22]

Results of plain radiograph imaging can guide treatment decisions and determine the risks of associated injuries. Radiographic indications for surgery include lateral fractures with more than 5 degrees of valgus tilt, medial plateau fractures, bicondylar fractures, articular depression greater than 3 mm, and condylar widening greater than 5 mm.[23] The AP radiograph may show articular surface depression and dense-appearing subchondral bone, which are indicative of a compression injury. The alignment of the knee joint and the fracture pattern can also be assessed from the AP view. Fractures that split and depress the lateral plateau have a higher incidence of associated lateral meniscus tears.[24] Medial tibial plateau fractures usually require high-energy mechanisms; thus, the suspicion of a fracture-dislocation in these cases should be high. Medial tibial plateau fractures demand a careful neurovascular examination, and ABI measurements may be needed.

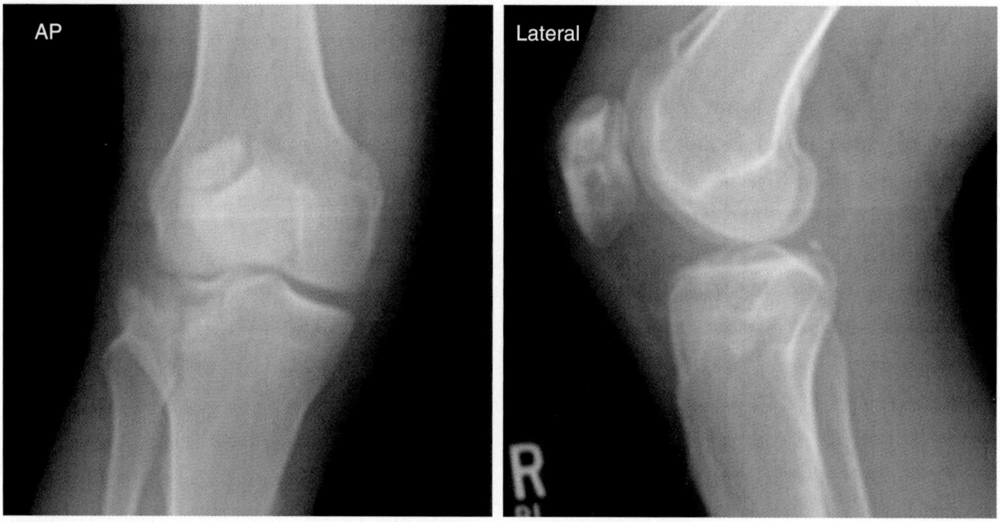

Fig. 2.1 Anterior-posterior (*left*) and lateral (*right*) radiographs of a lateral tibial plateau fracture that is comminuted, split, and depressed.

Additionally, fractures of the medial plateau are associated with a high incidence of medial meniscal tears and ACL rupture. ACL rupture has also been shown to have a significant association with fracture patterns including metaphyseal-diaphyseal separation.[25,26] Lateral radiographs are used to evaluate the medial plateau and may reveal coronal split fractures. Coronal split fractures are more common within the medial plateau and are often missed on the AP view.[26] A fracture with a large posteromedial fragment may necessitate a posteromedial approach for appropriate fixation.

Somewhat counterintuitively, patients with fractures with up to 10 mm of articular depression and joint stability have acceptable functional outcomes in long-term studies; however, joint instability in the context of certain other factors such as articular step-offs and central joint depression results in poor outcomes.[27] Additionally, more than 5 degrees of limb malalignment may triple the rate of posttraumatic degenerative arthritis.[28]

When there is substantial displacement, traction radiographs can be used to assess the fracture anatomy in both plain radiographs and CT scans. This can be obtained by manual traction or spanning external fixators. In severely comminuted fractures, contralateral radiographs may provide a template for reduction including condylar width, coronal alignment, and the posterior slope of the plateau in the sagittal plane.

Computed Tomography

CT scans have become a routine part of the assessment of tibial plateau fractures (Fig. 2.2). Axial CT cuts are especially helpful in visualizing posteromedial fracture lines not evident on plain radiographs. Axial CT and reconstructions provide important insight into fracture anatomy and serve as an aid in preoperative planning. It has been demonstrated in numerous studies that the use of CT scans in addition to plan films allows surgeons to more reliably classify fractures, which aids in providing the most appropriate treatment.[29–34] CT reveals articular displacement and comminution more readily than plain radiographs.[34] CT also allows for better assessment of the location and orientation of fracture lines, the degree of depression, and the size of articular segments, which provide important information in preoperative planning.

As in the interpretation of plain radiographs, one should evaluate CT imaging studies systematically. The appearance of lipohemarthrosis on CT indicates an intraarticular fracture and is most commonly seen with occult tibial plateau fractures. Complex fracture patterns are more clearly delineated on CT. One should rule out the presence of posterolateral and posteromedial fracture fragments, which often require adjunct fixation. These fragments sometimes occur in bicondylar tibial plateau fractures. The posterolateral fragment may appear as an inverted conical shape that is vertically oriented and

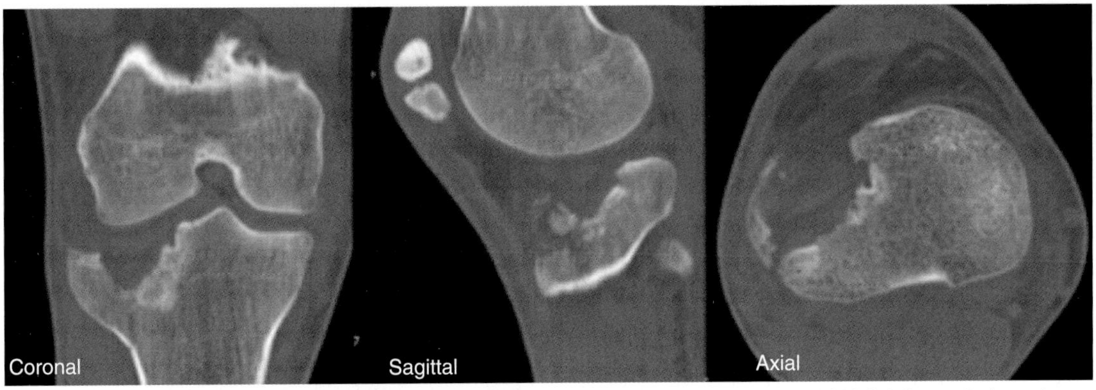

Fig. 2.2 Computed tomography scan of select coronal *(left)*, sagittal *(center)*, and axial *(right)* views of a lateral split-depression fracture of the tibial plateau. The medial condyle is unaffected.

occupies one-third of the lateral plateau surface.[35] The posteromedial fragment is often defined by any posteriorly based articular fracture that exits the medial cortex and is often best visualized on axial CT images. Failure to address these fragments can result in fracture malreduction and postoperative complications.[36]

Magnetic Resonance Imaging

MRI is increasingly used to evaluate tibial plateau fractures. Some argue that only MRI can adequately show soft-tissue injuries, especially those associated with high-energy fractures, which often cause ligamentous and meniscal pathology.[37] MRI is more sensitive than CT in detecting ligamentous and meniscal injuries that are both common occurrences in tibial plateau fractures.[38] Like CT, MRI (Fig. 2.3) will detect lipohemarthrosis. MRI is the gold standard when it comes to detecting occult fractures not seen on plain radiographs.

Compartment Syndrome

CS is a limb- and sometimes life-threatening condition that can lead to devastating outcomes if not appropriately diagnosed and treated. CS is often associated with trauma or other conditions that cause bleeding, edema, or vascular compromise and causes increased pressure within a myofascial compartment of the body. Because the fascia and connective tissue are inelastic, increased intracompartmental pressure eventually compresses the thin-walled veins, leading to venous hypertension and eventual tissue ischemia. Muscle necrosis can occur as quickly as 2 hours after onset of CS.[39] Irreversible nerve damage occurs 6 to 8 hours after onset. Given the high-energy nature of the injuries, tibial plateau fractures are often associated with CS. The reported incidence varies, though one study reports a 53% incidence of CS in Schatzker type IV tibial plateau fractures.[40] The overall incidence of CS following tibial plateau fractures varies in the literature from 1% to 11%.[41–43] Several studies on tibial plateau fractures suggest that acute CS contributes to postoperative complications such as nonunion and infections.[44–48] Acute CS needs to be appropriately recognized, diagnosed, and managed to prevent both acute and long-term complications for patients.

Early recognition and diagnosis of CS is critical to the overall outcome. The diagnosis is often clinical, although this can be challenging at times. The common clinical signs of CS include worsening pain out of proportion to the situation, pain with passive stretch (passive plantar flexion of the big toe), paresthesias, pulselessness, and poikilothermia. However, these clinical signs have been shown to have low sensitivity for diagnosing CS.[49–52] Additionally, clinical diagnosis can be difficult in polytrauma patients with distracting injuries or those too obtunded to report symptoms or show clinical signs (e.g., those who are intubated or sedated). Intracompartmental pressure measurement can be another useful diagnostic tool to diagnose CS. CS is diagnosed when the difference between diastolic blood pressure and compartment pressure is less than 30 mmHg (delta P). However, it is important to note that patients under anesthesia can have falsely decreased diastolic pressures, which may lead to overdiagnosis of CS and unnecessary

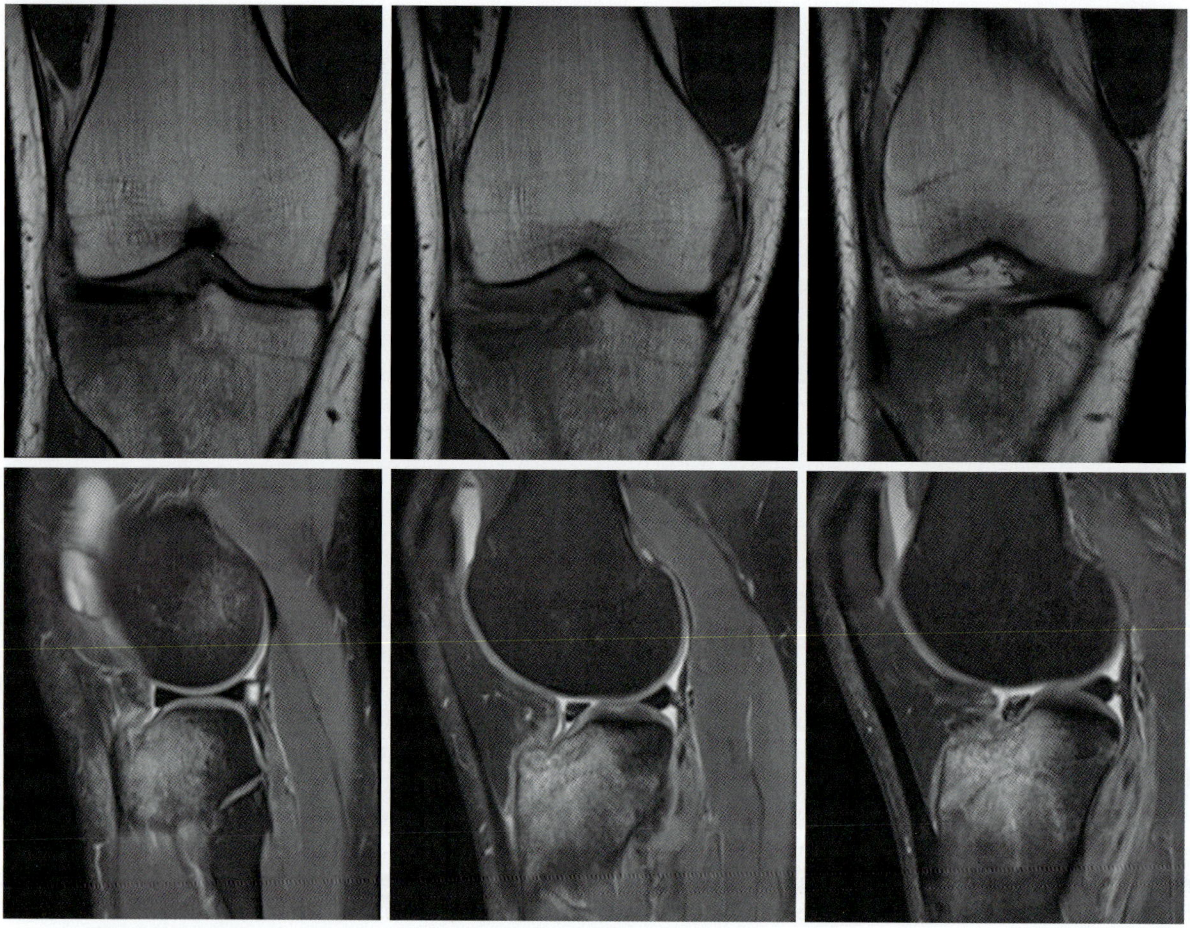

Fig. 2.3 Coronal and sagittal proton density-weighted magnetic resonance images demonstrate a depressed lateral tibial plateau fracture with associated meniscus tear.

fasciotomies, as described by Kakar et al.[53] It has also been shown that a single compartment pressure measurement with delta P < 30 mmHg may not be clinically significant.[54] One study showed that measuring delta P < 30 mmHg for 2 or more consecutive hours has a sensitivity of 94% for CS.[55] Compartment pressures can also vary based on the proximity to the fracture site and the depth of measurement. Studies have shown that the highest pressure measurements will be obtained within 5 cm of the fracture[56] and centrally in the muscle.[57] Surgeons must have a high index of suspicion for CS in tibial plateau fractures. When it is diagnosed, emergent fasciotomies are necessary to prevent irreversible limb and life-threatening complications (Fig. 2. 4).

Technique

In the case of CS associated with tibial plateau fractures, the authors recommend four compartment fasciotomies performed through medial and lateral incisions (two-incision technique). An anterolateral longitudinal incision is made from the proximal tibial metaphyseal-diaphyseal junction to the distal tibial metaphyseal-diaphyseal junction. The incision is centered between the lateral border of the tibia and the anterior border of the fibula. Subcutaneous tissue is incised down to fascia. In the midportion of the wound, a transverse incision is then made in the fascia and the intermuscular septum is identified and palpated. The anterior compartment fascia is then incised along the entire length of the tibia

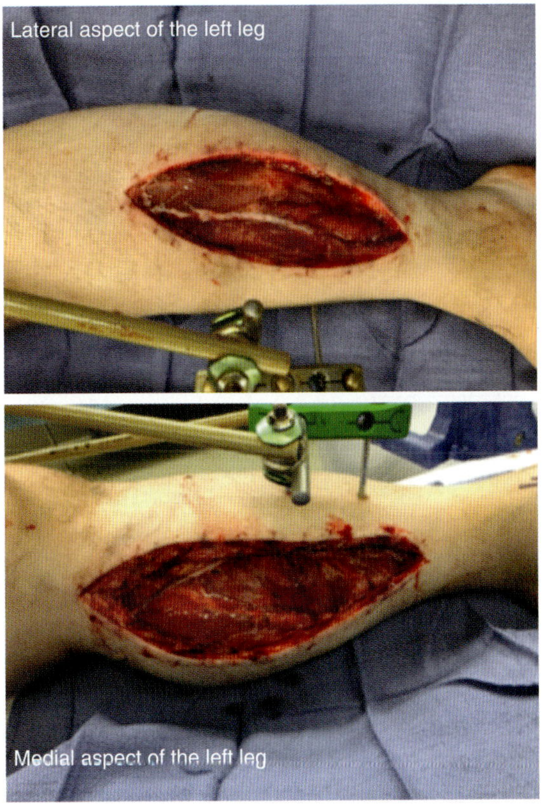

Fig. 2.4 Tibial plateau fracture with associated compartment syndrome treated with temporary external fixation and lateral *(top)* and medial *(bottom)* fasciotomies.

with an incision of the fascia anterior to the intermuscular septum. A fascial incision posterior to the intermuscular septum along the length of the tibia releases the lateral compartment while taking care to avoid injuring the superficial peroneal nerve. Fascial release can be performed with a scalpel, scissors, or a combination thereof (Fig. 2.5).

To release the posterior compartments, a posteromedial incision is made approximately 2 cm posterior to the posteromedial border of the tibia, again along nearly the entire length of the tibia. During subcutaneous dissection, care is taken to avoid injury to the saphenous vein and nerve. Fascia is then incised along the length of the tibia, releasing the superficial posterior compartment. The deep posterior compartment is then released by first incising fascia overlying the soleus muscle and flexor digitorum longus at the midtibia. A Cobb elevator is then used to release the entire deep posterior compartment by sliding it proximally and distally along the length of the posterior tibia, staying up against bone the entire time (Fig. 2.6).

Once compartments are released, muscle is inspected for color, consistency, contractility, and capacity to bleed (the four Cs) to bleed. Muscle that is suspected to be nonviable is debrided, although it is important to note that the four Cs and the surgeon's overall impression correlate poorly with histological findings regarding muscle viability, and attempts

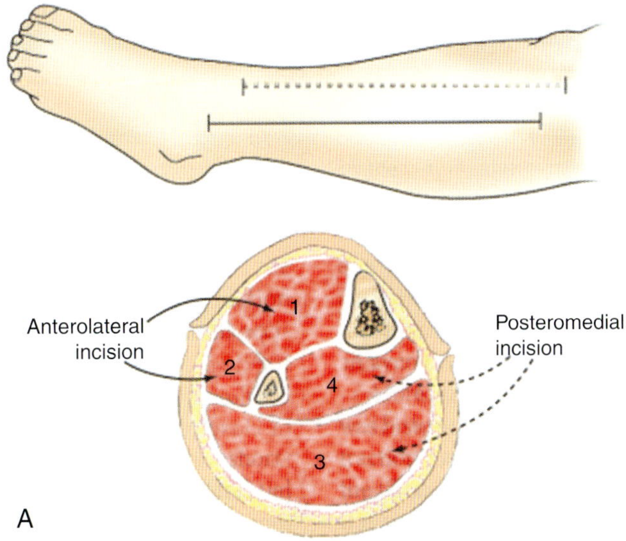

Fig. 2.5 Anterior and lateral compartment release. Longitudinal incision located halfway between the tibia and fibula extending from the proximal tibial metaphysis to the distal metaphysis (A). (Essential Orthopaedics, Stephen Shaheen, Jeffrey R. Bytomski, Elsevier, 2020).

Continued

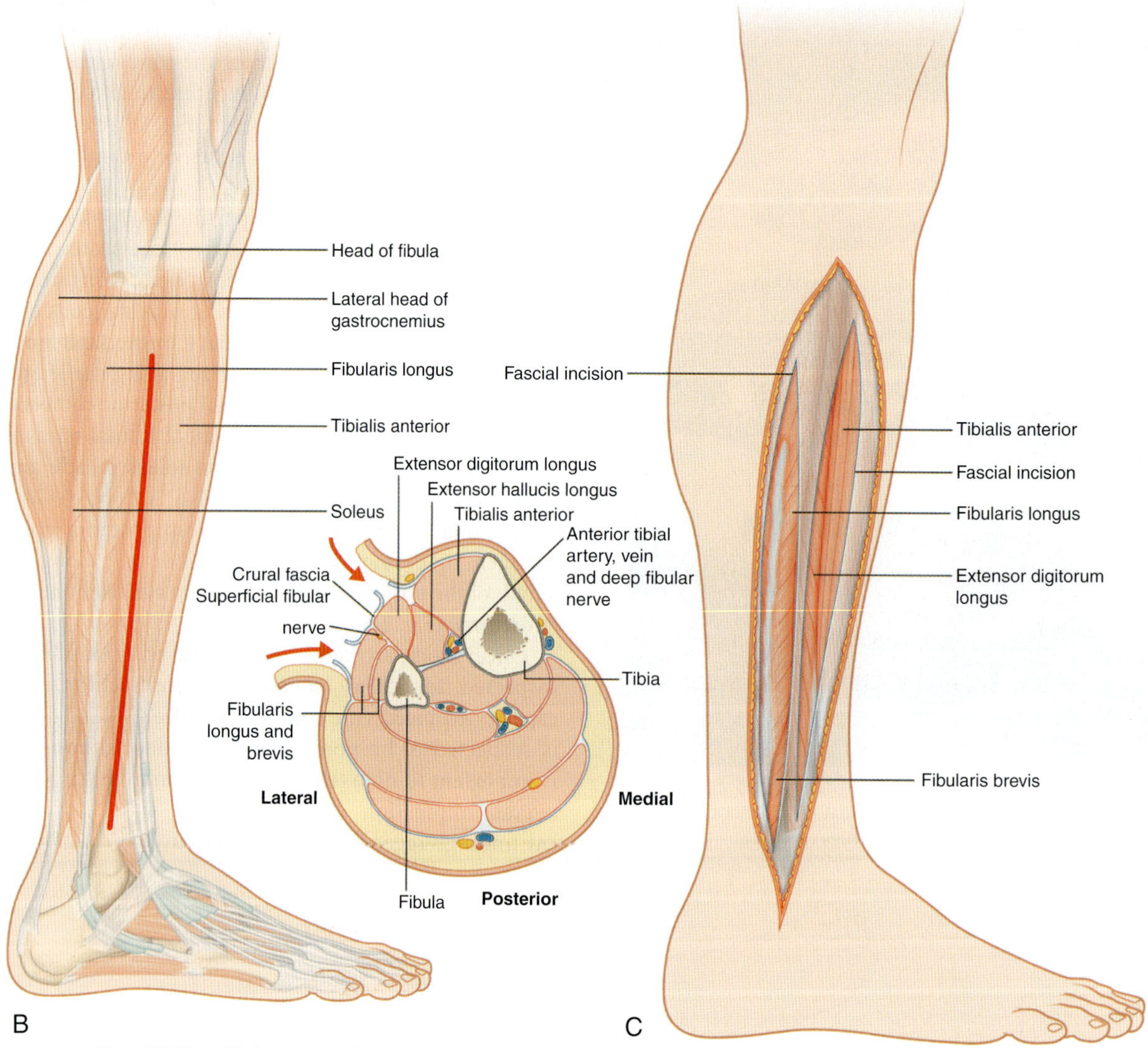

Fig. 2.5 Cont'd Intermuscular septum is identified and anterior and lateral compartments are released along their entire length (B and C). (Gray's Surgical Anatomy, Thomas A Schildhauer, Christian Fisahn, Elsevier, 2020).

should be made to avoid overly aggressive debridement.[58] Wounds can then be managed via wet to dry dressings, antibiotic bead pouch dressings, or negative pressure wound therapy. When utilizing negative pressure wound therapy, the surgeon should avoid placement of a wide sponge that causes the skin and subcutaneous tissue to adhere to the tissue below in a wide open position as this may lead to a higher incidence of the need for split-thickness skin grafting. The authors recommend cutting a sponge no more than approximately 3 cm in width when swelling allows and stapling the sponge directly to skin. When soft-tissue swelling does not allow for bringing the wound edges in close proximity to each other, it is imperative that the dressing be changed within 24 to 48 hours to try to provide further approximation of skin as muscle swelling subsides. Vessel loops and/or tension sutures may be used in an attempt to reapproximate and close skin as time progresses, and often skin can be closed from the proximal and distal ends of the wounds in stages.

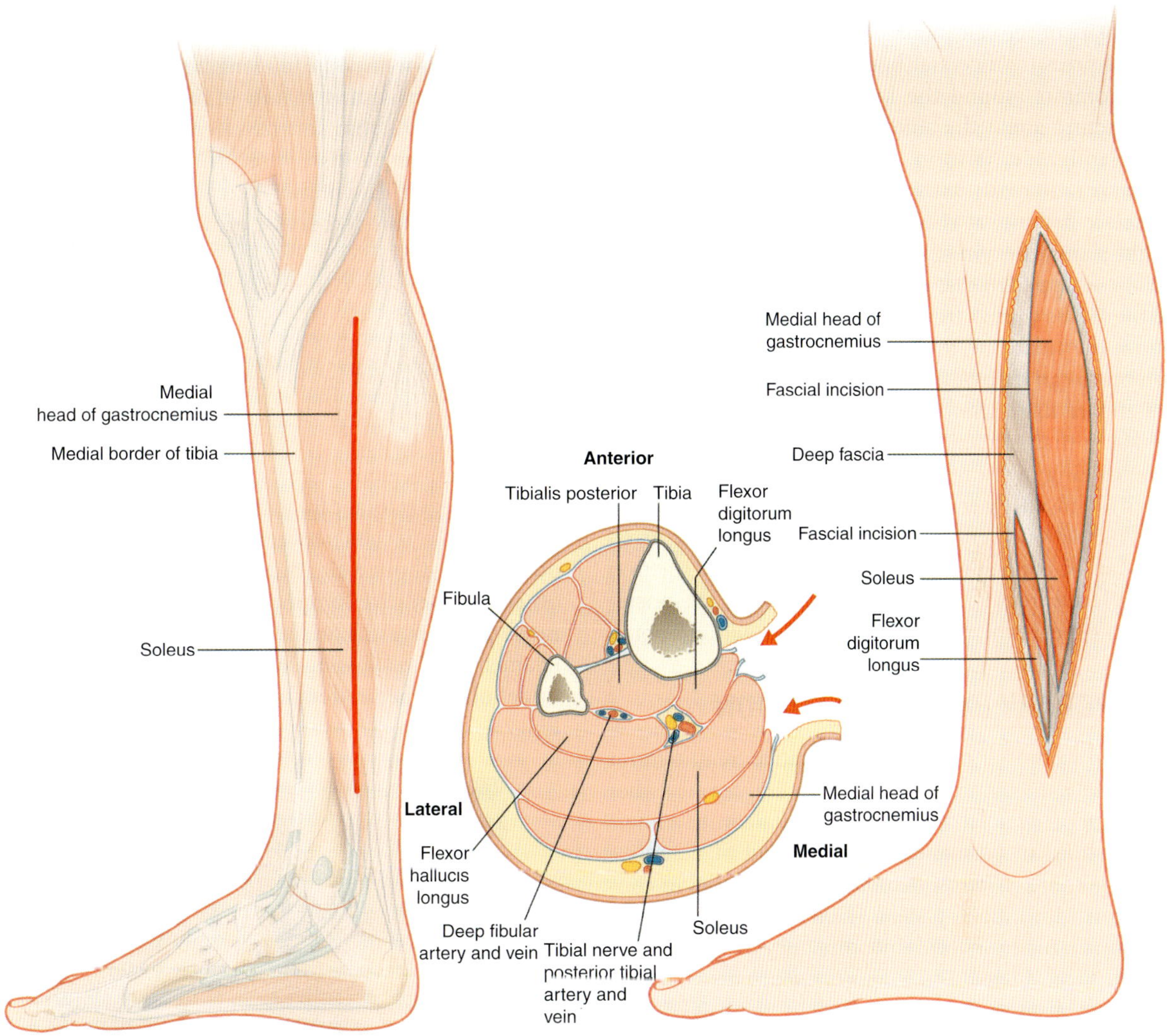

Fig. 2.6 Deep and superficial posterior compartment release. Longitudinal incision located 2 cm posterior to the tibia extending from the proximal tibial metaphysis to the distal metaphysis (A). Superficial posterior compartment is released by incising fascia along its entire length. Deep fascia is incised, and a Cobb elevator is used to elevate the flexor digitorum longus and soleus from the posterior tibia. (Gray's Surgical Anatomy, Thomas A Schildhauer, Christian Fisahn, Elsevier, 2020).

Finally, skin grafting is unavoidable in some cases and can be performed when closure is not possible.

TEMPORARY SPLINTING AND BRACING

Injury to the tibial plateau should not be left without proper immobilization and stabilization. This is important to prevent fracture displacement and soft-tissue tension and to control pain. One should place a temporary splint, brace, or traction/external fixator.

Fractures that will require acute surgical intervention can be treated by immobilizing the knee in extension through the use of a long leg splint or a knee immobilizer brace. A long leg splint should span from the gluteal crease of the thigh to the metatarsal heads of the foot. The knee can be positioned in a position of comfort with approximately 20 degrees to 30 degrees of flexion. The lower extremity should be sufficiently wrapped with cast padding using the half-overlapping technique. Ensure adequate padding near bony prominences, especially including the posterior tuberosity of the calcaneus. These measures reduce the risk of pressure ulcers at bony prominences and provide comfort around the knee. To avoid an equinus contracture about the ankle, it is typically splinted in the plantigrade position. However, leg compartment pressures increase with dorsiflexion, and therefore, in select patients at risk of CS, splinting the ankle in slight plantar flexion is preferred. Alternatively, the leg can be wrapped in cast padding and medial and lateral plaster slabs placed from the level of the groin to just above the ankle and overwrapped. An ankle dorsiflexion brace can then be applied if desired. Application of a standard knee immobilizing brace is often less cumbersome than placing a splint. Braces can be used as temporizing measures when splints cannot be applied or prior to an external fixator placement. Finally, in some situations, temporary traction may be preferred and can be applied either through a calcaneal traction pin (placed from medial to lateral through the posterior calcaneal tuberosity) or through a traction boot.

TEMPORARY EXTERNAL FIXATION

External fixation is one form of operative treatment for tibial plateau fractures. External fixation can be either temporary (often used as a bridge until definitive internal fixation) or permanent (as a method of definitive fixation itself). When soft-tissue trauma occurs in conjunction with a tibial plateau fracture, there is enough energy to incite a local inflammatory response that causes local edema and venous compromise, dermal hypoxia, blisters, and rarely, muscle necrosis.[59] Soft-tissue injury ensues, and therefore, the main goal of treatment is the prevention of any additional insults that could exacerbate existing damage. This often requires staged fixation of a tibial plateau fracture to allow the soft tissues to heal and recover. External fixation can be used as a temporary treatment when applied as a knee-spanning external fixator. This allows the surgeon to realign and restore length while allowing for soft-tissue recovery prior to definitive treatment with internal fixation. Soft tissues adjacent to the proximal tibia are commonly injured, especially when the injury is the result of a high-energy mechanism. Successful management of an associated soft-tissue injury is a prerequisite to a good outcome.[60,61] Injuries may occur to the nearby ligaments and menisci or to the surrounding soft-tissue envelope. The soft-tissue coverage over the proximal medial and lateral tibia as well as the full length of the anteromedial tibia is thin, consisting mainly of only skin and subcutaneous tissue. A thin soft-tissue envelope is more susceptible to complete disruption, from both extrinsic and intrinsic forces. The anterior, lateral, and posterior compartments of the leg otherwise provide robust soft-tissue coverage around the leg.

Prior studies have shown minimal soft-tissue complications when staged fixation with a temporary external fixator is used for high-energy tibial plateau fractures.[62] Following the results of this study, this group recommended staged treatment for all high-energy tibial plateau fractures due to better wound and blister management. Conversely, other studies have compared early total care with staged management and found similar results between the two treatment methodologies without a significant difference in wound or other postoperative complications.[63,64] The staged technique involves using an external fixator for temporary ligamentotaxis, allowing for soft-tissue recovery prior to definitive open reduction and internal fixation (see Fig. 2.7).

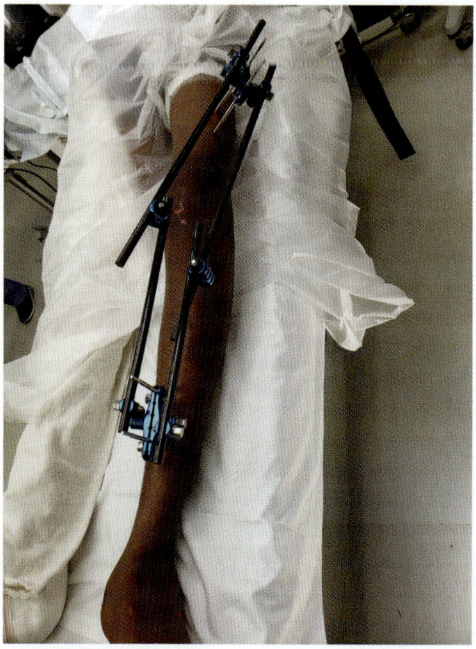

Fig. 2.7 Knee spanning external fixator for temporary stabilization of tibial plateau fracture.

Technique

The traditional knee-spanning external fixator used for these fractures consists of two 5.0-mm pins placed laterally or anterolaterally into the femur (femoral pin cluster) and two more pins in the middle or distal third of the tibial shaft (tibial pin cluster). The tibial shaft pins are generally placed anteriorly/anteromedially. The authors recommend predrilling for the tibial pins to prevent thermal necrosis in this subcutaneous location, while predrilling is not necessary for femoral pin placement. Insertion drill sleeves should be used for drilling and pin placement. Bars or large multipin clamps can then be configured to connect pin clusters. The farther these pins are placed from each other prior to connecting them into each pin cluster, the more stable the fixator construct will be. Stability will also be increased by bringing the connections between pins and between pin clusters closer to the bone/skin surface. Pin sites should be placed outside the zone of injury when possible in the case of temporary external fixation. Additionally, if it is necessary to place pins closer to the plateau, they should be placed at least 14 mm distal to the joint line, and care should be taken to avoid penetrating the joint space.[65] There is, however, no definitive evidence that penetrating the joint capsule increases the infection rate, as different studies have shown contradicting results.[66] Bars are then connected to pin clusters with clamps, and traction is pulled through the leg restoring gross alignment, length, and rotation. The knee can be slightly flexed (approximately 20 degrees) and clamps tightened down. When a large hemarthrosis is present, aspiration of the knee may help relieve patient discomfort. The goals of external fixation are to restore length, alignment, and stability of the fracture until definitive fixation can take place.

CASE 2.1

A 19-year-old male was involved in a motorcycle collision. He presented to the emergency department with a chief complaint of right knee pain that was associated with swelling, deformity, and pain. The initial physical examination demonstrated soft and compressible leg compartments and his neurovascular status was intact. Radiographs were obtained for further evaluation (Fig. 2.8)

Because isolated medial tibial plateau fractures can have a high association with vascular compromise and injury, further work up including Ankle-Brachial Index (ABI) measurements and a CT angiogram study were obtained. The ABI was found to be 0.85 (Fig. 2.9)

The CT angiogram was negative for vascular injury and the patient did not have any signs or symptoms of compartment syndrome. Due to the instability of the tibial plateau fracture-dislocation and significant soft tissue swelling and blistering, the decision was made to treat the patient in a staged fashion (Fig. 2.10).

Following the placement of temporary external fixation, a CT scan of the fracture was obtained to for preoperative planning (Fig. 2.11).

Once the patient's soft tissue swelling resolved, he underwent removal of external fixation followed by open reduction and internal fixation via a dual (anterolateral and posteromedial) incision approach (Fig. 2.12).

Post operatively, the patient was placed into a hinged knee brace locked into full knee extension. The long-term protocol for this patient was to maintain non weight bearing for a total of 3 months with progressive knee range of motion beginning at 2 weeks from the date of his procedure.

Key points of this case include having a high index of suspicion of vascular injury in a fracture/dislocation pattern and ruling out vascular injury with ABI's plus or minus CTA. Additionally, unstable fracture patterns with associated soft tissue injury can be treated safely in a staged manner with temporary external fixation, restoring length and alignment while placing pins outside of the zone of injury. Finally, goals of ORIF include restoration of articular congruity with absolute stability in addition to overall restoration of length, alignment, and condylar width, and stability allowing early range of motion.

Continued

CASE 2.1—CONT'D

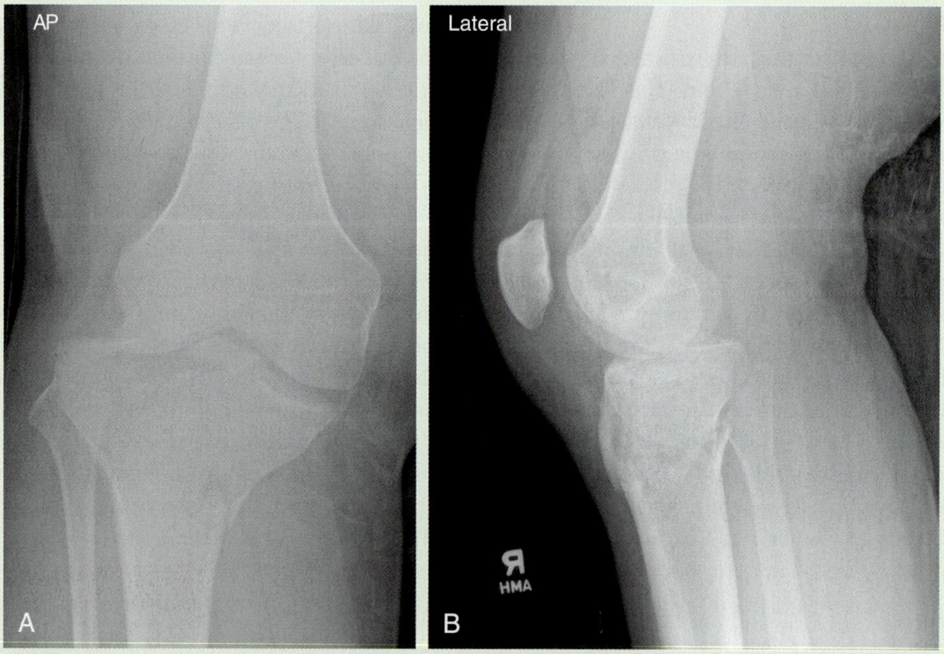

Fig. 2.8 Anterior-posterior and lateral radiographs of the right knee demonstrate a bicondylar tibial plateau fracture with metaphyseal-diaphyseal separation and associated lateral knee dislocation. Additionally, there is condylar widening, articular depression of the lateral tibial plateau and soft tissue swelling of the knee consistent with a lipohemarthrosis.

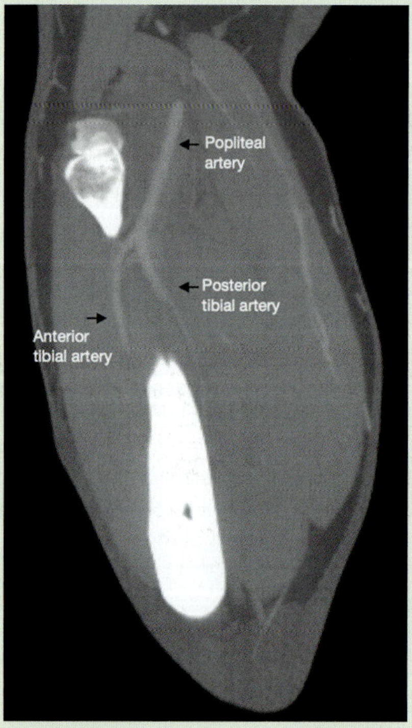

Fig. 2.9 Selected sagittal view of the CT angiogram demonstrates a normal appearing popliteal artery branching into the anterior and posterior tibial arteries. Complete evaluation of the lower extremity vasculature was negative for injury.

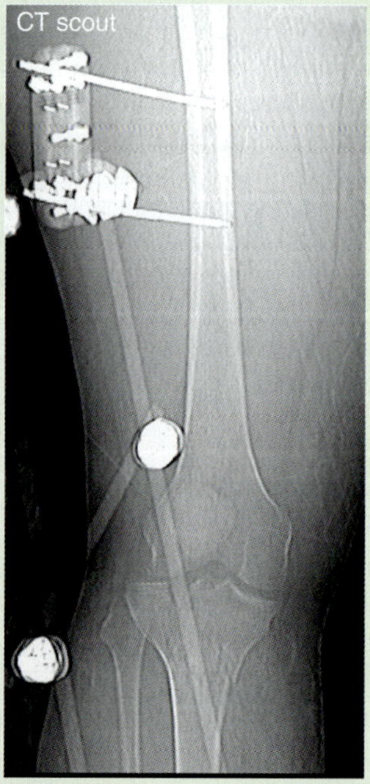

Fig. 2.10 Temporary External fixation spanning the tibial plateau fracture dislocation. Proximal pins are seen here in the femoral shaft and distal pins were placed in the distal tibial shaft. All external fixation pins were placed outside of the zone of injury to prevent contamination and future interference with internal hardware.

CASE 2.1—CONT'D

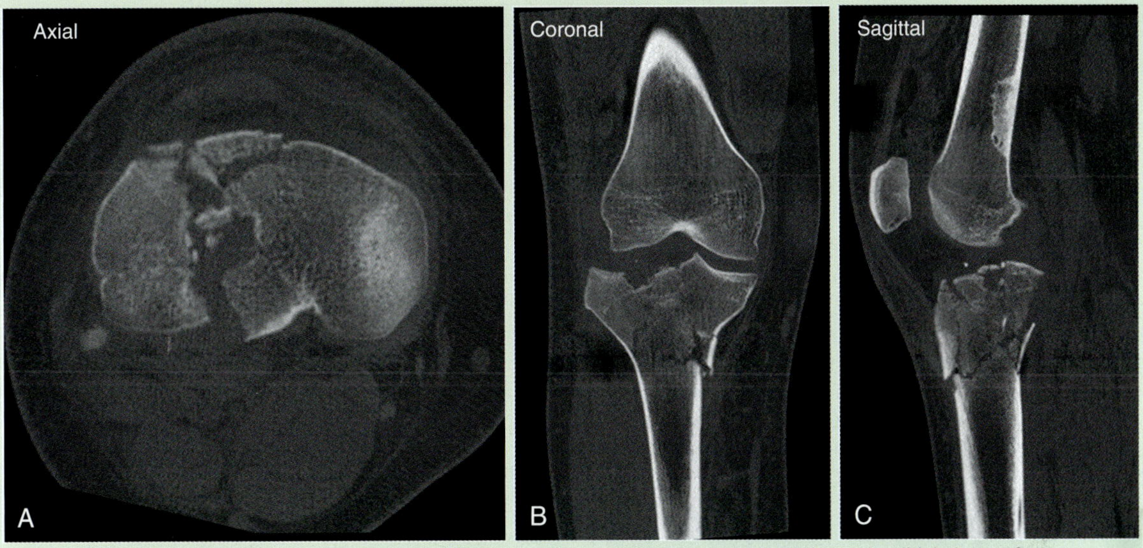

Fig. 2.11 Following temporary external fixation, a CT scan was obtained to evaluate the tibial plateau fracture under ligamentotaxis. There is a comminuted, split-depressed fracture of the lateral condyle as well as transverse meta-diaphyseal separation. The overall length, alignment, and rotation are well preserved.

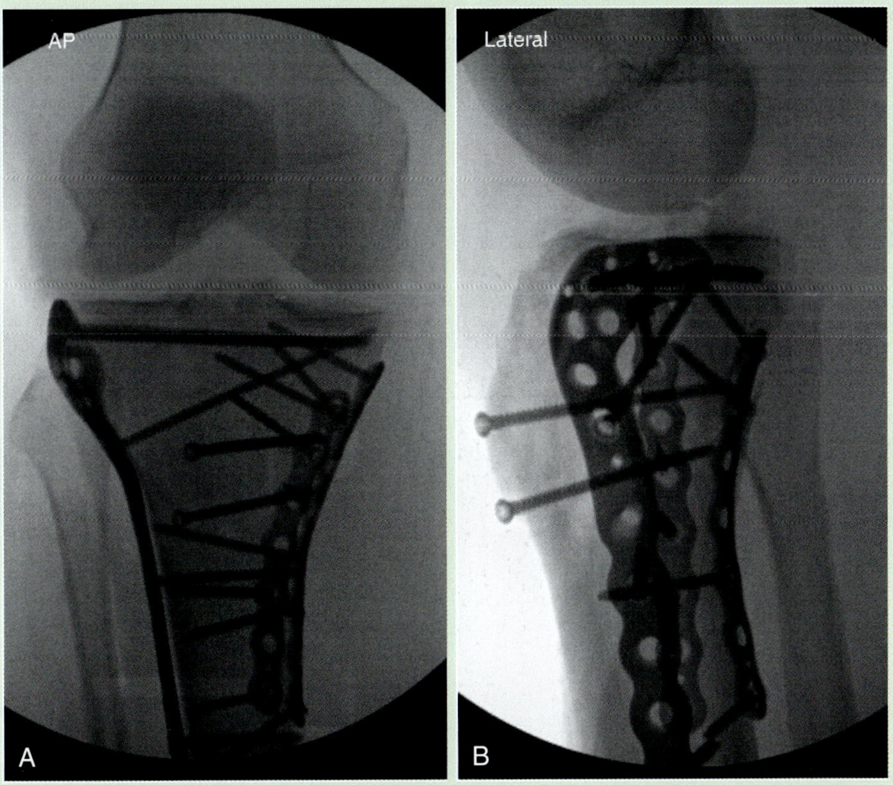

Fig. 2.12 Tibial plateau fracture status post open reduction and internal fixation. The articular surface, mechanical alignment, length, and rotation were restored.

CASE 2.2

27-year-old male involved in a high-speed motorcycle accident transferred to our trauma center. He was noted to have an open injury to the left proximal tibia and deformity to the right wrist. His past medical, surgical, and social history were significant for daily 1 pack per day smoking, otherwise noncontributory.

On physical exam two linear lacerations over the anterior proximal tibia were seen with slow oozing of blood. No obvious gross contamination was noted. The lower leg was grossly unstable through the tibia. Motor function and sensation were intact throughout the lower leg. Pulses were not palpable but present on doppler with sluggish capillary refill.

ABI was performed and recorded as 0.60

He was given intravenous cefazolin and an updated tetanus booster and imaging was obtained (Fig. 2.13).

Because of the ABI of 0.60 and concern for vascular injury, a CTA was obtained (Fig. 2.14).

Given the vascular injury seen on CTA and the high energy nature of the patient's injury, the patient was taken to the OR emergently for vascular repair followed by temporary stabilization of his fracture. Vascular surgery performed a repair of the popliteal artery and orthopedic intervention followed.

As this was an open fracture, a thorough debridement was initially performed with several bony fragments that were deemed nonviable removed from the wounds. Four compartment fasciotomies were performed. There was a large metadiaphyseal defect noted which was filled with antibiotic cement (Fig. 2.15).

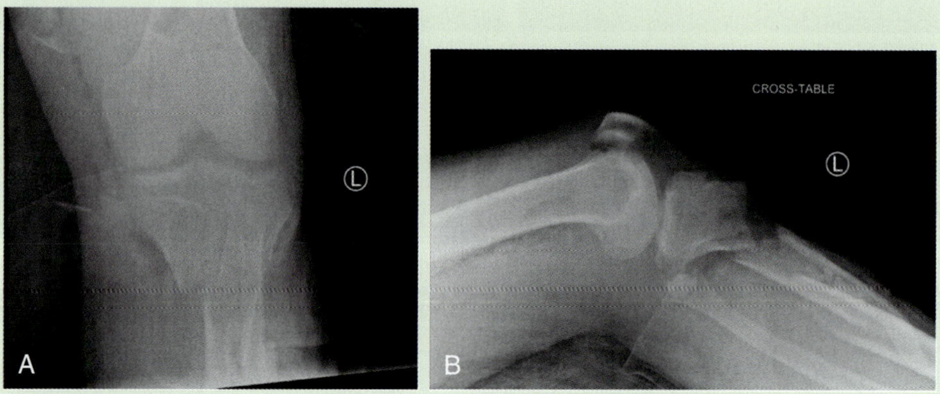

Fig. 2.13 Initial radiographs of the left knee demonstrating a bicondylar tibial plateau fracture with metadisphyseal dissociation (AP view (A) and Lateral (B) view of tibial plateau fracture).

CASE 2.2—CONT'D

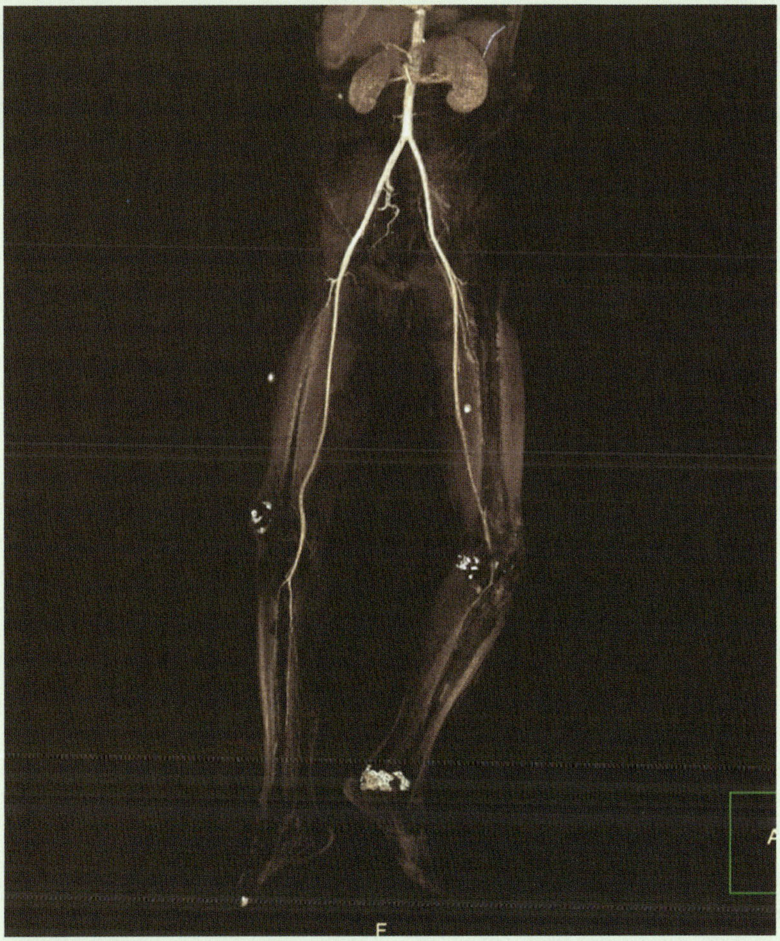

Fig. 2.14 CTA of the lower extremities demonstrating injury to the popliteal artery at the level of the tibial plateau with poor vascular flow seen distally.

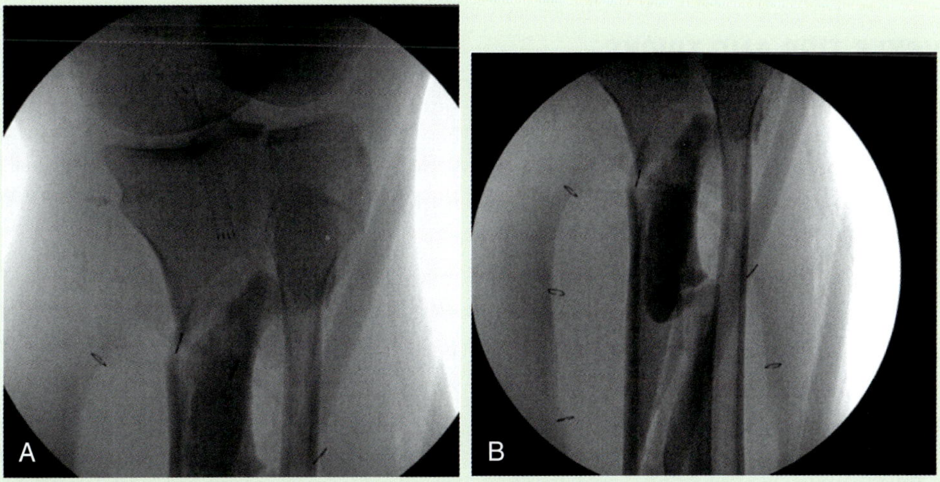

Fig. 2.15 Intra-operative fluroscopic images taken during initial debridement and irrigation and ex-fix application. A knee-spanning ex-fix was applied with pins placed into the distal femur and tibial shaft. Antibiotic cement spacer was placed to fill the metadiaphyseal bone void.

Continued

CASE 2.2—CONT'D

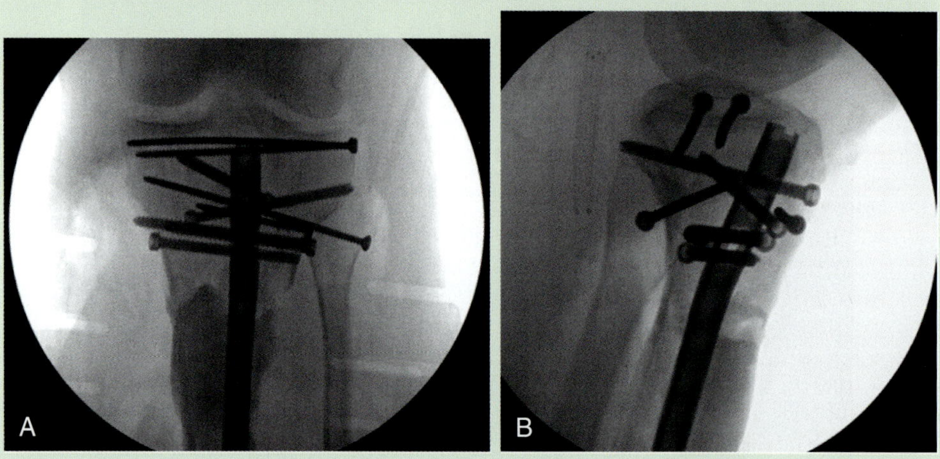

Fig. 2.16 Intra-operative fluoroscopic Xrays demonstrating fixation of the articular surface with peri-articular screws and insertion of tibial nail to regain alignment, length, and rotation of the tibia. The contralateral, uninjured tibia was used as a guide to determine appropriate length.

The patient was taken back to the operating room the next day intramedullary nailing and tibiofibular joint fixation (Fig. 2.16), as well as for flap coverage with the plastic surgery team, who covered the wound using a gastrocnemius flap and split-thickness skin graft. The remainder of his hospital stay was uncomplicated and he did not require any further trips to the operating room. He was discharged from the hospital 7 days after his definitive fixation (6 days after flap coverage). He was made toe-touch weight bearing to the left lower extremity following fixation.

Key points to this case include providing antibiotics and tetanus booster upon presentation in conjunction with thorough debridement due to the open fracture. Additionally, having a high index of suspicion for vascular injury with this fracture pattern, performing ABI and CT scan, which led to early vascular repair and four compartment fasciotomies. Finally, this case provides an example where staged fixation including temporary external fixation was appropriate to allow for stabilization with vascular repair and care of the soft tissues while administering local and systemic antibiotics and planning for definitive fixation and flap coverage.

SZATKOWSKI'S TIPS AND TRICKS

- Provide antibiotic and tetanus prophylaxis as soon as possible in open fractures.
- With fracture-dislocation patterns, check ABI; if abnormal, obtain CTA and/or vascular consult.
- Maintain a high index of suspicion for CS with tibial plateau fractures.
- In unstable fracture patterns with soft-tissue injury, consider temporary external fixation prior to definitive fixation.
- When placing temporary external fixation, place pins outside of the zone of injury and anticipated hardware placement.
- The goal of temporary external fixation is to restore length, gross alignment, and stability.

REFERENCES

1. Court-Brown CM, Caesar B. Epidemiology of adult fractures: a review. *Injury*. 2006;37(8):691–697.
2. Moore TM, Patzakis MJ, Harvey JP. Tibial plateau fractures: definition, demographics, treatment rationale, and long-term results of closed traction management or operative reduction. *J Orthop Trauma*. 1987;1(2):97–119.
3. Albuquerque RP, Hara R, Prado J, Schiavo L, Giordano V, do Amaral NP. Epidemiological study on tibial plateau fractures at a level I trauma center. *Acta Ortop Bras*. 2013;21(2):109–115.
4. Yuwen P, Lv H, Chen W, et al. Age-, gender- and Arbeitsgemeinschaft für Osteosynthesefragen type-specific clinical characters of adult tibial plateau fractures in eighty three hospitals in China. *Int Orthop*. 2018;42(3):667–672.

5. Elsoe R, Larsen P, Nielsen NP, Swenne J, Rasmussen S, Ostgaard SE. Population-based epidemiology of tibial plateau fractures. *Orthopedics*. 2015;38(9):e780–e786.
6. Ebraheim NA, Sabry FF, Haman SP. Open reduction and internal fixation of 117 tibial plateau fractures. *Orthopedics*. 2004;27(12):1281–1287.
7. Blokker CP, Rorabeck CH, Bourne RB. Tibial plateau fractures: an analysis of the results of treatment in 60 patients. *Clin Orthop Relat Res*. 1984;(182):193–199.
8. Kugelman DN, Qatu AM, Strauss EJ, Konda SR, Egol KA. Knee stiffness after tibial plateau fractures: predictors and outcomes (OTA-41). *J Orthop Trauma*. 2018;32(11):e421–e427.
9. He QF, Sun H, Shu LY, et al. Tibial plateau fractures in elderly people: an institutional retrospective study. *J Orthop Surg Res*. 2018;13(1):276.
10. Kugelman D, Qatu A, Haglin J, Leucht P, Konda S, Egol K. Complications and unplanned outcomes following operative treatment of tibial plateau fractures. *Injury*. 2017;48(10):2221–2229.
11. Kennedy JC, Bailey WH. Experimental tibial-plateau fractures: studies of the mechanism and a classification. *J Bone Joint Surg Am*. 1968;50(8):1522–1534.
12. Wilkins J, Patzakis M. Choice and duration of antibiotics in open fractures. *Orthop Clin North Am*. 1991;22(3):433–437.
13. Hoff WS, Bonadies JA, Cachecho R, Dorlac WC. East Practice Management Guidelines Work Group: update to practice management guidelines for prophylactic antibiotic use in open fractures. *J Trauma*. 2011;70(3):751–754.
14. Carver DC, Kuehn SB, Weinlein JC. Role of systemic and local antibiotics in the treatment of open fractures. *Orthop Clin N Am*. 2017;48(2):137–153.
15. Schatzker J, McBroom R, Bruce D. The tibial plateau fracture: the Toronto experience 1968–1975. Clin Orthop Rel Res. 1979(138):94-104.
16. Halvorson JJ, Anz A, Langfitt M, et al. Vascular injury associated with extremity trauma: initial diagnosis and management. *J Am Acad Orthop Surg*. 2011;19(8):495–504.
17. Green NE, Allen BL. Vascular injuries associated with dislocation of the knee. *J Bone Joint Surg Am*. 1977;59(2):236–239.
18. Stayner LR, Coen MJ. Historic perspectives of treatment algorithms in knee dislocation. *Clin Sports Med*. 2000;19(3):399–413.
19. Rasmussen PS. Tibial condylar fractures. Impairment of knee joint stability as an indication for surgical treatment. *J Bone Joint Surg Am*. 1973;55(7):1331–1350.
20. Lansinger O, Bergman B, Körner L, Andersson GB. Tibial condylar fractures: a twenty-year follow-up. *J Bone Joint Surg Am*. 1986;68(1):13–19.
21. Moore TM, Harvey Jr JP. Roentgenographic measurement of tibial-plateau depression due to fracture. *J Bone Joint Surg Am*. 1974;56(1):155–160.
22. Prasad N, Murray JM, Kumar D, Davies SG. Insufficiency fracture of the tibial plateau: an often missed diagnosis. *Acta Orthop Belg*. 2006;72(5):587–591.
23. Honkonen SE. Indications for surgical treatment of tibial condyle fractures. *Clin Orthop Rel Res*. 1994;(302):199–205.
24. Gardner MJ, Yacoubian S, Geller D, et al. Prediction of soft-tissue injuries in Schatzker II tibial plateau fractures based on measurements of plain radiographs. *J Trauma*. 2006;60(2):319–323. discussion 324.
25. Gardner MJ, Yacoubian S, Geller D, et al. The incidence of soft tissue injury in operative tibial plateau fractures: a magnetic resonance imaging analysis of 103 patients. *J Orthop Trauma*. 2005;19(2):79–84.
26. Berkson EM, Virkus WW. High-energy tibial plateau fractures. *J Am Acad Orthop Surg*. 2006;14(1):20–31.
27. Marsh JL, Buckwalter J, Gelberman R, et al. Articular fractures: does an anatomic reduction really change the result? *J Bone Joint Surg Am*. 2002;84(7):1259–1271.
28. Rademakers MV, Kerkhoffs GM, Sierevelt IN, Raaymakers EL, Marti RK. Operative treatment of 109 tibial plateau fractures: five- to 27-year follow-up results. *J Orthop Trauma*. 2007;21(1):5–10.
29. Chan PS, Klimkiewicz JJ, Luchetti WT, et al. Impact of CT scan on treatment plan and fracture classification of tibial plateau fractures. *J Orthop Trauma*. 1997;11(7):484–489.
30. Wicky S, Blaser PF, Blanc CH, Leyvraz PF, Schnyder P, Meuli RA. Comparison between standard radiography and spiral CT with 3D reconstruction in the evaluation, classification and management of tibial plateau fractures. *Eur Radiol*. 2000;10(8):1227–1232.
31. Macarini L, Murrone M, Marini S, Calbi R, Solarino M, Moretti B. Tibial plateau fractures: evaluation with multidetector-CT. *Radiol Med*. 2004;108(5-6):503–514.
32. Brunner A, Horisberger M, Ulmar B, Hoffmann A, Babst R. Classification systems for tibial plateau fractures; does computed tomography scanning improve their reliability? *Injury*. 2010;41(2):173–178.
33. Molenaars RJ, Mellema JJ, Doornberg JN, Kloen P. Tibial plateau fracture characteristics: computed tomography mapping of lateral, medial, and bicondylar fractures. *J Bone Joint Surg Am*. 2015;97(18):1512–1520.
34. Liow RY, Birdsall PD, Mucci B, Greiss ME. Spiral computed tomography with two- and three-dimensional reconstruction in the management of tibial plateau fractures. *Orthopedics*. 1999;22(10):929–932.
35. Sohn HS, Yoon YC, Cho JW, Cho WT, Oh CW, Oh JK. Incidence and fracture morphology of posterolateral fragments in lateral and bicondylar tibial plateau fractures. *J Orthop Trauma*. 2015;29(2):91–97.
36. Higgins TF, Kemper D, Klatt J. Incidence and morphology of the posteromedial fragment in bicondylar tibial plateau fractures. *J Orthop Trauma*. 2009;23(1):45–51.
37. Stannard JP, Lopez R, Volgas D. Soft tissue injury of the knee after tibial plateau fractures. *J Knee Surg*. 2010;23(4):187–192.

38. Mui LW, Engelsohn E, Umans H. Comparison of CT and MRI in patients with tibial plateau fracture: can CT findings predict ligament tear or meniscal injury? *Skelet Radiol*. 2007;36(2):145–151.
39. Vaillancourt C, Shrier I, Vandal A, et al. Acute compartment syndrome: how long before muscle necrosis occurs? *CJEM*. 2004;6(3):147–154.
40. Stark E, Stucken C, Trainer G, Tornetta 3rd P. Compartment syndrome in Schatzker type VI plateau fractures and medial condylar fracture-dislocations treated with temporary external fixation. *J Orthop Trauma*. 2009;23(7):502–506.
41. Ziran BH, Becher SJ. Radiographic predictors of compartment syndrome in tibial plateau fractures. *J Orthop Trauma*. 2013;27(11):612–615.
42. Park S, Ahn J, Gee AO, Kuntz AF, Esterhai JL. Compartment syndrome in tibial fractures. *J Orthop Trauma*. 2009;23(7):514–518.
43. Andrews JR, Tedder JL, Godbout BP. Bicondylar tibial plateau fracture complicated by compartment syndrome. *Orthop Rev*. 1992;21(3):317–319.
44. Shao J, Chang H, Zhu Y, et al. Incidence and risk factors for surgical site infection after open reduction and internal fixation of tibial plateau fracture: a systematic review and meta-analysis. *Int J Surg*. 2017;41:176–182.
45. Norris GR, Checketts JX, Scott JT, Vassar M, Norris BL, Giannoudis PV. Prevalence of deep surgical site infection after repair of periarticular knee fractures: a systematic review and meta-analysis. *JAMA Netw Open*. 2019;2(8):e199951.
46. Blair JA, Stoops TK, Doarn MC, et al. Infection and nonunion after fasciotomy for compartment syndrome associated with tibia fractures: a matched cohort comparison. *J Orthop Trauma*. 2016;30(7):392–396.
47. Colman M, Wright A, Gruen G, Siska P, Pape HC, Tarkin I. Prolonged operative time increases infection rate in tibial plateau fractures. *Injury*. 2013;44(2):249–252.
48. Ruffolo MR, Gettys FK, Montijo HE, Seymour RB, Karunakar MA. Complications of high-energy bicondylar tibial plateau fractures treated with dual plating through 2 incisions. *J Orthop Trauma*. 2015;29(2):85–90.
49. Allmon C, Greenwell P, Paryavi E, Dubina A, O'Toole RV. Radiographic predictors of compartment syndrome occurring after tibial fracture. *J Orthop Trauma*. 2016;30(7):387–391.
50. Marchand LS, Working ZM, Rane AA, et al. Compartment syndrome in tibial plateau fractures: do previously established predictors have external validity? *J Orthop Trauma*. 2020;34(5):238–243.
51. Schmidt AH. Acute compartment syndrome. *Injury*. 2017;48(suppl 1):s22–s25.
52. Ulmer T. The clinical diagnosis of compartment syndrome of the lower leg: are clinical findings predictive of the disorder? *J Orthop Trauma*. 2002;16(8):572–577.
53. Kakar S, Firoozabadi R, McKean J, Tornetta 3rd P. Diastolic blood pressure in patients with tibia fractures under anaesthesia: implications for the diagnosis of compartment syndrome. *J Orthop Trauma*. 2007;21(2):99–103.
54. Prayson MJ, Chen JL, Hampers D, Vogt M, Fenwick J, Meredick R. Baseline compartment pressure measurements in isolated lower extremity fractures without clinical compartment syndrome. *J Trauma*. 2006;60(5):1037–1040.
55. McQueen MM, Duckworth AD, Aitken SA, Court-Brown CM. The estimated sensitivity and specificity of compartment pressure monitoring for acute compartment syndrome. *J Bone Joint Surg Am*. 2013;95(8):673–677.
56. Heckman MM, Whitesides Jr TE, Grewe SR, Rooks MD. Compartment pressure in association with closed tibial fractures: the relationship between tissue pressure, compartment, and the distance from the site of the fracture. *J Bone Joint Surg Am*. 1994;76(9):1285–1292.
57. Nakhostine M, Styf JR, van Leuven S, Hargens AR, Gershuni DH. Intramuscular pressure varies with depth: the tibialis anterior muscle studied in 12 volunteers. *Acta Orthop Scand*. 1993;64(3):377–381.
58. Sassoon A, Riehl J, Rich A, et al. Muscle viability revisited: are we removing normal muscle? A critical evaluation of dogmatic debridement. *J Orthop Trauma*. 2016;30(1):17–21.
59. Giordano CP, Koval KJ, Zuckerman JD, Desai P. Fracture blisters. *Clin Orthop Rel Res*. 1994;307:214–221.
60. Barei DP, Nork SE, Mills WJ, Henley MB, Benirschke SK. Complications associated with internal fixation of high-energy bicondylar tibial plateau fractures utilizing a two-incision technique. *J Orthop Trauma*. 2004;18(10):649–657.
61. Papagelopoulos PJ, Partsinevelos AA, Themistocleous GS, Mavrogenis AF, Korres DS, Soucacos PN. Complications after tibia plateau fracture surgery. *Injury*. 2006;37(6):475–484.
62. Egol KA, Tejwani NC, Capla EL, Wolinsky PL, Koval KJ. Staged management of high-energy proximal tibia fractures (OTA types 41): the results of a prospective, standardized protocol. *J Orthop Trauma*. 2005;19(7):448–455. discussion 456.
63. Benirschke SK, Agnew SG, Mayo KA, Santoro VM, Henley MB. Immediate internal fixation of open, complex tibial plateau fractures: treatment by a standard protocol. *J Orthop Trauma*. 1992;6(1):78–86.
64. Borade A, Kempegowda H, Richard R, Graham J, Suk M, Horwitz DS. Is "early total care" a safe and effective alternative to "staged protocol" for the treatment of Schatzker IV-VI tibial plateau fractures in patients older than 50 years? *J Orthop Trauma*. 2017;31(12):e400–e406.
65. Reid JS, Van Slyke MA, Moulton MJ, Mann TA. Safe placement of proximal tibial transfixation wires with respect to intracapsular penetration. *J Orthop Trauma*. 2001;15(1):10–17.
66. Shah CM, Babb PE, McAndrew CM, et al. Definitive plates overlapping provisional external fixator pin sites: is the infection risk increased? *J Orthop Trauma*. 2014;28(9):518–522.

3

Nonoperative Treatment of Tibial Plateau Fractures

James C. Widmaier Jr., MD and Cassandra A. Ricketts, MD

INTRODUCTION

Tibial plateau fractures have been documented in the literature as early as the 1820s, and the mainstay of treatment was nonoperative until the 1950s.[1] Many reports in the 1970s and beyond suggest that open reduction and internal fixation is indicated for most displaced tibial plateau fractures.[2–4] With modern advances in fracture treatment principles, techniques, imaging methods, and implants, operative intervention has become the standard treatment for the majority of tibial plateau fractures.

Over the years, operative treatment of tibial plateau fractures has shown improved outcomes, which has led to expanding indications. Advanced imaging techniques allow surgeons to better visualize fracture morphology in three dimensions, creating a better understanding of applied anatomy. With the development of medial, lateral, and posterior approaches to the proximal tibia, surgeons can safely reduce and apply fixation to almost any fracture pattern. Furthermore, specialty plates and bone graft substitutes that may obviate the need for autograft have made surgery a more attractive option with less morbidity. While the current mainstay for the treatment of tibial plateau fractures involves surgical intervention, nonoperative treatment may be indicated in certain fractures and patient populations. Techniques of conservative treatment, including historical methods and modern immobilization devices, can lead to good outcomes when applied appropriately. In this chapter, we describe the selection criteria, historical treatment methods with modern adaptations, as well as outcomes of nonoperative treatment.

INDICATIONS

Indications for nonoperative treatment are driven by patient factors, socioeconomic factors, and fracture characteristics.

Patient Factors

Patient-specific factors, including ambulatory status, medical comorbidities, risk of anesthesia, and patient's ability to receive transfusion, must be taken into consideration. For example, nonsurgical treatment should be considered in a low-demand, nonambulatory, or minimally ambulatory patient who uses the affected limb for transfers or short distances only. This low-demand scenario may be seen in patients with hemiplegia or paraplegia, morbid obesity, advanced age, or severe deconditioning.

Nonoperative treatment may be considered in patients with multiple medical comorbidities, who are at high risk of complications from anesthesia and surgery. Medical comorbidities, such as diabetes (especially uncontrolled) and renal failure, may drive treatment decisions. A markedly elevated hemoglobin A1c (HbA1c) indicates poor diabetic control and is associated with other conditions such as malnutrition with hypoalbuminemia and anemia. Patients with a poor host classification grade, initially described by Cierny et al., may be at extremely high risk for complication from acute intervention, and conservative treatments should be strongly considered.[5] The host classification indicates the number of Immune system-compromising factors include diabetes, renal disease requiring dialysis, malnutrition, nicotine use, Age >80, malignancy, alcoholism, and more. (Fig. 3.1).[6] Additionally, a systematic review indicated that diabetes increased rates of

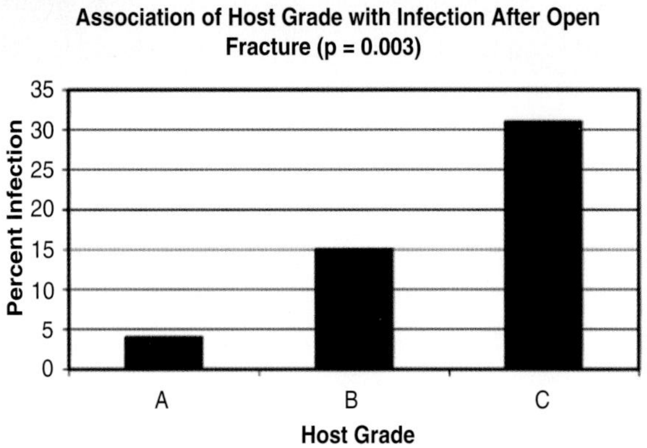

Fig. 3.1 The graph shows the relationship between Host Grade and infection after open fracture. (From Bowen TR, Widmaier JC. Host classification predicts infection after open fracture. *Clin Orthop Relat Res.* 2005;(433):205–211.)

malunion, infection, and reoperation rates in operative lower extremity fractures and increased rates of nonunion in fractures below the knee.[7]

While a set point for HbA1c has not been universally established for fracture care, the arthroplasty literature uses a benchmark of 7% as an agreed-upon preoperative target.[8] A recent study in the *Journal of Arthroplasty* found that a threshold of 7.7 was a specific risk factor that could predict periprosthetic joint infection.[9] This threshold may be considered as a reference point in fracture care to predict infection risk and can be used as a tool in the decision-making process. In patients with uncontrolled diabetes, tibial plateau fractures may be treated initially nonoperatively, and once glucose control is established, patients may then become candidates for procedures such as arthroplasty in a delayed fashion.

Similarly, patients with renal failure have poor wound and fracture healing as well as an increased risk of mortality when undergoing noncardiac surgery and should be considered for nonoperative modalities.[10] In a recent metaanalysis of the joint arthroplasty literature, Kim et al. found that patients with chronic kidney disease (CKD) have a higher rate of mortality and periprosthetic joint infection based on the unadjusted odds ratio. After total hip arthroplasty, the risk of periprosthetic joint infection was higher in patients who were on dialysis than in CKD patients not on dialysis.[11] Other medical conditions that may influence treatment decisions include active infection, recent myocardial infarction, or stroke, especially when high doses of anticoagulants are required, leading to a high risk of bleeding complications.

Socioeconomic Considerations

Various socioeconomic scenarios can affect the surgeon's ability to provide optimal operative treatment, such as in the setting of a contagious pandemic or in areas of conflict or poverty where resources can be limited. During the unexpected COVID-19 pandemic, some patients opted for nonoperative treatment, limiting their visits and exposure to a large hospital system and utilizing telehealth and home therapy. In underdeveloped countries, orthopedic surgeons may encounter limited access to sterile operating rooms and may elect to proceed with nonoperative treatment of tibial plateau fractures. In these unusual circumstances, surgical treatment may not be an option. Lastly, the religious and cultural beliefs of patients may indicate nonoperative management. For example, if the patient's belief system precludes them from receiving a transfusion, the surgeon may choose nonoperative treatment, especially in the setting of polytrauma.

Fracture Characteristics

The characteristics of the fracture provide the basis for nonoperative versus operative treatment decision making. Historically, the most stringent criteria for operative intervention are articular step-off more than 3 mm, condylar widening of more than 5 mm relative to contralateral side, and lateral tilt or valgus malalignment of more than 5 degrees.[12] Other authors indicate that up to 10 mm of step-off and 10 degrees of malalignment can be treated nonoperatively, and beyond this cutoff, surgery is almost universally indicated.[13] Specifically, for lateral plateau fractures, up to 3 mm of articular step-off, 5 mm of condylar widening, and 5 degrees of valgus malalignment are well tolerated without adverse effects.[12] Bicondylar fractures and displaced medial plateau fractures likely require operative intervention. Additionally, knee instability will require surgical treatment.[12] Preexisting arthritis of a severe nature may also be a reason to strongly consider closed fracture treatment and then delayed arthroplasty without fear of surgical site infection, multiple incisions, and stress risers from preexisting hardware. Lastly, closed treatment with systemic and/or local antibiotics may be considered in the setting of open injury and significant contamination where the presence of a metallic foreign body may drive infection.

PATIENT EVALUATION

The decision to operate or not may be easy in the healthy, uncomplicated patient, but in a chronically ill patient with multiple comorbidities, the adage "the decision is more important than the incision" applies. To make the best decision on how a fracture should be treated, a thorough patient workup should be completed, including history and physical examination, appropriate basic and advanced imaging studies, and risk-benefit discussion between the surgeon and the patient. This complete approach will mitigate risk and allow for optimization of the patient's function and overall outcome.

History and Physical Examination

A comprehensive history and physical examination should be performed on all patients with tibial plateau fractures. Investigation of the patient's medical comorbidities, ambulatory and functional status, allergies including metal allergy, previous anesthesia complications, social history including occupation, tobacco, and other drug use must be completed. A complete neurovascular examination should be performed, including palpation of pulses, Doppler examination, and ankle-brachial index assessment in high-energy trauma. Sensory examination involves evaluating the injured limb as well as the contralateral limb for preexisting neuropathy. A visual inspection of the skin should be completed, looking for any preexisting skin conditions, including signs of vascular disease or cellulitis. The location of open wounds and compromised skin should be noted in the context of proposed incisions.

Stability of the knee should be checked, as it is paramount in the decision-making process of operative versus nonoperative treatment. As described by Lansinger et al., stability is tested by examination of the knee with the leg in full extension.[13] Often after tibial plateau fractures, knee hemarthrosis creates a painful distension of the knee and can be aspirated to allow the patient to tolerate a clinical examination better. Anesthesia may be required for stability examination, such as with a peripheral nerve block (if compartment syndrome is not suspected), spinal anesthesia, or general anesthesia in the operating room. According to a 20-year follow-up study by Lansinger et al., a 10-degree increase in lateral or medial deviation of the mechanical axis of the involved knee compared with the uninjured side is defined as unstable and a clear indication for surgery.[13] The authors also concluded that instability measured with a knee flexed more than 20 degrees was clinically irrelevant. Using this simple physical examination maneuver to screen patients, Lansinger was able to select surgical candidates and achieve excellent or good results in over 90% of patients over the 20-year follow-up. The 10% of patients who achieved fair or poor results were those with depressed fractures where the articular surface was depressed more than 10 mm. They concluded that patients with stability of the extended knee should be treated nonoperatively irrespective of the roentgenographic appearance of the fracture.[13]

Clinically, 10 degrees can be hard to assess, so we recommend using radiographic stress views. In the patient with tibial plateau fracture, full-length standing films are not an option. However, alignment decisions are best made with a large field of view; thus, stress radiographs should be taken on large cassettes (14 inches or larger if possible). Alignment assessment can be completed on a flat top imaging table, with a reaming rod for an intramedullary nail that is prebent to 10 degrees positioned over the top of the examined limb with the bend at the joint line while the image is being captured (Fig. 3.2).

Imaging

After a complete history and physical examination, standard radiographs, including anteroposterior (AP), lateral, and plateau view, should be performed. Contralateral limb radiographs should be considered for comparison if nonoperative treatment is an option. While findings such as depression of the articular surface and fracture lines may be visible on plain radiographs, computed tomography (CT) imaging shows a more accurate assessment of the fracture morphology, location of each fragment, and occult fracture lines. CT will also better represent the amount of depression and its location.

Care should be taken to identify medial fractures, especially medial and posterior shear fractures, on CT scans as these are inherently unstable unless proven otherwise. In a recent cadaveric imaging study, Immerman et al. demonstrated that if a posteromedial fracture is present, the size of the fragment and the fracture line orientation to the posterior edges of the femoral condyles can be used as a reference for stability. They found that medial fragments occupying over 60% of the medial plateau were loaded at all flexion angles. However, fragments involving 30% of the medial plateau would contact the femoral condyle in the range of 70 to 90 degrees with high load. Fracture lines oriented between 0 and 20 degrees of external rotation to the posterior femoral condylar axis (PFCA) also allowed fragments to remain unloaded. For example, based on their cadaveric model,

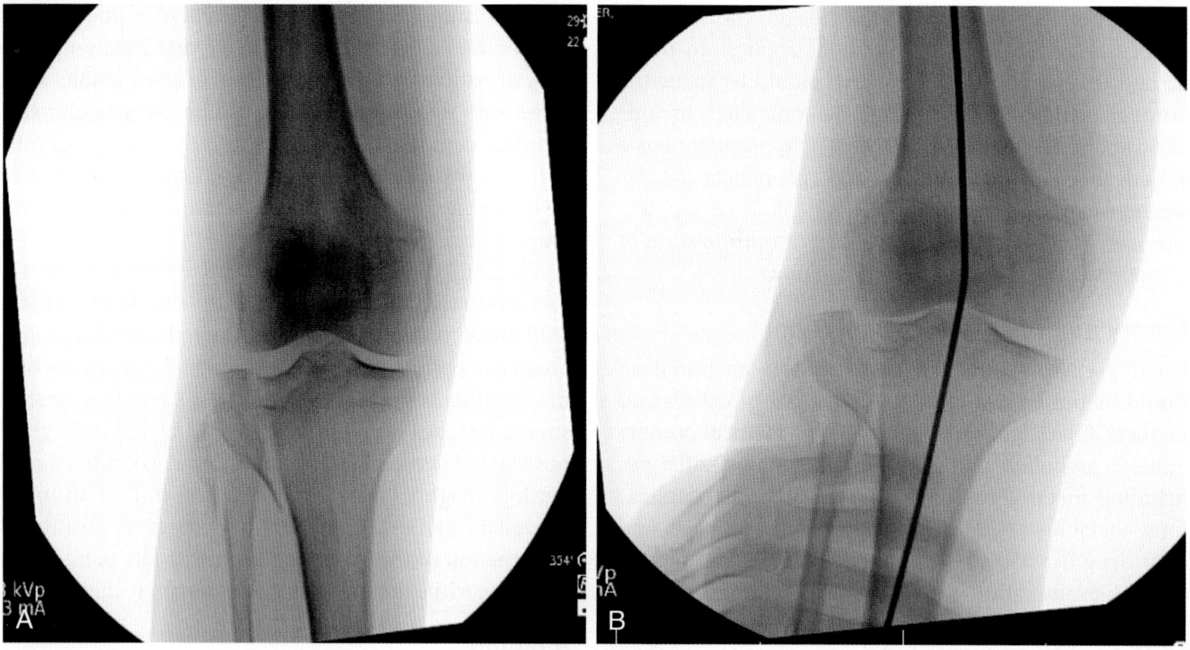

Fig. 3.2 Fluoroscopic imaging to evaluate coronal alignment. (A) This is a lateral split-depressed tibial plateau fracture. (B) A reaming rod for an intramedullary nail is prebent to 10 degrees in the middle and positioned over the top of the examined limb at the joint line as a guide for alignment. The knee is examined in full extension and shows a valgus deformity of 10 degrees or more when compared with the rod. This shows an unstable fracture that is indicated for operative treatment.

a fracture oriented at neutral to 20 degrees external rotation relative to the PFCA that occupies less than 30% of the medial tibial plateau would be stable from 0 to 90 degrees of flexion, allowing for early motion.[14]

In cases where an accurate stability examination is not possible and the mechanism is suspicious for ligamentous injury, magnetic resonance imaging (MRI) may be indicated to objectively determine the stability of the knee. Numerous authors cite ligamentous stability as paramount for a successful outcome.[4,15–17] For instance, a medically unstable patient with 5 mm of lateral depression and intact ligaments on MRI can be treated nonoperatively with confidence in an acceptable outcome.

TECHNIQUES

Techniques of nonoperative treatment have evolved from strict immobilization in a spica cast to early range of motion with removable bracing.[18] Most historical nonoperative treatment methods may not be tolerated by today's patients; however, they may be required in unique circumstances. We also call on the techniques of the past to create modern nonoperative treatment options.

Cast Immobilization and Modern Bracing

In the past, fractures deemed stable on examination, were treated in a long leg plaster cast from the groin to the toes with the knee flexed 20 degrees for 4 to 16 weeks, followed by gradual range of motion exercises.[12,19,20] While a long leg plaster cast may no longer be advisable, a long leg fiberglass cast or splint may be more durable in minimally displaced fractures, especially in unreliable patients. A simple Velcro knee immobilizer can be employed, especially in more reliable patients, but requires frequent adjustment and inevitably runs the risk of sliding inferiorly on the injured limb. A modern fracture brace, either locked in extension or slight flexion, can also be substituted for a traditional cast.

Modern fracture braces have improved upon the cast brace with lighter, water-resistant cuff material and the ability to modulate flexion and remove and replace the brace easily. For fractures that meet nonoperative criteria, the authors prefer application of the brace for 2 weeks in extension, followed by incremental increases in flexion at 2-week intervals until 90 degrees is reached. Ideally, 90 degrees of flexion would be achieved by 6 weeks. For distal fractures or to limit

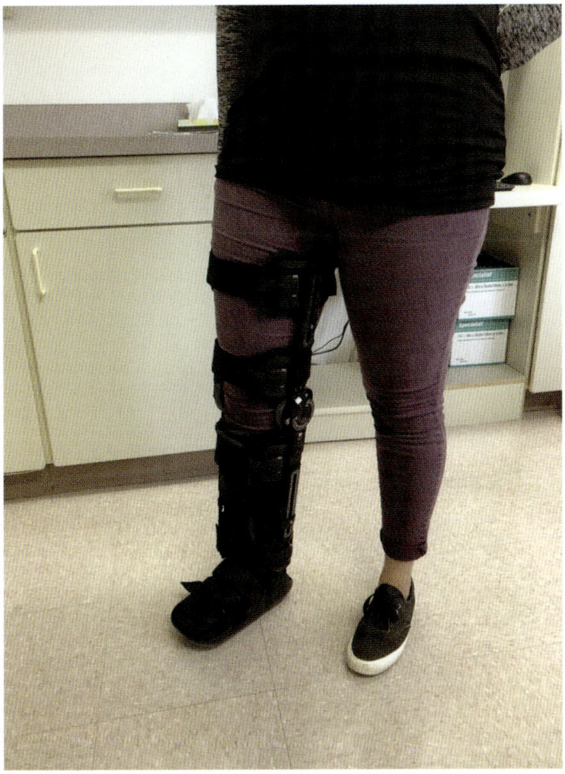

Fig. 3.3 A hinged knee brace, locked in extension, incorporated into a CAM (controlled ankle motion) boot, or walking boot to prevent inferior translation of ill-fitting hinged braces.

inferior translation of the brace, a modern adaptation of the cast brace can be made by incorporating the hinged knee brace to the metallic uprights of a fracture boot. As in traditional cast bracing, the hinges can be "massaged" to unload certain fracture patterns or an unloader style brace (if long enough) can be utilized. We have found that incorporating the knee brace to a foot orthosis or an articulated ankle attachment alleviates the inferior translation seen with typical knee immobilizers or ill-fitting hinged braces (Fig. 3.3). This option lessens the chances of heel pressure wounds and loss of motion from the brace when the hinged axis of rotation accidentally slips below the knee joint level.

Cast Brace

Traditionally, the cast brace consisted of a plaster short-leg walking cast attached to a plaster circumferential thigh cuff using metal hinges (Fig. 3.4).[21] The hinges could be contoured into varus or valgus alignment to offload the affected condyle while allowing early range of motion.[22] In their study of nonoperative treatment of tibial plateau fractures, Segal et al. recommended frequent follow-up every 2 weeks for the first 2 months and then monthly until the brace was removed. This allowed the plaster portions to be changed to accommodate for atrophy of the fractured limb and ensure good fit. Motion and weight bearing were encouraged immediately as tolerated after the brace was applied.[22]

Traction and Plaster Knee Exerciser

Traction can also be utilized in the form of skin traction (Buck's traction) or skeletal traction. Today's method of Buck's traction involves applying a foam boot to the patient's foot and ankle and attaching weight to a pulley system, allowing a longitudinal pull on the leg through skin traction. Moore et al. defined Buck's traction as usage of any form of skin traction applied to the leg, utilizing a pulley at the foot of the bed.[23] Weight is limited to 8 to 10 lbs. (3.5–4.5 kg). Patients were encouraged to perform active straight leg raises, as well as active range of motion of the knee as tolerated. According to Moore's treatment method, Buck's traction was continued until the patient could actively flex to at least 90 degrees, which took, on average, 1 week. Once this degree of flexion was met, traction was discontinued. The patient was discharged with instructions to remain non–weight bearing and work on antigravity knee range of motion three times daily to the point of muscle fatigue. This method was utilized for "minor" fractures of the plateau, which included fractures that were stable to varus-valgus examination in extension, and the articular surface is depressed to less than the thickness of the involved cartilage (roughly 2.5 mm).[23]

Closed reduction can also be performed using skin traction. In 1987, Duwelius and Connolly described a closed reduction technique for fractures that proved stable after examination. Heavy longitudinal traction was applied with the patient on a fracture table while an assistant used a strap to apply a reduction force, such as varus force for a laterally compressed fracture. The authors found that in stable fractures, 89% of patients had satisfactory results based on functional outcomes at an average of a 5-year follow-up.[24]

More invasive than Buck's traction, skeletal traction was historically used as a nonoperative technique. Skeletal traction was applied via a threaded Steinman pin, placed in the tibial diaphysis below the fracture site. This technique was employed when more weight was needed to reduce a fracture by ligamentotaxis. The pin was placed 7.5 to 10 cm below the most distal fracture line. The typical traction weight was anywhere from 4.4 lbs (2 kg) up to 30 lbs (13.5

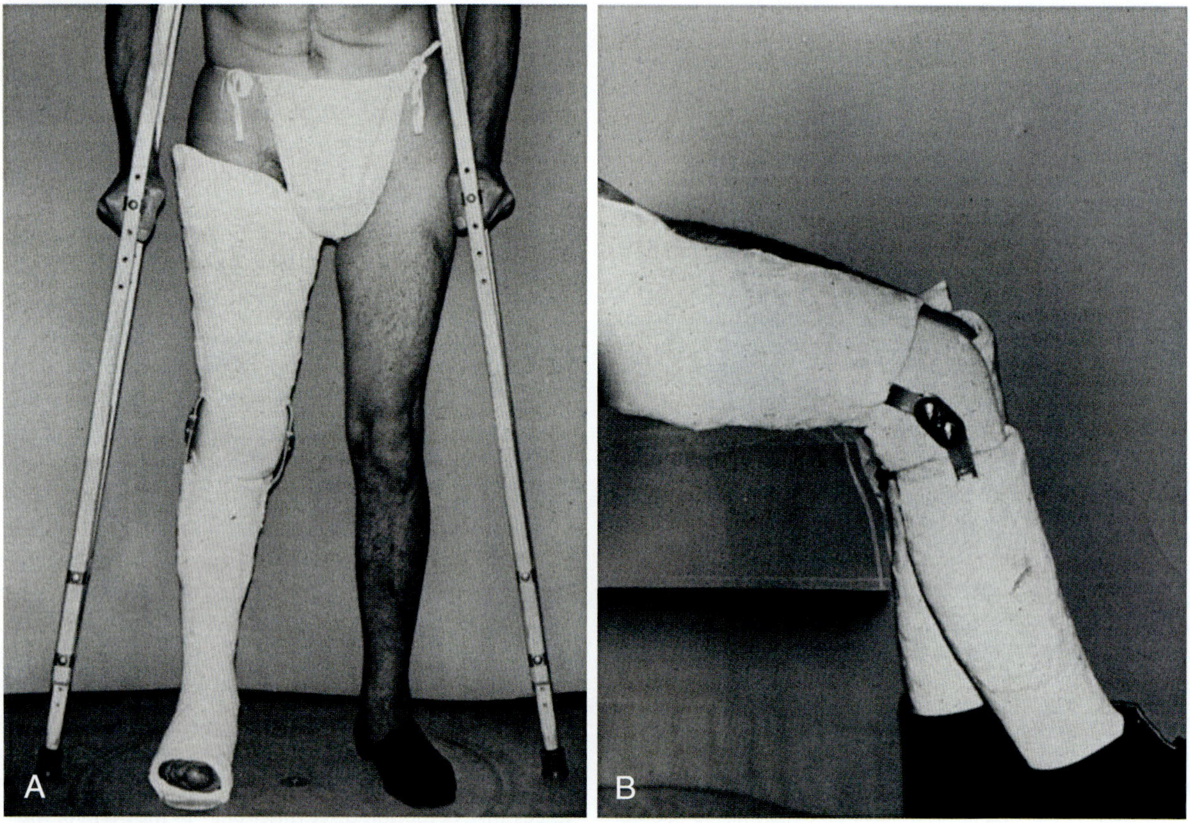

Fig. 3.4 Cast brace showing the short leg walking cast attached to a plaster circumferential thigh cuff, by means of metal hinges. (From Wardlaw D. The cast-brace treatment of femoral shaft fractures. *J Bone Joint Surg Br*. 1977;59-B(4):411-416.)

kg) for a few days.[25] Skeletal traction can be employed for varying amounts of time. In their study of skeletal traction, Marwah et al. treated patients in traction for roughly 6 weeks. The patients were initially treated in extension with quadriceps exercises for 10 to 12 days and then began range of motion exercises until the patient was able to flex to 90 degrees. Traction was then discontinued, and the patient began protected weight bearing with crutches for up to 3 months.[25] Similar methods were employed by Jensen et al., except that skeletal traction was applied through a calcaneal pin with 5% of the patient's body weight, exercises beginning after 1 week, and 4 to 6 weeks of traction followed by delayed weight bearing until 3 months.[26] Typically, if shorter intervals of traction were employed, patients were converted to either a cast brace or a plaster knee exerciser after an initial period of 1 week.[22,23,27–29]

The plaster knee exerciser described by Moore et al. incorporates tibial skeletal traction into a short leg cast with a plaster thigh cylinder. With this setup, a rope and pulley system has balanced suspension to maintain heavy traction and allow motion to occur at the knee. Side clamps allow for adjustment of varus or valgus alignment. The intricate knee exerciser was maintained for 6 weeks only if the fracture could maintain reduction, and if not, surgery was performed.[23,30]

RESULTS

Cast Immobilization

Lansinger et al. found that fractures stable on examination with either a split-depressed or simple split fracture pattern, with depression of the articular surface less than 10 mm (especially if not centrally located), could be treated nonoperatively. These patients were managed in a cast for 2 weeks followed by range of motion exercises. Patients achieved excellent to good results.[13] In comminuted bicondylar fractures and fractures with a large central depression, reconstruction was recommended.[13] Moore et al. also found similar poor results with bicondylar and medially based fractures. These fracture patterns were less likely to maintain reduction, and the authors recommended surgical stabilization.[23] Honkonen also used cast immobilization for an average of 7.4 weeks and allowed weight bearing after an average of 9.8 weeks. Fracture types treated by closed or open means were not delineated. Upon follow-up, 95% of patients achieved flexion exceeding 109 degrees and 82% came within 5 degrees of full extension. However, the author indicated that prolonged immobilization of nonoperative patients was less likely to affect range of motion compared with operatively treated patients. The author also found that condylar widening of up to 5 mm showed no adverse effect on the results, but the results deteriorated when the widening became greater. Additionally, severe instability was found in 18% of the knees even after casting, leading to only 31% acceptable results in the face of instability.[12] Residual alignment also affected results. Fractures aligned in varus or with more than 5 degrees of lateral tilt compared to the contralateral side fared less well and markedly worse with over 10 degrees of lateral tilt. Functional and subjective scores also declined when articular step-off exceeded 3 mm.[12]

Cast Brace

After cast brace treatment, as described by Duwelius and Connolly, posttreatment radiographic findings did not always correlate with functional results. However, those fractures with medial plateau involvement led to varus and worse outcomes.[24] Complications specific to cast brace treatment include peroneal and sciatic palsy, venous thromboses, and pulmonary embolism from prolonged inactivity. According to Segal et al., fractures with 5 mm or less of depression or displacement also had good functional outcomes when treated with the combination of cast bracing with early weight bearing.[22] Cast bracing was shown to unload 50% of the weight at the fracture site while ambulating. While the authors found that no fracture incurred more than 2 mm of further depression with weight bearing in the brace, split-depressed fractures were prone to further development of valgus deformity.[22]

Traction and Plaster Knee Exerciser

Isolated traction described by Marwah et al. has the intended goal of molding the fractured tibial condyle into the shape of the femur and allowing the depressed area of the plateau to fill in with fibrocartilage if the joint is protected for a sufficient period of time. While excellent results were achieved in 64% of patients, the patient remained in traction for 6 weeks, and complications of pressure wounds and pin tract infection occurred. The authors acknowledge that anatomic reduction of fragments is unlikely, and the patient must be kept from weight-bearing before 12 weeks.[25] Jensen et al. surmised that in stable knees, treatment by traction and early motion provided functional results equal to surgery. However, the method was found to be very time-consuming for patients and also required hospitalization.[31] In the technique described by Moore et al., those "minor" fractures treated with Buck's traction or the plaster knee exerciser had 71% return to their previous activity level compared with 77% return for operative fractures. The authors stressed that only major fractures were advised to have surgery, so the baseline groups were not equivalent or randomized. Complications discussed from closed treatment were nonunion in fractures with metaphyseal-diaphyseal involvement and fractures with a fragment of the tibial tuberosity that could not be maintained in reduction.[23]

CASE 3.1

Our patient is a 47-year-old healthy male. He is a nonsmoker, very active, and notably runs approximately 40 to 50 miles per week. The patient works as a physician assistant at the hospital. The patient presented to the clinic status post-twisting injury to his left knee. He was found to have significant lateral proximal tibial pain on examination, with associated swelling and mild knee effusion. His knee was stable to varus and valgus stress in full extension. He was neurovascularly intact. CT scan showed a split-depressed tibial plateau fracture, with approximately 3 mm of depression and 3 mm of widening. The patient underwent MRI of the knee, which showed intact anterior cruciate ligament/posterior cruciate ligament, medial collateral ligament/lateral collateral ligament, with a medial meniscal tear and lateral meniscal degeneration (Fig. 3.5A–D).

The patient was treated non–weight bearing for 6 weeks, initially in a hinged knee brace, locked from 0 to 45 degrees for the first 2 weeks, and then unlocked for another 4 weeks. After 6 weeks, the patient's weight bearing was slowly advanced, the brace was discontinued, and he began gentle biking. He returned to running and full activity without complaint by 3 months

Continued

CASE 3.1—CONT'D

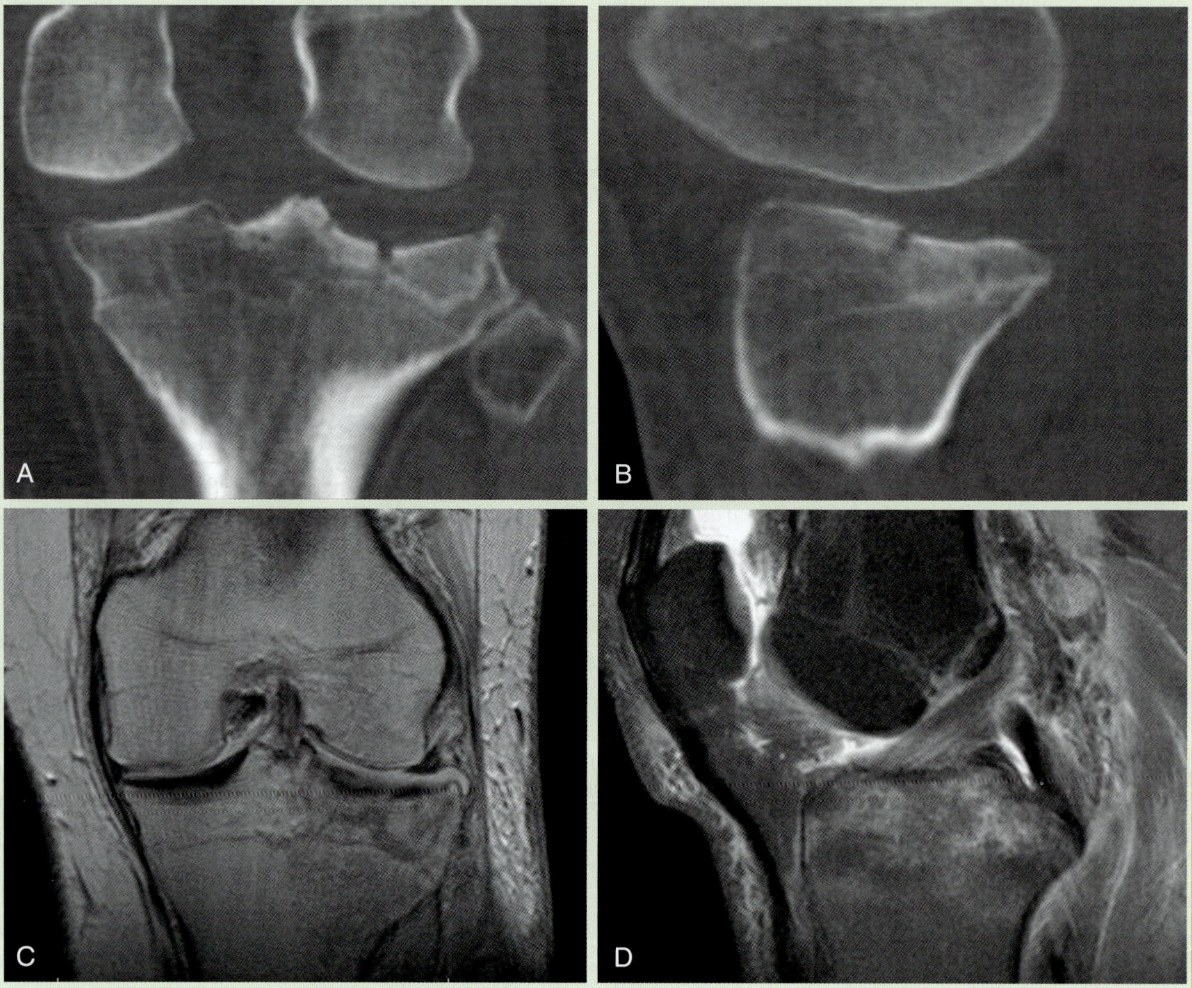

Fig. 3.5 Computed tomography (CT) and magnetic resonance imaging (MRI) of lateral split-depressed tibial plateau fracture. (A) Coronal CT scan showing less than 3 mm of depression and 3 mm of widening. (B) Sagittal CT scan showing no significant displacement. (C) Coronal MRI showing intact medial collateral ligament. (D) Sagittal MRI showing intact anterior cruciate ligament and posterior cruciate ligament.

post injury. Two-year follow-up radiographs show maintained alignment of the tibial plateau fracture (Fig. 3.6). This case is a great example of nonoperative treatment in a healthy, active patient using modern bracing and early mobilization. Factors that may have improved this patient's outcome include his medical literacy and compliance with brace wear and non–weight-bearing restrictions.

CASE 3.1—CONT'D

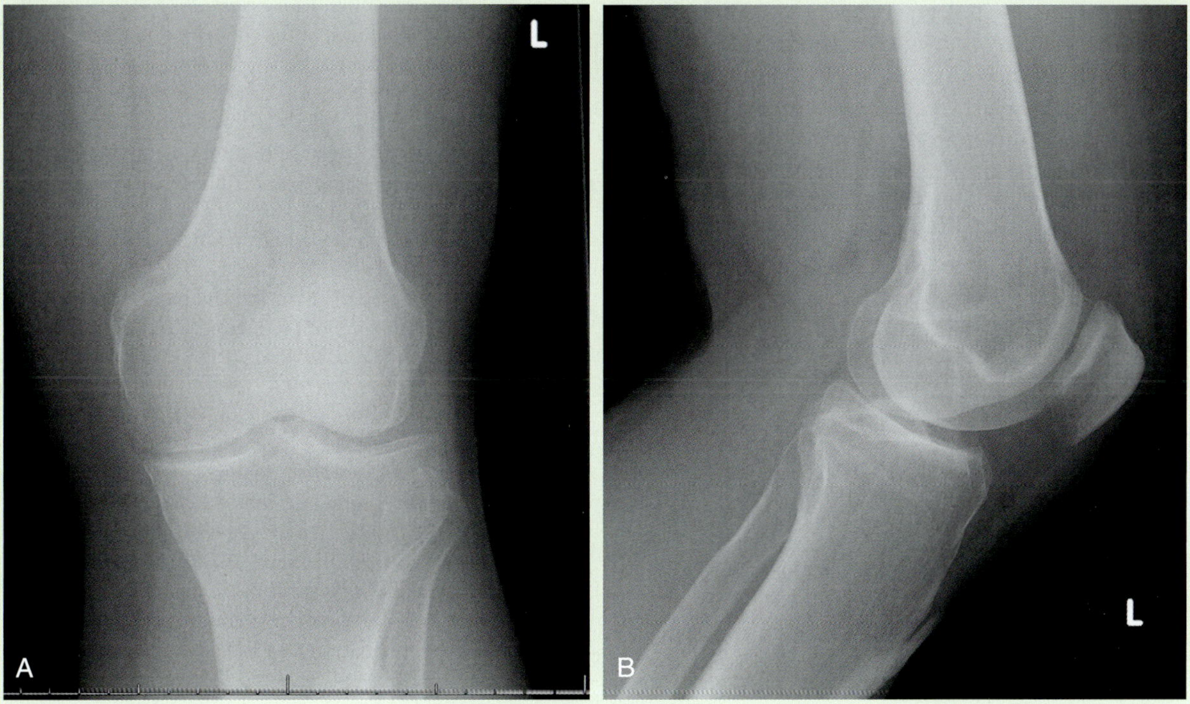

Fig. 3.6 Two-year post operative follow up imaging (A) AP radiograph of the Left knee and (B) lateral radiograph of the Left knee, showing a well-healed tibial plateau fracture with maintained alignment of the knee and no significant joint line depression.

CONCLUSIONS

While operative treatment has evolved to become the mainstay for treating tibial plateau fractures, nonoperative treatment has also adapted. The body of literature for nonoperative treatment has helped refine our indications for both surgical and nonsurgical management.

Some plateau fractures are amenable to nonoperative treatment, and this chapter aids in identifying those fracture patterns that can be treated nonoperatively. Until proven otherwise, bicondylar fractures and those fractures with metaphyseal and diaphyseal comminution should be considered surgical indications. Other fracture patterns may be considered for nonsurgical care if they are stable to stress in full extension, ligamentously stable, with articular step-off 3mm or less, and with condylar widening less than 5 mm. Coronal alignment should be scrupulously evaluated. Up to 5 degrees of lateral tilt is acceptable, and between 5 and 10 can be considered for nonoperative treatment. However, greater than 10 degrees of lateral tilt or varus angulation should forgo closed treatment in most circumstances.

The historical nonoperative treatment methods may not be practical. However, adaptations to these methods certainly have their place given the changes in our patients over the years, including the aging population and increase in medical conditions, such as morbid obesity, diabetes, and other medical comorbidities that make patients high risk for surgery. An increasing number of patients may be considered inappropriate for surgery, and fracture patterns proven to maintain reduction with acceptable functional outcomes should be treated nonoperatively.

WIDMAIER'S TIPS AND TRICKS

- A reaming rod prebent 10 degrees can be used as an overlay during radiographic stress examination to determine the degree of varus/valgus instability.
- While the overwhelming majority of medial fractures should be considered operative, there may be

a subset of medial fractures that occupy a small area of the joint (less than 20%), with specific fracture orientations (0–20 degrees external rotation (ER) to PFCA), that may be treated nonoperatively.

- Hinged knee braces can be used for nonsurgical treatment to gradually increase knee range of motion while protecting the fracture. An Cam walking boot may be used below the knee brace to prevent inferior translation of the brace, which could lead to decreased knee range of motion and pressure wounds.
- Hinged knee braces can be contoured to help unload the affected plateau.

REFERENCES

1. A treatise on dislocations and fractures of the joints. *Med Chir Rev J Med Sci Anal Ser*. 1823;3(12):832–857.
2. Blokker CP, Rorabeck CH, Bourne RB. Tibial plateau fractures. An analysis of the results of treatment in 60 patients. *Clin Orthop Relat Res*. 1984;182:193–199.
3. Bakalim G, Wilppula E. Fractures of tibial condyles. *Acta Orthopaedica*. 1973;44(3):311–322.
4. Schatzker J, McBroom R, Bruce D. The tibial plateau fracture. The Toronto experience 1968–1975. *Clin Orthop Relat Res*. 1979;(138):94–104.
5. Cierny G, Mader JT, Pennick JJ. A clinical staging system for adult osteomyelitis. *Contemp Orthop*. 1985;10:17–37.
6. Bowen TR, Widmaier JC. Host classification predicts infection after open fracture. *Clin Orthop Relat Res*. 2005;433:205–211.
7. Gortler H, Rusyn J, Godbout C, Chahal J, Schemitsch EH, Nauth A. Diabetes and healing outcomes in lower extremity fractures: a systematic review. *Injury*. 2018;49(2):177–183.
8. Aggarwal VK, Tischler EH, Lautenbach C, et al. Mitigation and education. *J Orthop Res*. 2014;32(S1):S16–S25.
9. Tarabichi M, Shohat N, Kheir MM, et al. Determining the threshold for HbA1c as a predictor for adverse outcomes after total joint arthroplasty: a multicenter, retrospective study. *J Arthroplast*. 2017;32(9):S263–S267. e1.
10. Mathew A, Devereaux PJ, O'Hare A, et al. Chronic kidney disease and postoperative mortality: a systematic review and meta-analysis. *Kidney Int*. 2008;73(9):1069–1081.
11. Kim C, Kim H, Lee C, Wang L, Rhee SJ. Effect of chronic kidney disease on outcomes of total joint arthroplasty: a meta-analysis. *Knee Surg Relat Res*. 2020;32(1):12.
12. Honkonen SE. Indications for surgical treatment of tibial condyle fractures. *Clin Orthop Relat Res*. 1994;302:199–205.
13. Lansinger O, Bergman B, Körner L, Andersson G. Tibial condylar fractures. A twenty-year follow-up. *J Bone Joint Surg Am*. 1986;68(1):13–19.
14. Immerman I, Bechtel C, Yildirim G, Heller Y, Walker PS, Egol KA. Stability of the posteromedial fragment in a tibial plateau fracture. *J Knee Surg*. 2013;26(2):117–126.
15. Roberts JM. Fractures of the condyles of the tibia. An anatomical and clinical end-result study of one hundred cases. *J Bone Joint Surg Am*. 1968;50(8):1505–1521.
16. Rasmussen P. Tibial condylar fractures: impairment of knee joint stability as an indication for surgical treatment. *J Bone Joint Surg Am*. 1973;55(7):1331–1350.
17. Delamarter RB, Hohl M, Hopp Jr E. Ligament injuries associated with tibial plateau fractures. *Clin Orthop Relat Res*. 1990;250:226–233.
18. Drennan D, Locher F, Maylahn D. Fractures of the tibial plateau. Treatment by closed reduction and spica cast. *J Bone Joint Surg Am*. 1979;61(7):989–995.
19. Honkonen SE, Järvinen MJ. Classification of fractures of the tibial condyles. *J Bone Joint Surg Br*. 1992;74(6):840–847.
20. Waddell JP, Johnston DW, Neidre A. Fractures of the tibial plateau: a review of ninety-five patients and comparison of treatment methods. *J Trauma*. 1981;21(5):376–381.
21. Wardlaw D. The cast-brace treatment of femoral shaft fractures. *J Bone Joint Surg Br*. 1977;59-B(4):411–416.
22. Segal D, Mallik AR, Wetzler MJ, Franchi AV, Whitelaw GP. Early weight bearing of lateral tibial plateau fractures. *Clin Orthop Relat Res*. 1993;294(294):232–237.
23. Moore T, Patzakis M, Harvey J. Tibial plateau fractures: definition, demographics, treatment rationale, and long-term results of closed traction management or operative reduction. *J Orthop Trauma*. 1987;1(2):97–119.
24. Duwelius PJ, Connolly JF. Closed reduction of tibial plateau fractures. A comparison of functional and roentgenographic end results. *Clin Orthop Relat Res*. 1988;230:116–126.
25. Marwah V, Gadegone WM, Magarkar DS. The treatment of fractures of the tibial plateau by skeletal traction and early mobilisation. *Int Orthop*. 1985;9(4):217–221.
26. Jensen DB, Rude C, Duus B, Bjerg-Nielsen A. Tibial plateau fractures. A comparison of conservative and surgical treatment. *J Bone Joint Surg Br*. 1990;72(1):49–52.
27. Apley AG. Fractures of the lateral tibial condyle treated by skeletal traction and early mobilisation; a review of sixty cases with special reference to the long-term results. *J Bone Joint Surg Br*. 1956;38-B(3):699–708.
28. DeCoster TA, Nepola JV, el-Khoury GY. Cast brace treatment of proximal tibia fractures. A ten-year follow-up study. *Clin Orthop Relat Res*. 1988;231:196–204.
29. Brown GA, Sprague BL. Cast brace treatment of plateau and bicondylar fractures of the proximal tibia. *Clin Orthop Relat Res*. 1976;119:184–193.
30. Badgley CE, O'Connor SJ. Conservative treatment of fractures of the tibial plateau. *AMA Arch Surg*. 1952;64(4):508–515.

4

External Fixators for the Treatment of Proximal Tibia Fractures: Ringed and Standard

David Seligson, MD and Adam Kessler, DO

INTRODUCTION

Tibial plateau fractures come in many forms from the senile nursing home patient falling on the way to the bathroom to the young motorcyclist driving into a tractor-trailer. Similarly, external fixators range from simple uniplanar large pin frames to complex ring fixators that take hours to construct and "fine tune." This chapter is a guide to fitting the frame to the problem.

The treatment of bicondylar tibial plateau fractures can be a daunting undertaking. The orthopedic trauma surgeon must keep in mind that the amount of energy transferred to the bone also takes its toll on the soft tissues. Not only can the injury to the cartilage and the subchondral plate lead to arthrosis but the injury to the soft-tissue envelope can also cause many complications involved with open reduction and plate fixation of these fractures. Oftentimes, treatment requires dual plating, which in itself involves extensive mobilization of the already severely injured soft tissues from the comminuted bone with impaired blood supply, walking the fine line of being able to heal as well as not becoming infected.

Ringed external fixators have previously been utilized in the treatment of these high-energy injuries but have the potential for the added complication of a septic knee joint from intraarticular pins. Recent modifications to pin placement based on anatomic studies.[1] have led to a resurgence in the use of ringed fixators for the treatment of these devastating injuries. This chapter will guide you through pin placement and configuration for a ringed fixator as well as simple large pin external fixators.

BIOMECHANICS

The construction of the ring external fixator allows the surgeon to adjust the stiffness of the construct as well as to customize the fixation based on the injury pattern. With adjustments to the transfixion wire spread, the crossing angle, ring diameter, half-pin diameter, number of rings, and the ring symmetry the surgeon can adjust the stiffness of the construct. All of these variables can be used to increase or decrease the stiffness and, therefore, the overall stability of the construct.[2]

A crossing angle of the tensioned wires in the proximal tibia increased from 30 to 90 degrees will increase the axial, torsional, and bending stiffness by 75%.[3,4] Transfixion pin angles between 60 and 90 degrees allow appropriate stiffness and resistance to shear forces in the sagittal plane with knee range of motion[5,4,6] but can lead to the placement of pins outside of the soft-tissue safe corridors.[5] An additional half-pin placed in the anterior position in the proximal tibia will augment sagittal stability. Gellar et al. changed the pin configuration so that the pins did not all cross the tibia in the center, allowing for crossing angles of 80 degrees, while placing them more within the sagittal plane.[7] However, this places the pins outside the soft-tissue safe corridors[5,8] and can lead to impingement on the patellar tendon. Antoci et al. experimented with varying wire-crossing configurations while maintaining 60-degree crossing angles.[5] Wire placement with two pins crossing 1 cm posterior to the center of the plateau and the horizontal wire in the coronal plane passing 1 cm anteriorly and inferiorly

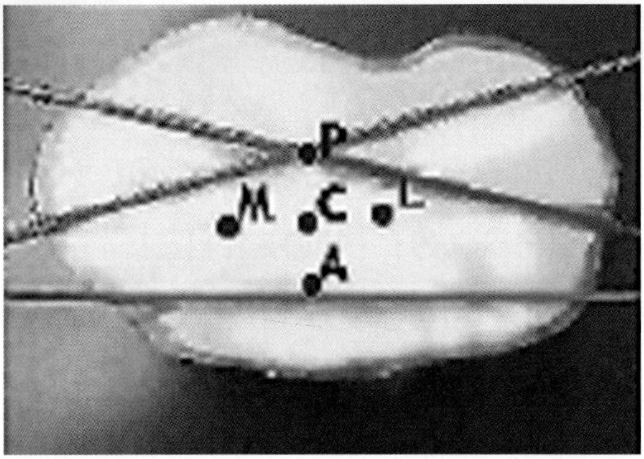

Fig. 4.1 Wire placement of proximal tibia. (From Antoci V, Raney EM, Antoci V, Voor MJ, Roberts CS. Transfixion wire positioning within the bone. *J Pediatr Orthop.* 2006;26(4):466-470.)

from the center of the tibia increased the sagittal plane stiffness without decreasing coronal or torsional stiffness (Fig. 4.1). Three wires are sufficient for weight bearing and stiffness of the construct, but more wires may be used if desired to further increase stability. Wires 1.8 mm in diameter are small enough to capture smaller fragments of comminution as well as stiff enough once tensioned to resist loads[14]; however, the larger the diameter, the greater the stability imparted. Tensioning olive wires on both sides of the fracture and placing them on the side of bending will also increase the bending stiffness of the external fixator. Tensioned wires cannot be placed in the anterior-posterior direction as this would place the posterior tibial artery, nerve, and muscles at risk of injury. The greatest deforming force is in the sagittal (anteroposterior [AP]) plane when walking, and half-pins apply greater frame stiffness in this plane and are therefore used to add to the stability in the sagittal plane.[9,10] A second ring added to the proximal segment as well as wires in two levels will also increase the stability of the construct.[11,12] Hybrid fixators follow similar principles with the addition of half-pins in the diaphysis where the half-pins have greater purchase. Using pins mounted on rings will also increase the overall stiffness.[11,9]

The stability of traditional knee-spanning constructs with half-pins and bars is less critical as they are, in general, temporary in nature.[13] Half-pin diameter, the number of half-pins, multiplanar half-pins, bar height relative to the bone, pin to fracture distance, and the working length of the fixator are all variables that can be adjusted to manage the stiffness of the montage.[14,15]

INDICATIONS

The general indication for external fixation of a proximal tibia fracture is a complex fracture with soft-tissue injury, which would make open plating unsafe due to increased risk of infection and/or further soft-tissue injury. Fracture patterns can be used as an indication for external fixation; more specifically, Schatzker type V and VI fractures, proximal tibia fractures with metaphyseal and subchondral comminution not amendable to routine plating, soft-tissue compromise (i.e., compartment syndrome), mangled limbs, fractures with soft-tissue defects, and fractures in the multiply injured pat ient.[3,16,17,18,19] Schatzker type IV fracture may also be considered for external fixation. These can be deceptively high-energy fractures with compromise of the soft tissue, knee dislocation, or neurovascular injury.[20,21]

X-ray clues that staged management may reduce complications include the following:

1. The mechanical axis of the tibia is not in line with the femur—there is significant varus, valgus, or displacement anteriorly or posteriorly.
2. The spread of the tibial condyles is wider than the spread of the distal femoral condyles.
3. The fibular head is disassociated from the tibia.
4. The tibial tuberosity is pulled anteriorly by the patella ligament.
5. There is air in the proximal tibia or the interosseous space.
6. A part of the plateau is displaced posteriorly.

TECHNIQUE

Ring Fixators

The patient is positioned supine on a radiolucent fracture table with fluoroscopic control. The operative thigh and leg is elevated on a bolster to allow 360 degree viewing and access to the operative limb. A tourniquet is in place and can be inflated when needed. Manual traction or a femoral distractor may be used to obtain length and use ligamentotaxis to reduce the fracture fragments. If there are areas of comminution blocking reduction, limited incisions over the major fracture line may be made and an elevator or a forceps used to manipulate the fragments into place.[8] Next, small and large bone clamps may be applied to assemble the fracture site.[8] If the articular surface is depressed, a bone tamp can be introduced through an incision over the major fracture line and under fluoroscopy used to elevate depressed bone into place where it can be held temporarily with a bone clamp or kept in position with k-wires (Fig. 4.2). Once an appropriate reduction is obtained and confirmed by good biplanar fluoroscopic views, one or more cancellous screws can be placed across the proximal tibia to compress the fracture and stabilize the joint (Fig. 4.3). It is important to ensure that the screw will not interfere with future wire placement in the proximal tibia. Any voids in the metaphyseal bone can be filled with autogenous bone graft or bone graft substitute.

The ring fixator construct begins with choosing appropriate size rings for the patient, ensuring two- to three-fingerbreadth clearance around the ring when in place. Generally, the tibia is in the anterior portion of the ring. An incomplete ring may be used to allow for better knee range of motion as it is open in the back (Fig. 4.4) or a full ring may be utilized for better fracture stabilization.[22] If a full ring is chosen, a stack of surgical towels should be placed under the calf so that the tibia does not sag within the ring (Fig. 4.5). This will maintain the two- to three-fingerbreadth distance between the ring and the limb,[23] preventing impingement on the soft tissues.

Due to the capsular extension of the knee (Fig. 4.6), the reference wire should be placed 14 mm distal to the joint line on the fluoroscopic AP and lateral views; this will ensure extra-articular placement of the wires.[8,9] The key is to ensure a true lateral of the joint with the femoral condyles superimposed to avoid inaccurate wire placement. Once the location for a wire is identified, we recommend utilizing a small stab incision and sweeping the soft tissue with a hemostat to clear away any neurovascular structures. The wire should also be placed approximately 1 cm anterior to the midportion of the proximal tibia (Fig. 4.7). The ring can then be attached to the reference wire to aid in positioning the two olive wires, one from posterolateral through the fibular head if necessary, angled 60 degrees so that the wire will cross with the following posteromedial wire 1 cm posterior to the midproximal tibia.[4,5,9] Although the ideal angle is 90 degrees, and a technique has been described by Geller et al.[7] that obtains a crossing angle of 80 degrees, the surgeon must keep in mind that this will bring the wires more anterior and they may then impinge on the patellar tendon, which needs 2 cm of clearance from the pins.[5,9] Again, the wires should be at least 14 mm distal to the joint line. It is important to not pass the lateral wire distal to the fibular neck as this may injure the common peroneal nerve. The knee can also be flexed to help protect the nerve by

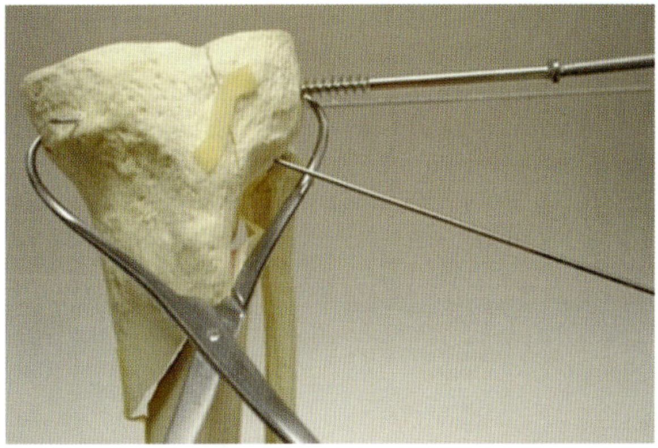

Fig. 4.2 Reduction. (Picture courtesy Smith & Nephew.)

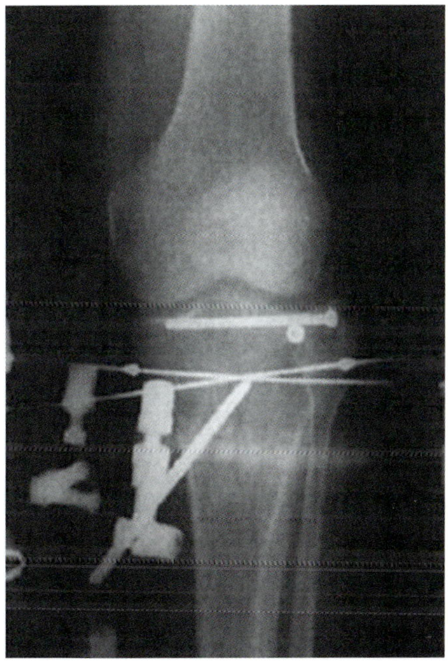

Fig. 4.3 Screw placement. (From Sirkin MS, Bono CM, Reilly MC, Behrens FF. Percutaneous methods of tibial plateau fixation. *Clin Orthop Relat Res.* 2000;(375):60-68.)

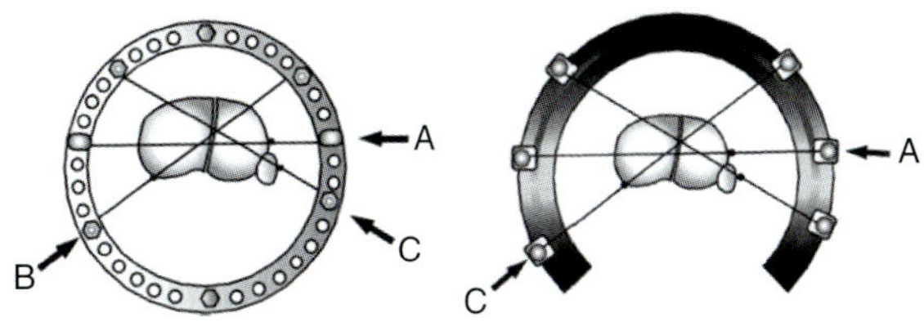

Fig. 4.4 Fine-wire placement through rings. (From Hutson JJ Jr. The centered lateral fluoroscopic image of the knee: the key to safe tensioned wire placement in periarticular fractures of the proximal tibia. *J Orthop Trauma.* 2002;16(3):196-200.)

moving it posteriorly.[9] The olive wires are then tensioned sequentially at 90 lbs. from the side opposite the olive. The olives are used to compress the fracture and should be checked with fluoroscopy after tensioning. Be certain that during tensioning, the olive is not pulled into the tibia. This can be avoided by tensioning partway, then fixing the wire to the ring on the olive side, and then completing the tensioning. A second ring placed 2 cm below the proximal ring may be needed to increase stability. This can be done with fine wires with or without olives. Again, ensuring that the safe corridors are maintained, the wires are passed in the same posterolateral and posteromedial fashion but may need to be slightly more anterior than the previous wires. A 5-mm half-pin can also be placed 10 to 15 degrees off the medial aspect of the tibia to add more sagittal stability,[9] especially if an oblique fracture is present.

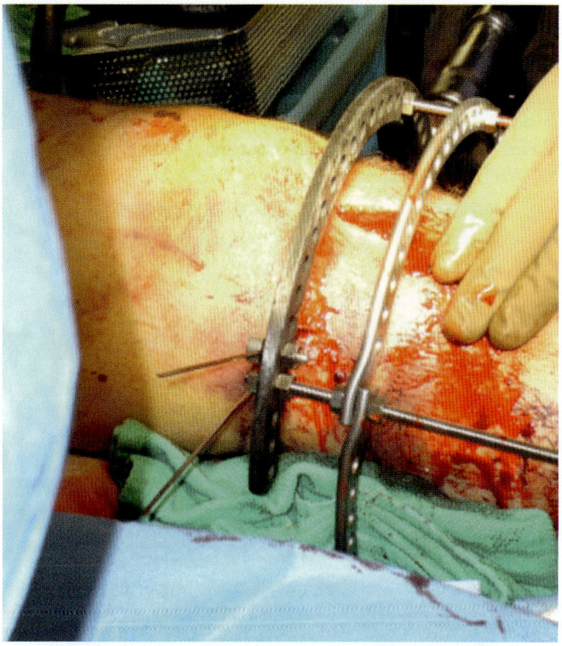

Fig. 4.5 Surgical towels to maintain space between frame and leg. (From Hall JA, Beuerlein MJ, McKee MD; Canadian Orthopaedic Trauma Society. Open reduction and internal fixation compared with circular fixator application for bicondylar tibial plateau fractures. Surgical technique. *J Bone Joint Surg Am.* 2009;91(suppl 2, pt 1):74-88.)

The distal portion of the frame can be attached by fine wires and rings, half-pins and rings, or a combination of wires and half-pins. The diaphyseal bone with

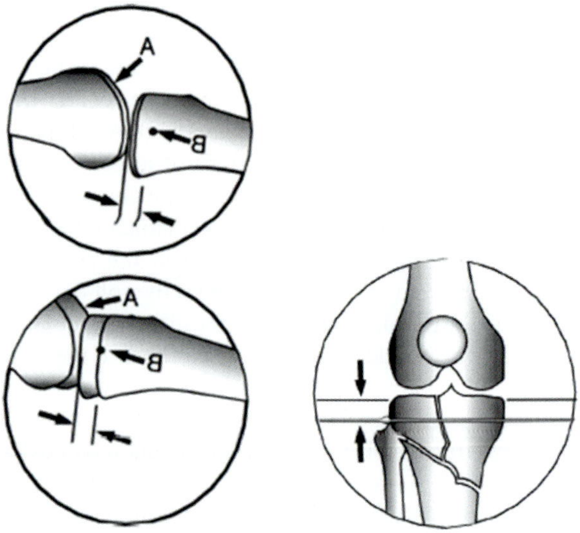

Fig. 4.7 Centered wire technique. (From Hutson JJ Jr. The centered lateral fluoroscopic image of the knee: the key to safe tensioned wire placement in periarticular fractures of the proximal tibia. *J Orthop Trauma.* 2002;16(3):196-200.)

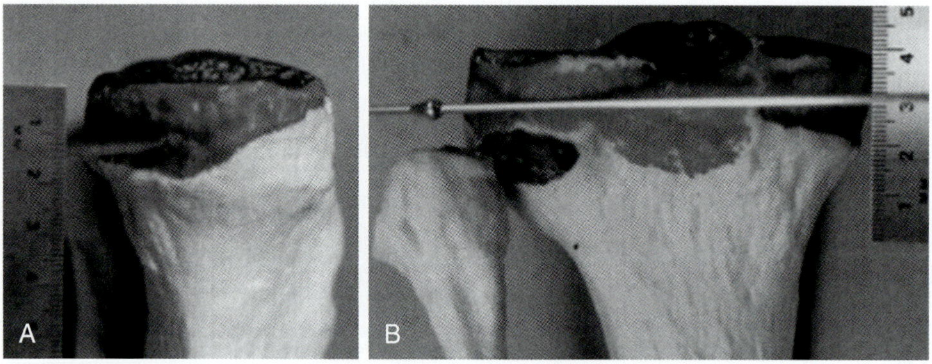

Fig. 4.6 Reference-wire placement. (From DeCoster TA, Crawford MK, Kraut MAS. Safe extracapsular placement of proximal tibia transfixation pins. *J Orthop Trauma.* 1999;13(4):236-240.)

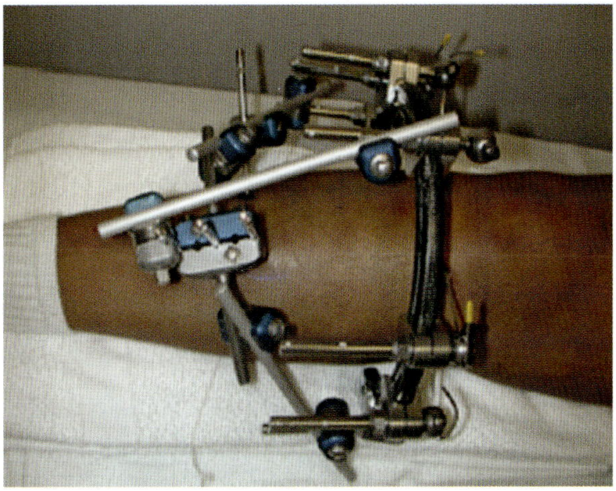

Fig. 4.8 Hybrid fixator.

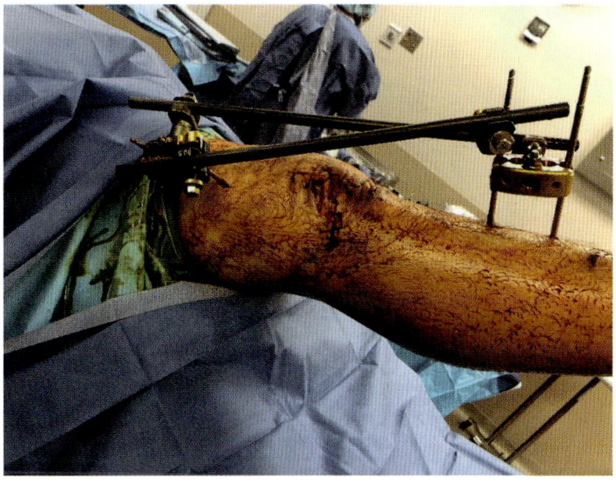

Fig. 4.9 Simple knee spanning external fixator.

its thicker cortices is able to maintain half-pins better than the metaphyseal bone; therefore, they can be used in the distal portion of the construct. Half-pins with rings[11,12] distally increase the stability of the overall construct compared to half-pins and bars or fine wires. Once overall mechanical alignment is confirmed with fluoroscopy, a smooth wire is passed 90 degrees to the distal tibia and tensioned. This is followed by additional smooth wires or a 5-mm half-pin 90 degrees to the distal reference wire. Another alternative is two half-pins per ring placed in the tibial shaft from the medial face in multiple planes. Once the alignment is confirmed by C-arm, three threaded rods are used to attach the distal and proximal rings (Fig. 4.8). Mechanical alignments can be confirmed using an electrocautery cord from the Anterior superior iliac spine (ASIS) passing through the femoral head, the center of the knee, and the ankle center down to the second ray.

Hybrid Construct

A hybrid construct is one that utilizes proximal periarticular tensioned wires and ring(s) connected to the tibial shaft by half-pins and bars.[24] These constructs are often used for the treatment of proximal tibial metaphyseal fractures.

The proximal portion is completed in the same manner as that previously described for the ringed fixator. The distal portion is attached to the diaphysis with multiple pin holding clamps with two parallel 5-mm half-pins and a third pin in another plane. Bars are then connected from the ring to the distal pin groups (Fig. 4.9).

Knee Spanning External Fixator

A simple, stable, and quickly applied uniplanar external fixator connects a pin group in the lateral distal femur with a pin group in the proximal medial tibia. The distal femoral pins are aimed a bit posteromedial and the medial tibia face pins start on the broad medial face of the proximal tibia and angle somewhat posterolateral. This usually allows a single bar to pass from the proximal to the distal group to complete the frame. This uniplanar frame works well unless there is appreciable instability about the knee (Fig. 4.10). For unstable patterns, a multiplanar frame with two lateral and one medial distal femoral pins works better. Knee spanning external fixators are generally temporary in nature; however, they can be used definitively if needed, and this should be kept in mind when constructing the fixator. With proximal tibia and tibial plateau fractures, the knee is spanned utilizing a standard pin and bar external fixator to avoid placing pins in the zones of injury.

The multiplanar frame is constructed as follows. Starting at the distal femur, a 5-mm half-pin is placed in the supracondylar femur laterally. A pin to bar clamp is attached followed by a "stop sign" style bar around the distal femur. Utilizing this bar, another pin to bar clamp is attached and used to guide an anterolateral pin into place. Again, utilizing the bar and pin clamp as a guide, an anteromedial pin is placed in the femur and secured with a pin to bar clamp.

Ensuring that the tibial pins will be outside the zone of injury and future fixation, a 5-mm half-pin is placed on the medial face of the tibia angled 10 to

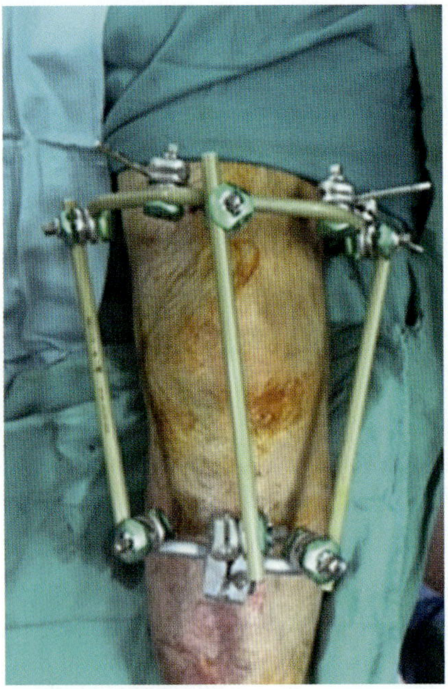

Fig. 4.10 Multiplanar external fixator.

15 degrees lateral. A pin clamp is attached to guide the next pin. Side rails are placed on the clamp with bar-to-bar clamps, with a pin-to-bar clamp attached to one of the tibial pins. Three spanning bars are attached to the bar-to-bar clamps. Utilizing bump and traction, the fracture is reduced under fluoroscopy and the clamps tightened. The knee should be slightly flexed when the construct is tightened to help prevent compartment syndrome. If the fracture pattern is such that there is a portion of the tibial condyle that is not reducing with traction and gentle manipulation, a half-pin can be placed into the fracture to maneuver the fragment into place and attach it to the construct to maintain the reduction. This overall construct allows multiple planes of reduction, which if necessary can be utilized as definitive treatment (Fig. 4.11).[25]

POSTOPERATIVE CARE

The postoperative course is based on the plan for management of the fracture. An external fixator can be placed to expedite patient care. In these cases, definitive fixation can be done a few days after injury during the initial hospitalization. If the external fixator was placed to allow soft-tissue swelling and skin damage to subside, the frame can be removed once the soft-tissue damage resolves, and then internal fixation performed at 1 to 3 weeks. Generally, external fixation is not used for definitive treatment. Patients with long-term external fixation need follow-up every 2 to 3 weeks to monitor healing and pin-track problems. Depending on the fracture pattern and the frame construct, the patient may be non–weight bearing to partial weight bearing for 6 to 8 weeks, with gradual increases in weight bearing based on healing. Every 2 to 3 weeks, x-rays will be obtained to check the alignment. The construct may need tightening in follow-up. Oral antibiotics are used to treat pin tract infections.[26] Patients and their families are instructed in pin care. Patients may shower with the external fixator, which encourages skin hygiene, but are discouraged from submerging the extremity in a bath. When patients can weight bear convincingly, the montage can be gradually disassembled. It is prudent to apply either a cast or a brace when the frame is finally removed.

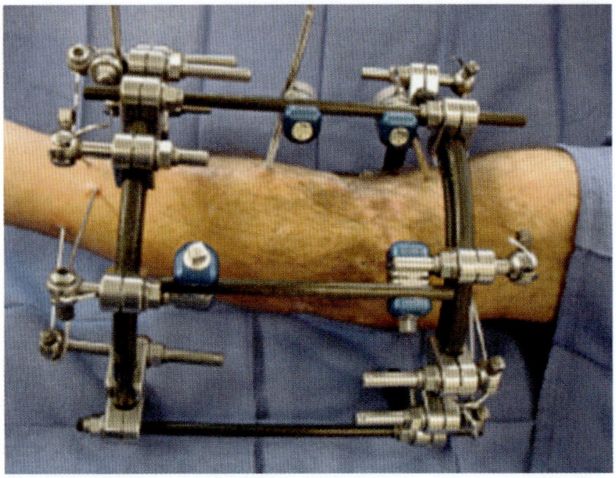

Fig. 4.11 Ring fixator.

COMPLICATIONS

Complications of proximal tibia external fixators include loss of fixation, pin tract infection, deep infections, nonunion, malunion, septic arthritis, arthrofibrosis, quadriceps atrophy, and posttraumatic arthrosis.[3]

Pin-tract infection is the major complication of external fixation: its incidence can range from 0.5% to 66%.[27,28,29] The incidence of pin-tract infections with the use of ring fixators has been reported as 3.9%, 12.9% for unilateral external fixators, and 20% for hybrid fixators.[30] Pin-tract infections are defined as signs and symptoms of infection around pins or wires that require a change in antibiotics, removal of pins or wires, or surgical debridement.[3] Although there is a pin tract grading system, it is more practical to think in terms of superficial and deep infections. Superficial infections are treated with local pin care, antibiotics, and if needed removal of the infected pin and debridement. Deep infections are treated similarly but may need overdrilling of the bone or even removal of the external fixator. The incidence of osteomyelitis after external fixation has been historically reported to be around 4%; more recent studies report an incidence of 0.4%.[31]

Septic knee has been reported after placement of tensioned wires and half-pins in the proximal tibia. Hutson and Zych reported an incidence of 2%.[30] With changes in technique based on anatomic studies defining a distance to avoid capsular reflections, Hutson et al. in a more recent study reported an incidence of 0.8%.[1,22,9] In the anterior plateau, 6 to 14 mm is considered safe. In our experience, the capsule is severely damaged with complex tibial plateau fractures; however, it is prudent to adhere to the described distance for pin placement. Whether or not the capsular reflections are disrupted, the key is to have a high index of suspicion when there is concern for a septic joint and prompt diagnosis and treatment implemented. Treatment for septic arthritis would be arthrotomy, specimen for culture, irrigation, and appropriate antibiotics.

Fracture malunion is more common with external fixation compared with locked plating for Schatzker type V and VI fractures. Krupp et al. reported a malunion rate of 14% in the locked plating group versus 43% in the external fixation group, with the main cause of malunion being a loss of articular reduction.[17]

Loss of knee motion is common after tibial plateau fractures and results from arthrofibrosis, as well as posttraumatic arthrosis. Extensor mechanism scarring is associated with prolonged knee spanning fixation. The Canadian Orthopedic Trauma Society study demonstrated superior arc of motion after treatment with a ring external fixator compared to open reduction and internal fixation.[32] In contrast, Bertrand et al. found no statistically significant difference in knee range of motion between the open reduction and internal fixation group and the external fixation group.[33] The goal of knee motion is 90 degrees of flexion at 4 weeks postoperatively. If motion is less than 90 degrees after 4 weeks, then an accelerated rehabilitation program may be warranted. Quadriceps weakness and atrophy are often the cause of the poor progress and may be associated with half-pin insertion through the quadriceps muscle.

Posttraumatic arthrosis after tibial plateau fractures was reported as 10.5% by Katsenis et al. in a 5-year follow-up.[34] Multiple studies have shown that articular incongruity and joint damage are the main causes of posttraumatic arthrosis. Occult meniscus tears are another cause of poor joint function. Although the initial articular reduction was appropriate in many cases in their study, significant articular damage may have occurred at the time of injury, leading to posttraumatic arthrosis.

CONCLUSION

External fixators have a significant role in the treatment of tibial plateau and proximal tibia fractures, especially high-energy Schatzker type V and VI fractures and some Schatzker type IV fractures with soft-tissue compromise. External fixators can be used as a temporary stopgap measure or as the definitive fixation when patient comorbidities, bony injury, and soft-tissue damage are all taken into account. With a larger number of the population who have renal disease, diabetes mellitus, and peripheral vascular disease sustaining these devastating injuries, the likelihood of a bad outcome with a large dissection to perform dual plating is sometimes inevitable. Although radiographically the fracture reduction and fixation may be noteworthy, the final outcome may not be if the patient ends up with a knee fusion or above-the-knee amputation.

Fine-wire circular external fixators and their hybrid counterpart may have a larger role to play in Schatzker type V and VI fractures in the future as our techniques, equipment, and knowledge improve. While the fine-wire frame may be time-consuming to construct, it does allow for continued correction as the patient heals, whereas internal fixation does not. It does take vigilance to monitor for infection, but with the external wires the patient and family can assist.

When a definitive treatment with a fine-wire frame is selected, the surgeon needs to ensure that the rings are symmetric and the pins are in the proper location for the best stability. Fine wires have a lower incidence of pin tract infection (3.9% vs 12%). Temporary or definitive external fixators are a powerful tool in the traumatologist's toolbox for the treatment of tibial plateau and proximal tibia fractures.

CASE 4.1

A 47-year-old female involved in a motor vehicle collision (MVC) with multiple fractures including a closed right knee injury (Fig. 4.12). The patient was hemodynamically unstable and intubated on arrival in the trauma bay. Severe displacement of the tibial plateau was causing pressure on the overlying skin. The patient was taken to the operating room for reduction with the use of a percutaneous "joystick" (Fig. 4.13) and temporary external fixation (Fig. 4.14) providing stabilization and allowing soft-tissue healing prior to definitive fixation (Fig. 4.15).

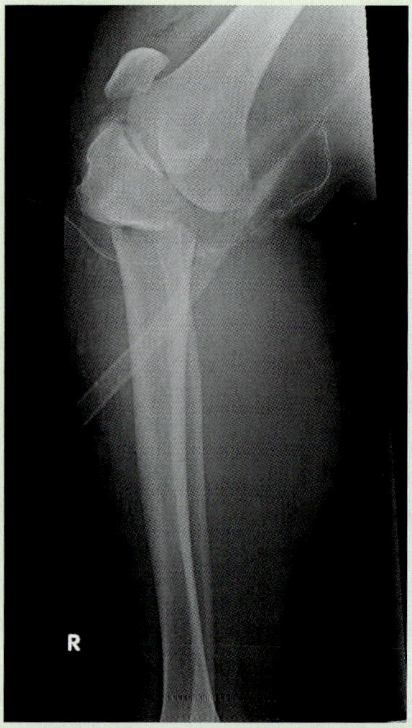

Fig. 4.12 X-ray at initial presentation demonstrating displaced tibial plateau fracture.

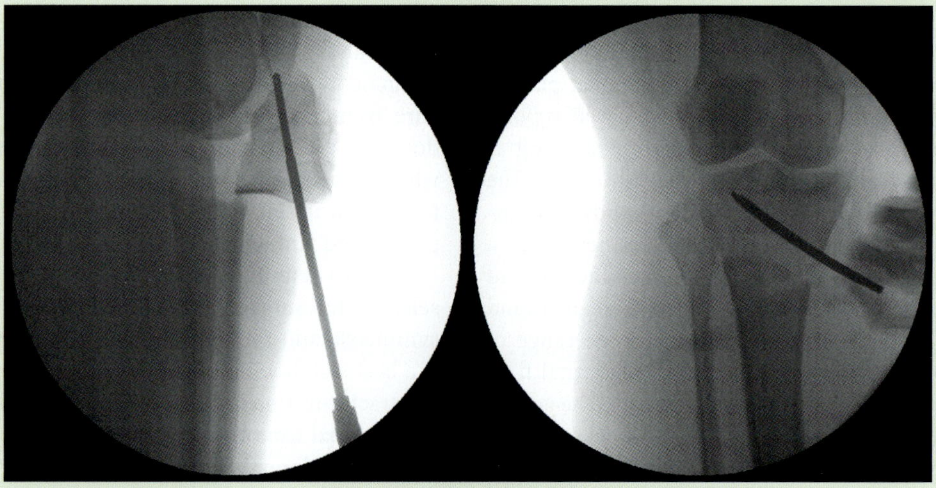

Fig. 4.13 Pin-assisted closed reduction of displaced tibial plateau fracture.

CASE 4.1—CONT'D

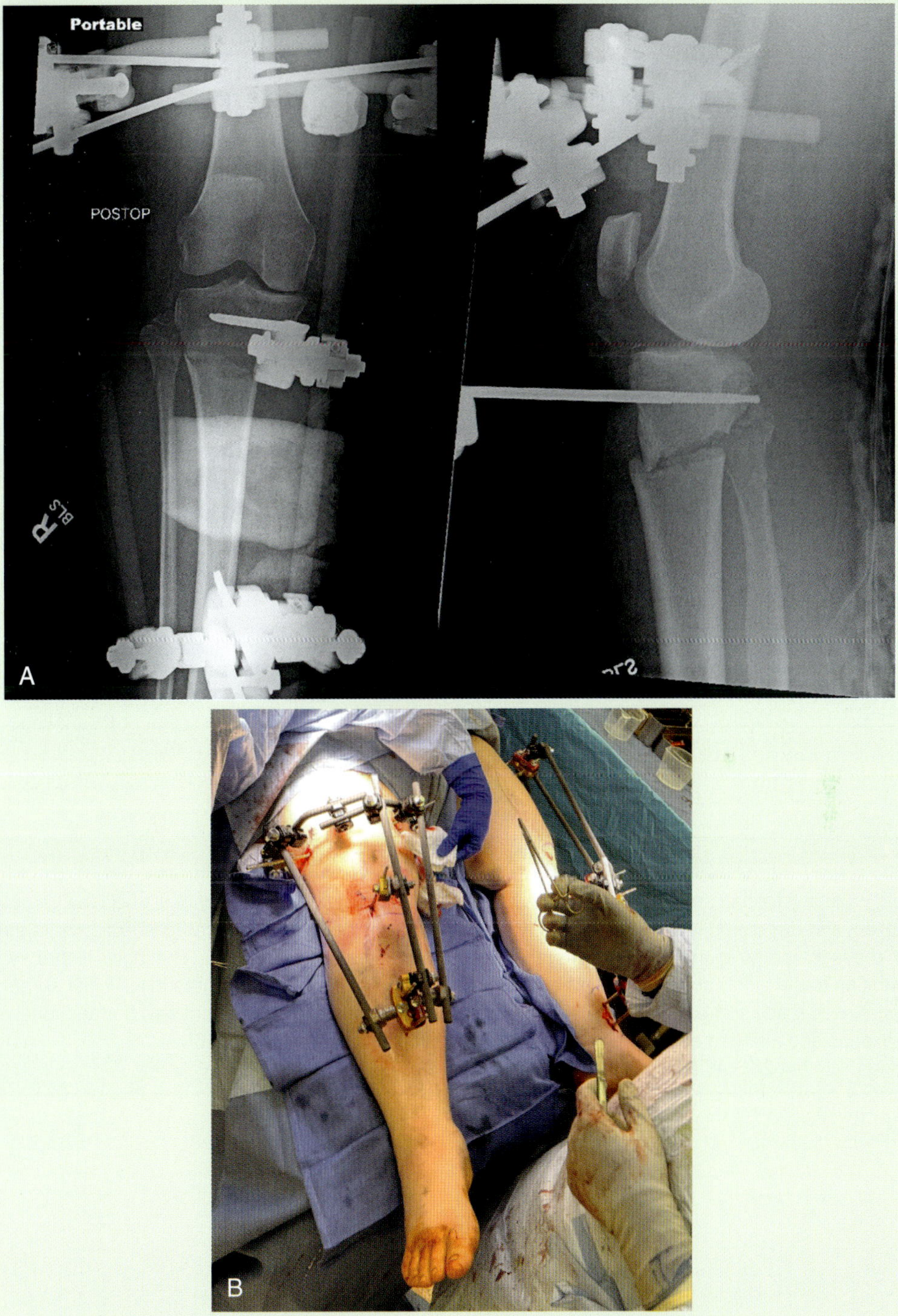

Fig. 4.14 Postoperative x-rays (A and B) and clinical photograph of large pin knee spanning frame.

Continued

CASE 4.1—CONT'D

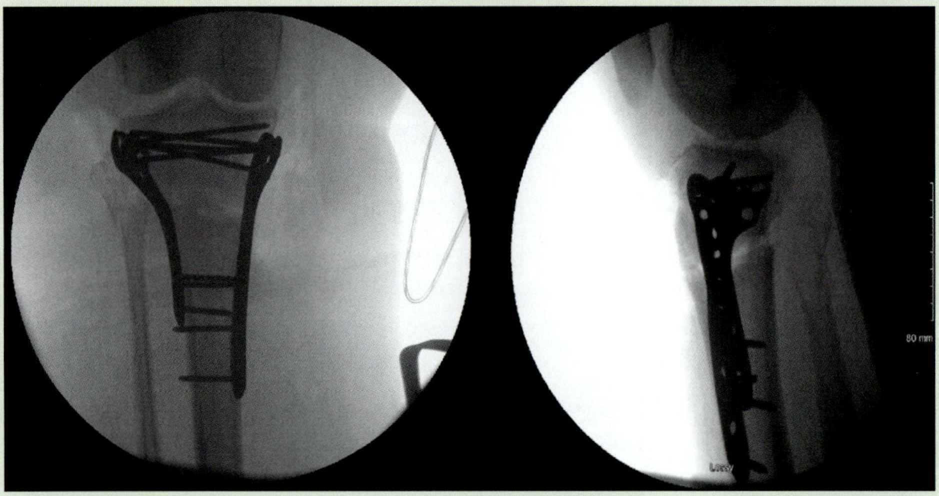

Fig. 4.15 Anteroposterior and lateral views showing definitive fixation with bicolumnar plating.

CASE 4.2

A 42-year-old male involved in an MVC presented with a painful, swollen, and discolored left lower extremity (Fig. 4.16). Given the high-energy injury compromising the soft tissues in addition to the highly comminuted articular fracture, a decision was made to treat definitively with limited internal fixation and a ringed external fixator spanning the knee (Figs. 4.17–4.24). At approximately 6 weeks postoperatively, the femoral ring was removed and full weight bearing as tolerated and active range of motion were begun (Fig. 4.25). The tibial fixator was removed at approximately 3 months after initial surgery, and at 1-year follow-up, the patient had no functional deficits with healed fracture (Fig. 4.26).

CASE 4.2—CONT'D

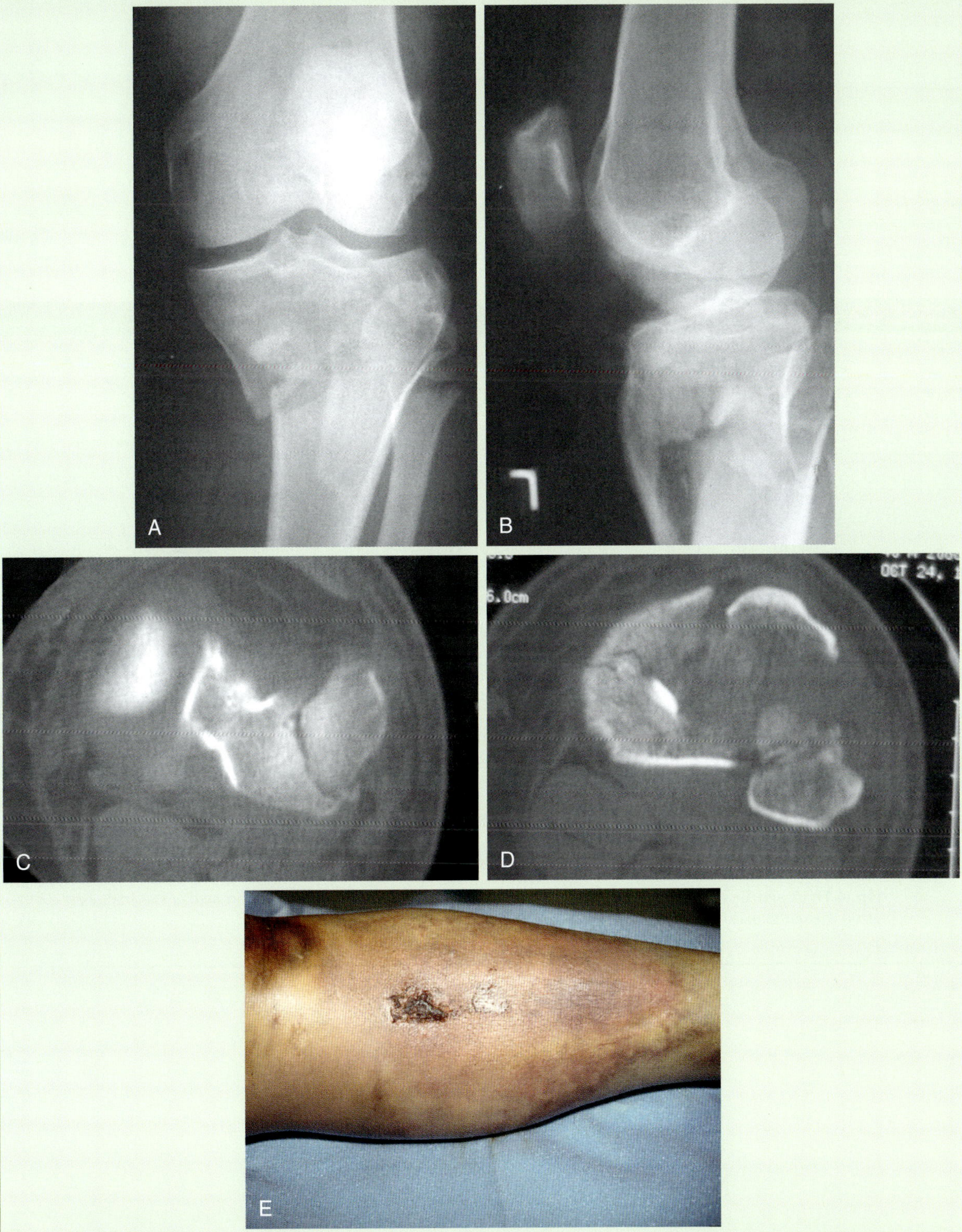

Fig. 4.16 Closed C3 bicondylar tibia plateau adult male. (A and B) Anterior posterior and lateral x-ray. (C and D) CT joint surface. (E) Discolored extremity with swelling.

Continued

CASE 4.2—CONT'D

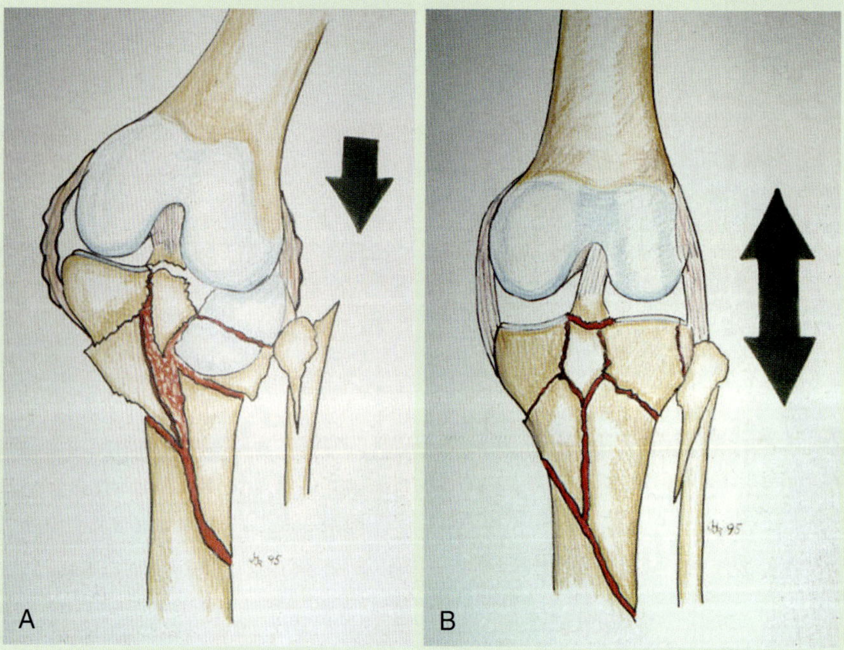

Fig. 4.17 (A and B) The basic reduction alignment is obtained initially with distraction across the fracture using ligamentotaxis.

CASE 4.2—CONT'D

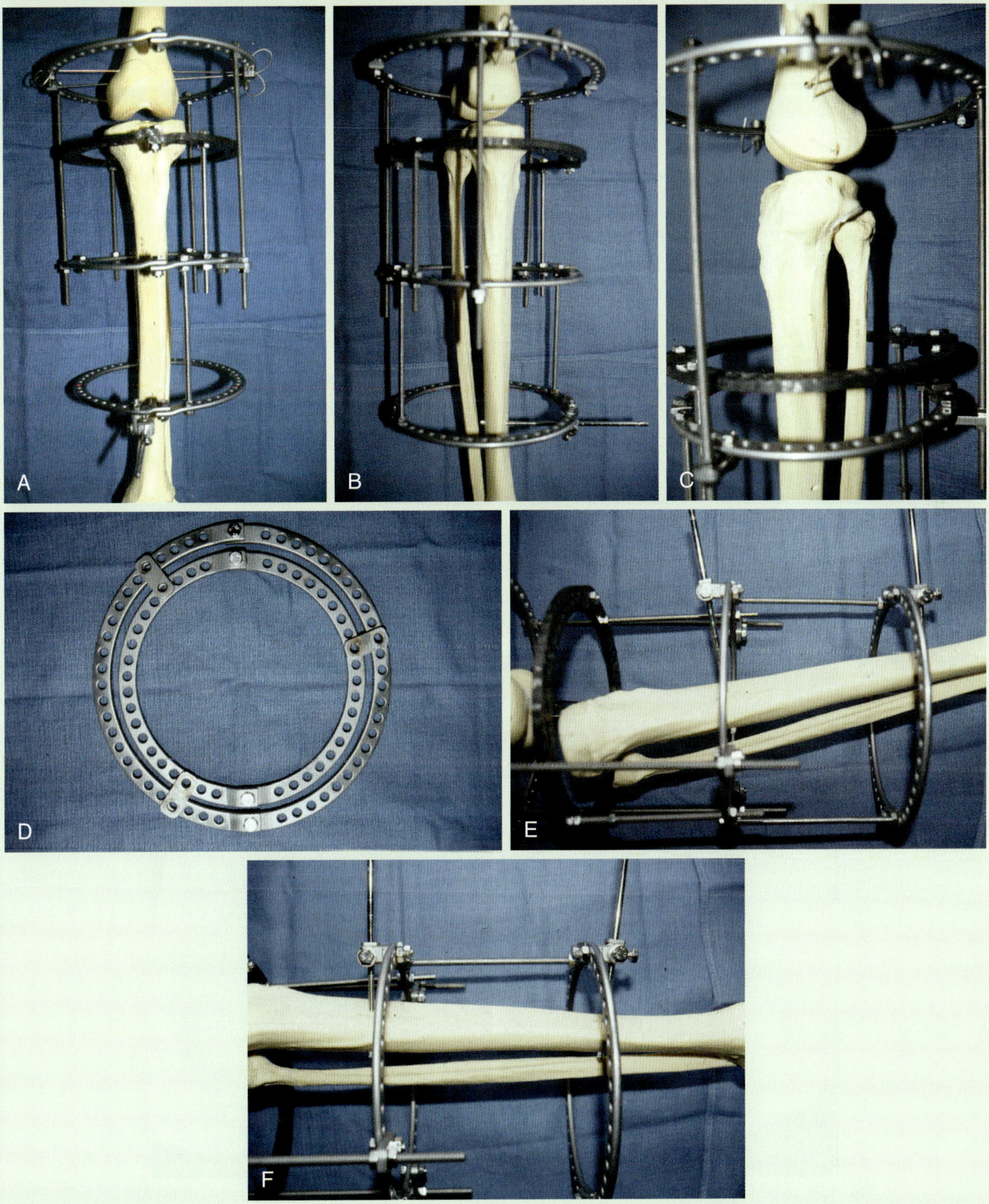

Fig. 4.18 (A) Anterior fixator model consisting of two ring fixation block on tibia shaft, femoral ring distraction through femoral condyles, and fracture fixation ring on the proximal tibial metaphysis. (B) The distal ring is fixated to the tibia shaft in the AP plane with a universal rancho cube. Two opposed olive wires in the femoral condyles and initial traction is placed across fracture. (C) The tibia plateau ring is initially dropped down on the two ring fixation block to allow access to the joint fracture. (D) The mid tibia ring has an accessory femoral ring attached with two hole plates. The fracture is first distracted between the tibia shaft fixation block and the femoral ring. (E and F) The shaft is then aligned orthogonal in the to the two ring fixation block.

CASE 4.2—CONT'D

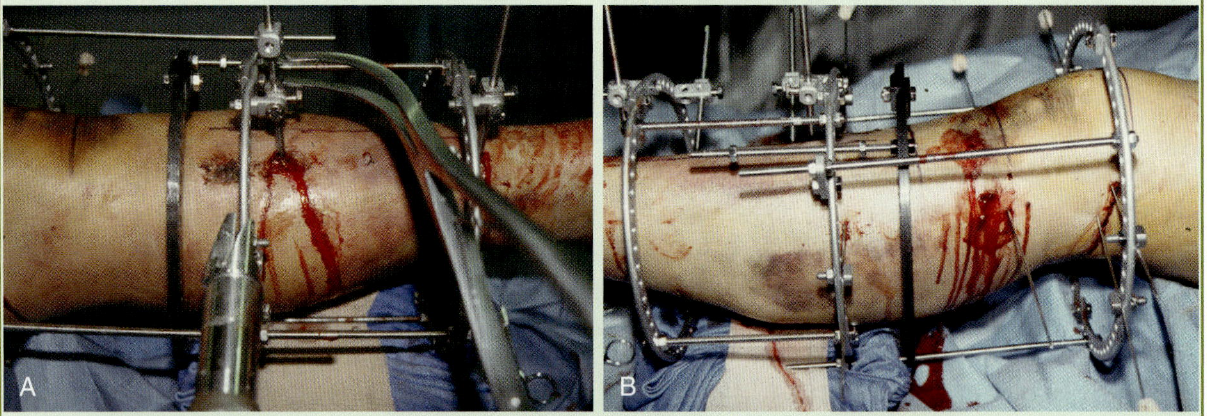

Fig. 4.19 (A, B) Clinical photograph of shaft alignment using AP half pin on universal Rancho Cube with draw wire technique combined with laminar spreader elevation technique. Notice proximal fracture carbon fiber ring position inferior in frame to provide access to plateau fracture. (B) Shaft aligned orthogonal to frame.

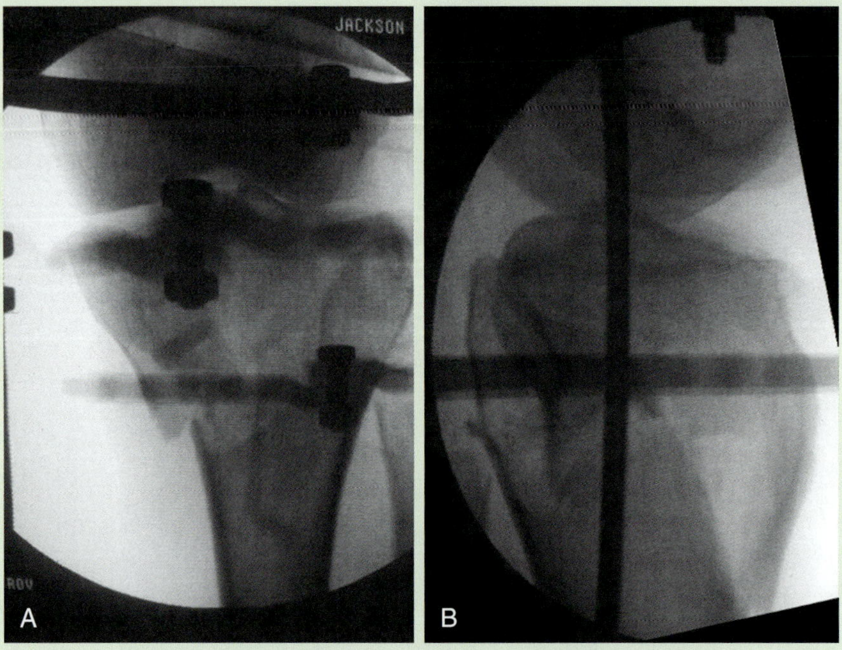

Fig. 4.20 (A and B) Plateau fracture before distraction applied across femoral condyles to tibia shaft.

CASE 4.2—CONT'D

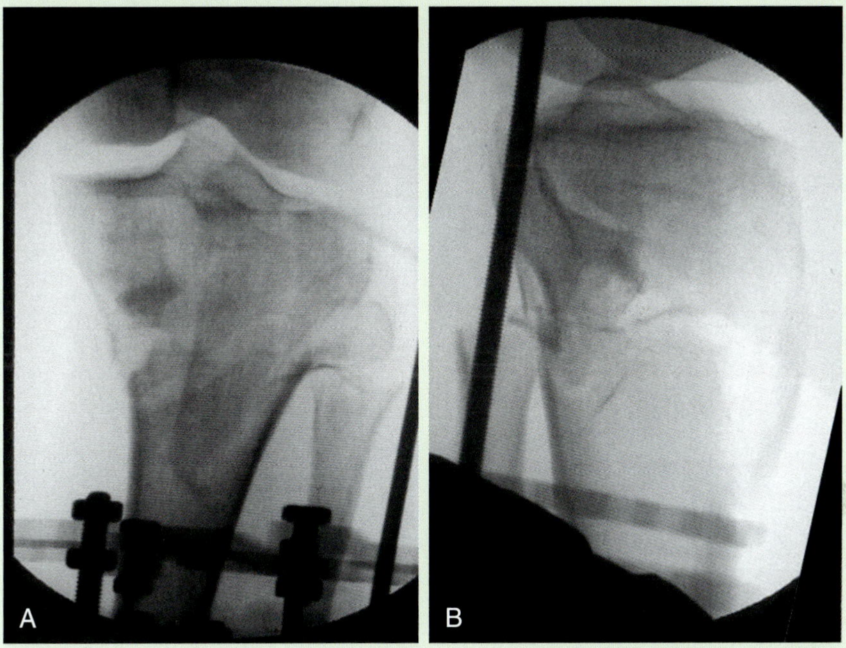

Fig. 4.21 (A and B) Reduction of plateau fracture to anatomic length from ligamentotaxis.

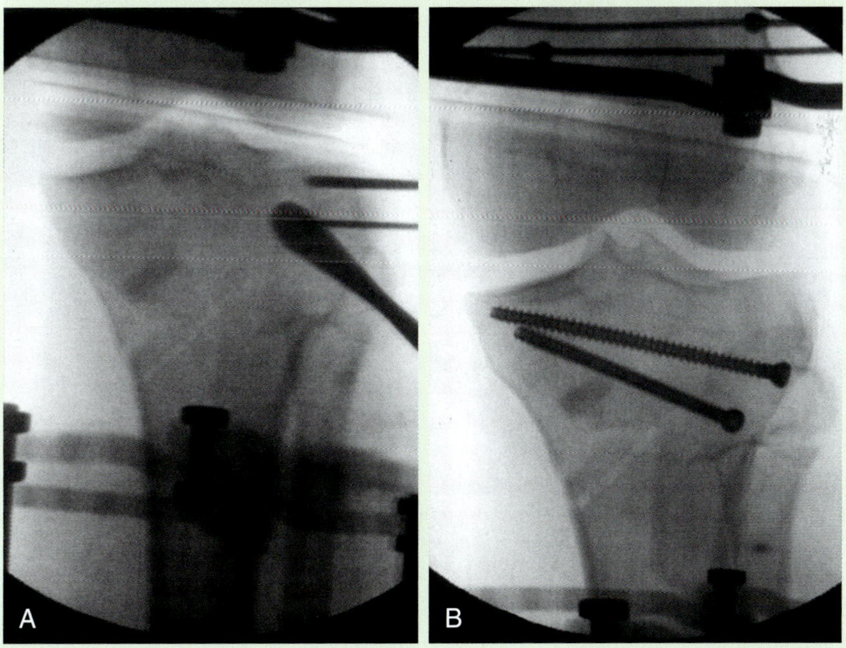

Fig. 4.22 (A and B) Percutaneous reduction of plateau fragments and limited internal fixation.

Continued

CASE 4.2—CONT'D

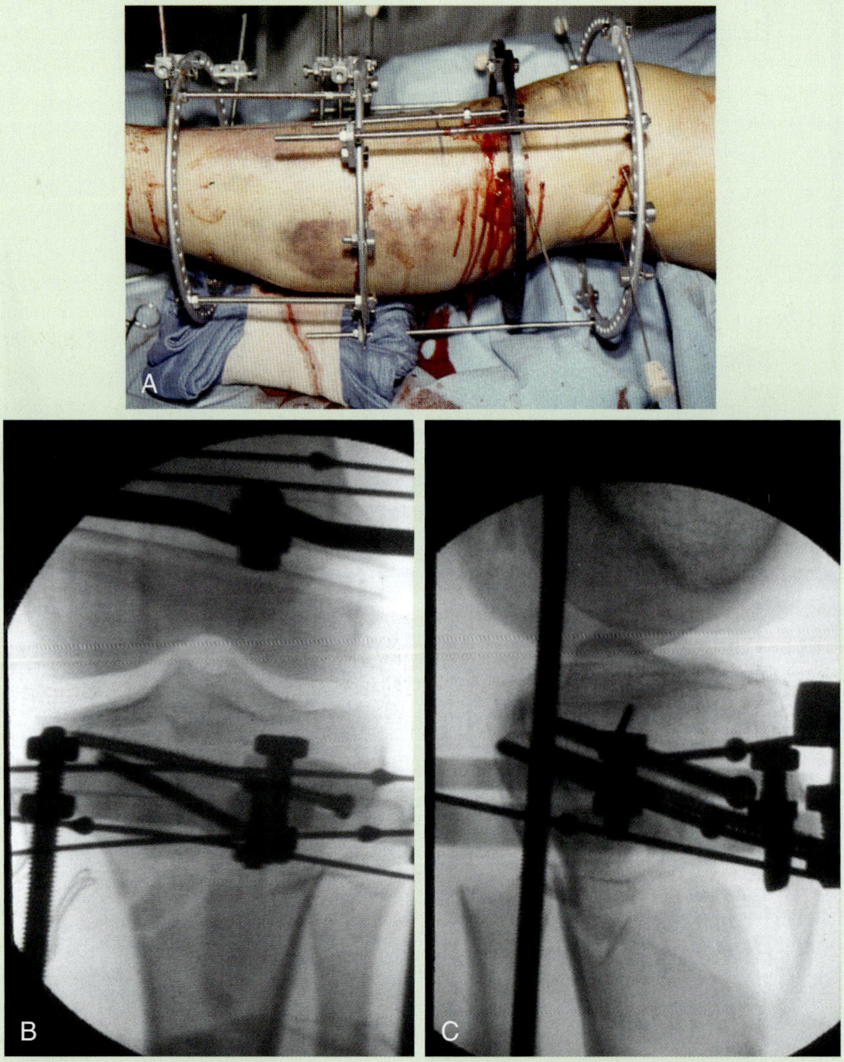

Fig. 4.23 (A–C) The carbon fiber fracture fixation ring is elevated to the metaphysis aligned on the horizontal reference wire. (B, C) Two additional opposed olive wires are added to the fracture fixation ring.

CASE 4.2—CONT'D

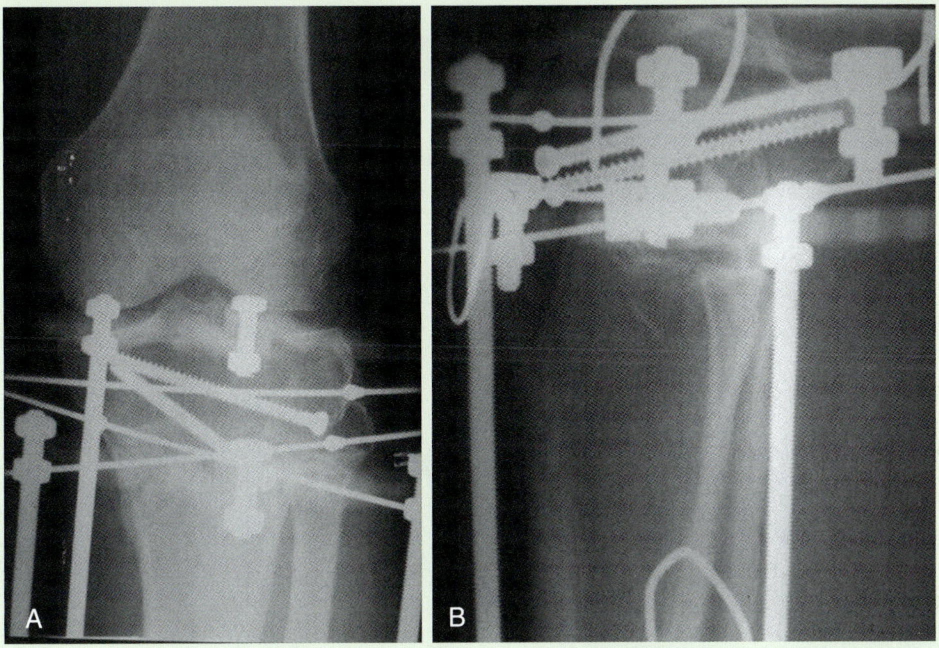

Fig. 4.24 (A and B) Four to six weeks post operatively the femoral ring is removed in clinic advancing to weight bearing as tolerated and active range of motion of the knee.

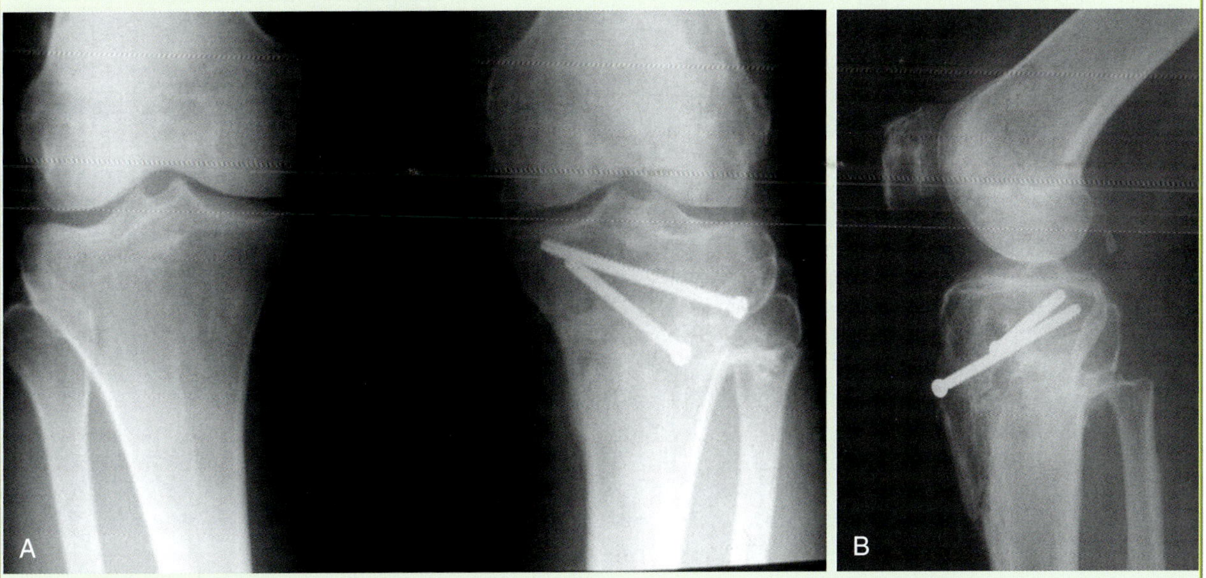

Fig. 4.25 (A and B) The Ilizarov fixator was removed 12-16 weeks post surgery. AP and lateral x-rays show mature healing of fracture one year post injury.

Continued

CASE 4.2—CONT'D

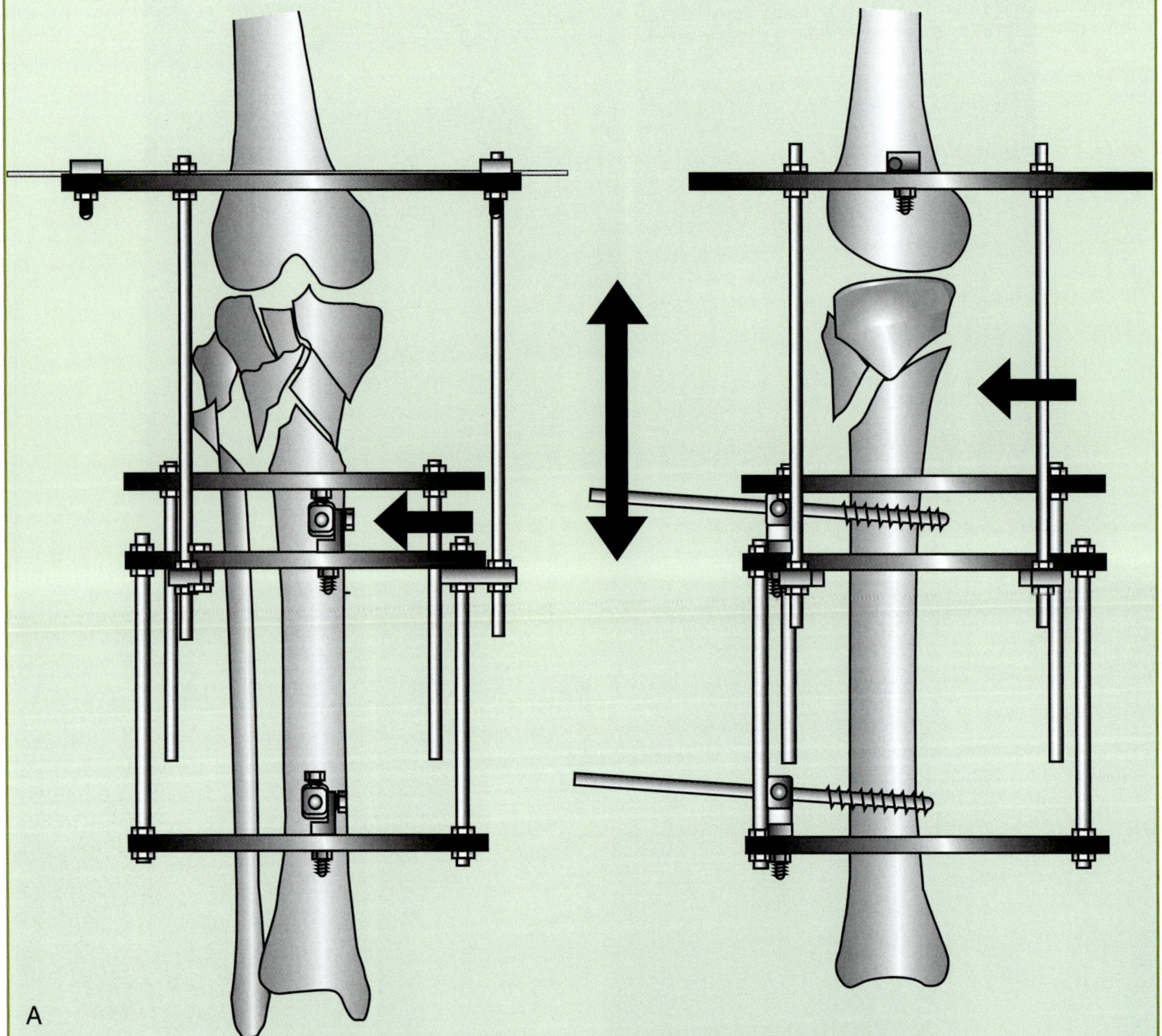

Fig. 4.26 Technical drawing technique. (A) Two ring fixation block and femoral fixation before distraction.

CASE 4.2—CONT'D

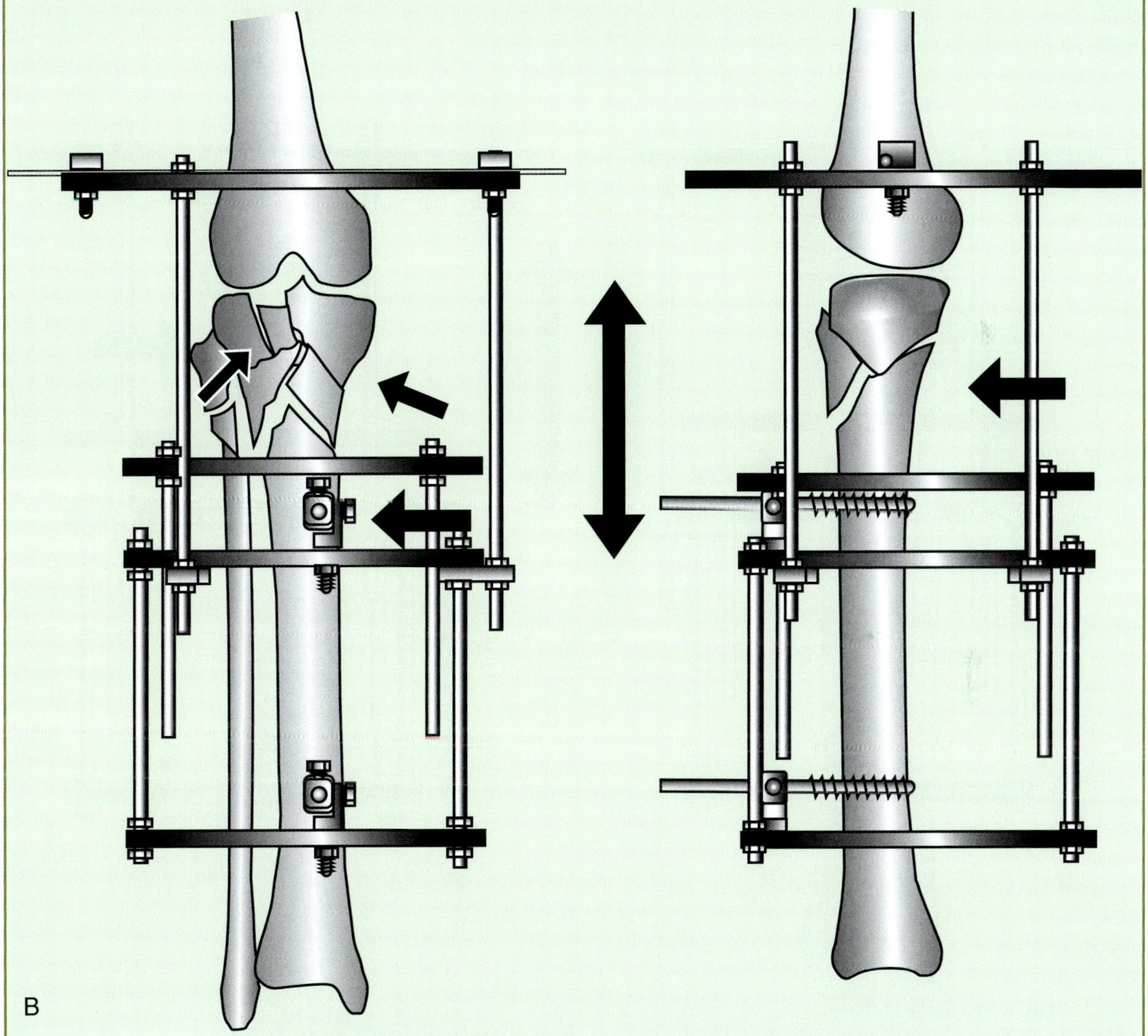

Fig. 4.26 cont'd (B) Fracture reduction by ligamentotaxis.

Continued

CASE 4.2—CONT'D

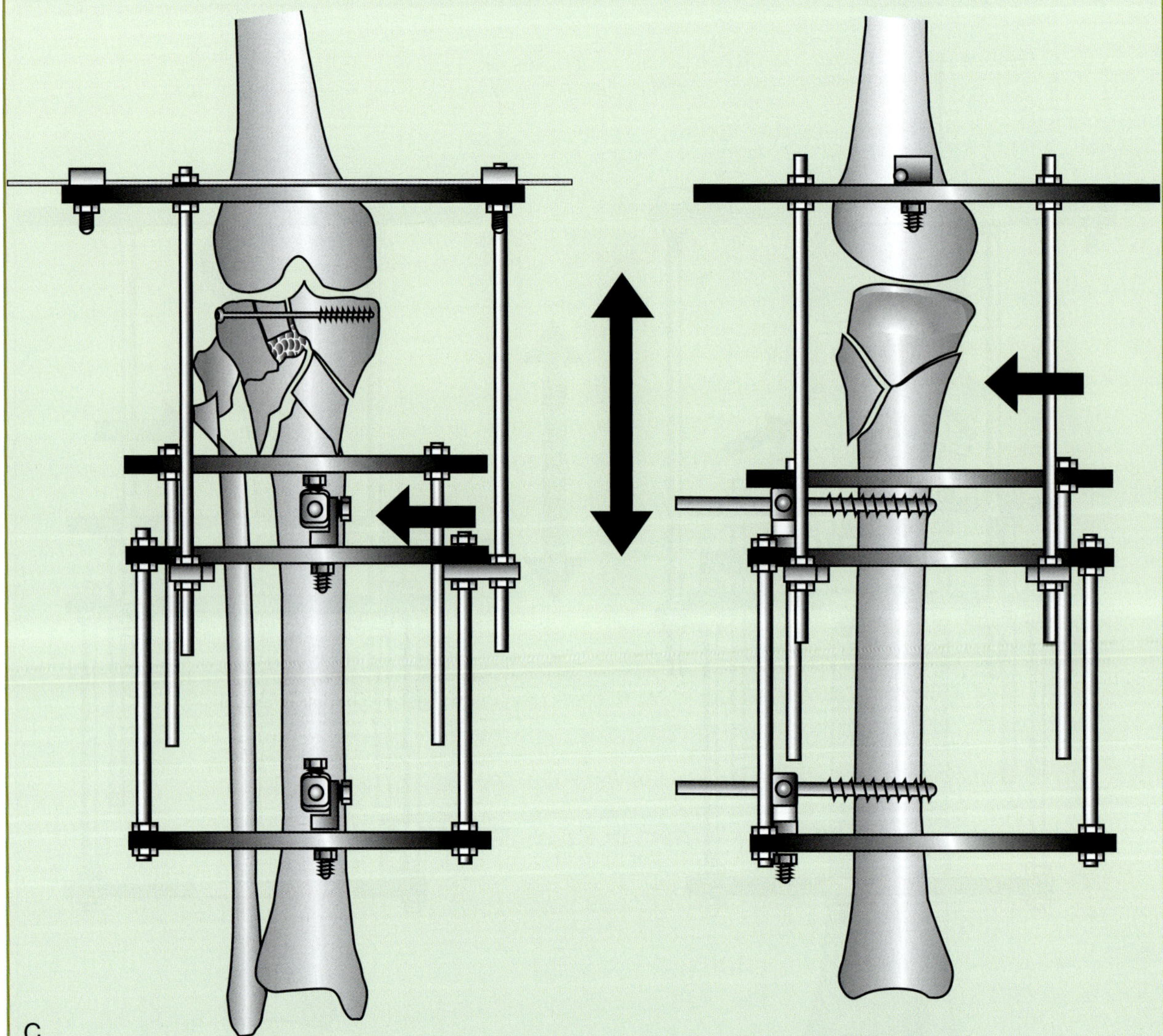

C

Fig. 4.26 cont'd (C) Limited internal fixation of joint surface. The joint can be reduced with percutaneous technique or limited open technique. The drawing shows a cancellous allograft support of joint.

CASE 4.2—CONT'D

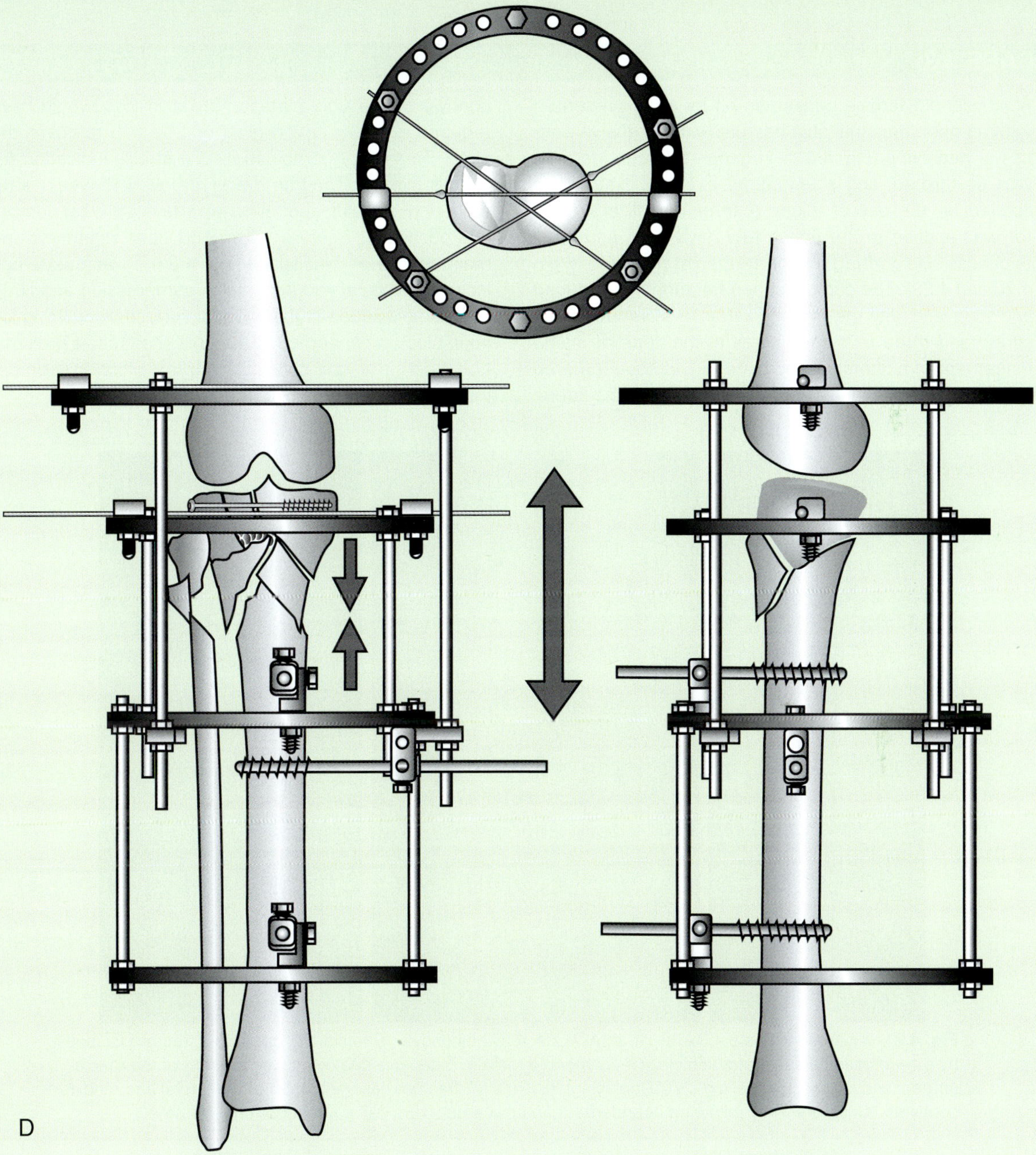

Fig. 4.26 cont'd (D) Elevation of fracture ring to support metaphysis reduction.

(Courtesy Dr. Hutson JJ Jr, MD, Professor Clinical Orthopedic Trauma Service, Ryder Trauma Center University of Miami Medical School, Miami, FL)

CASE 4.3

A 73-year-old female pedestrian hit by a car presented with an open proximal tibia fracture with extensive soft-tissue degloving (Fig. 4.27). Irrigation and debridement was performed, and a temporary external fixator was applied on the day of injury. A three-ring Ilizarov fixator was applied to the tibia a few days later, and split-thickness skin grafting was performed at that time (Figs. 4.28 and 4.29). The complex open fracture was reduced and stabilized with the limited fixation of a percutaneous screw and three tensioned wires in the zone of injury. Placement of a lateral locked plate would have required further soft-tissue injury to place the plate on the lateral condyle of the tibia plateau. The skin loss would have required a local rotation graft or free flap to cover the plate. This injury combination is a strong indication for circular fixation. The frame was removed 15 weeks after surgery (Fig. 4.30), and follow-up x-rays at 1 year demonstrated healed fracture with good tibial alignment and maintenance of joint space (Fig. 4.31). Fixation strategy includes articular reduction with compression and limited internal fixation at the articular surface. A two-ring fixation block is connected to the tibia shaft, and a proximal tibia fracture ring is connected to the articular segment with tensioned wires (Fig. 4.32).

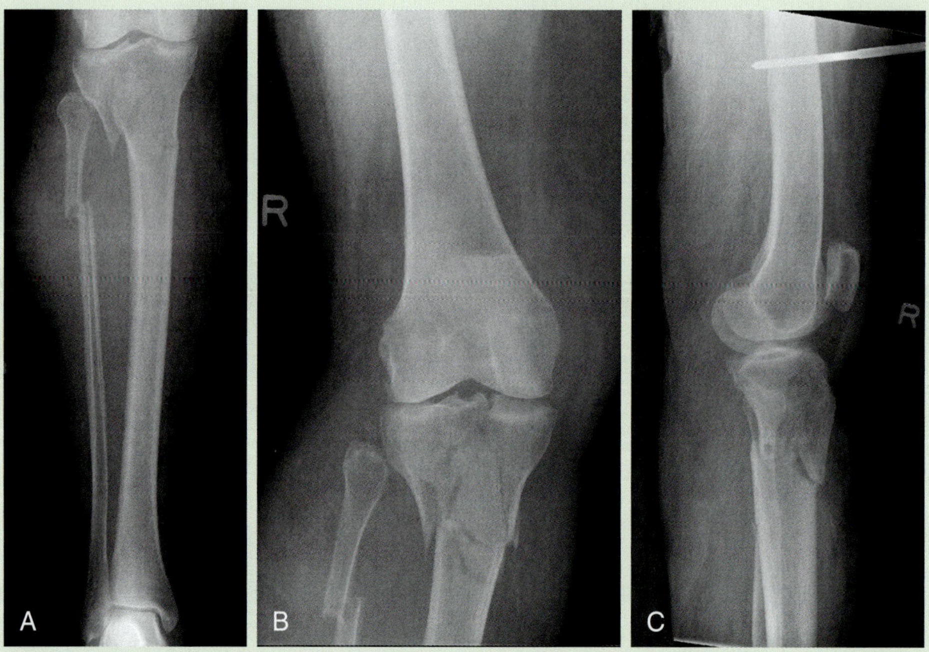

Fig. 4.27 (A) Anterior Posterior x-ray of an AO/OTA 41C2 bicondylar Gustillo IIIA open tibia fracture caused by a pedestrian versus motor vehicle in a 73 year old female. Extensive degloving was present of the medial, anterior and lateral proximal leg (270°Degloving). (B) This C2 fracture has separation of the lateral and medial condyles. (C) Lateral x-ray following debridement and placement of a half pin anterior bridge frame.

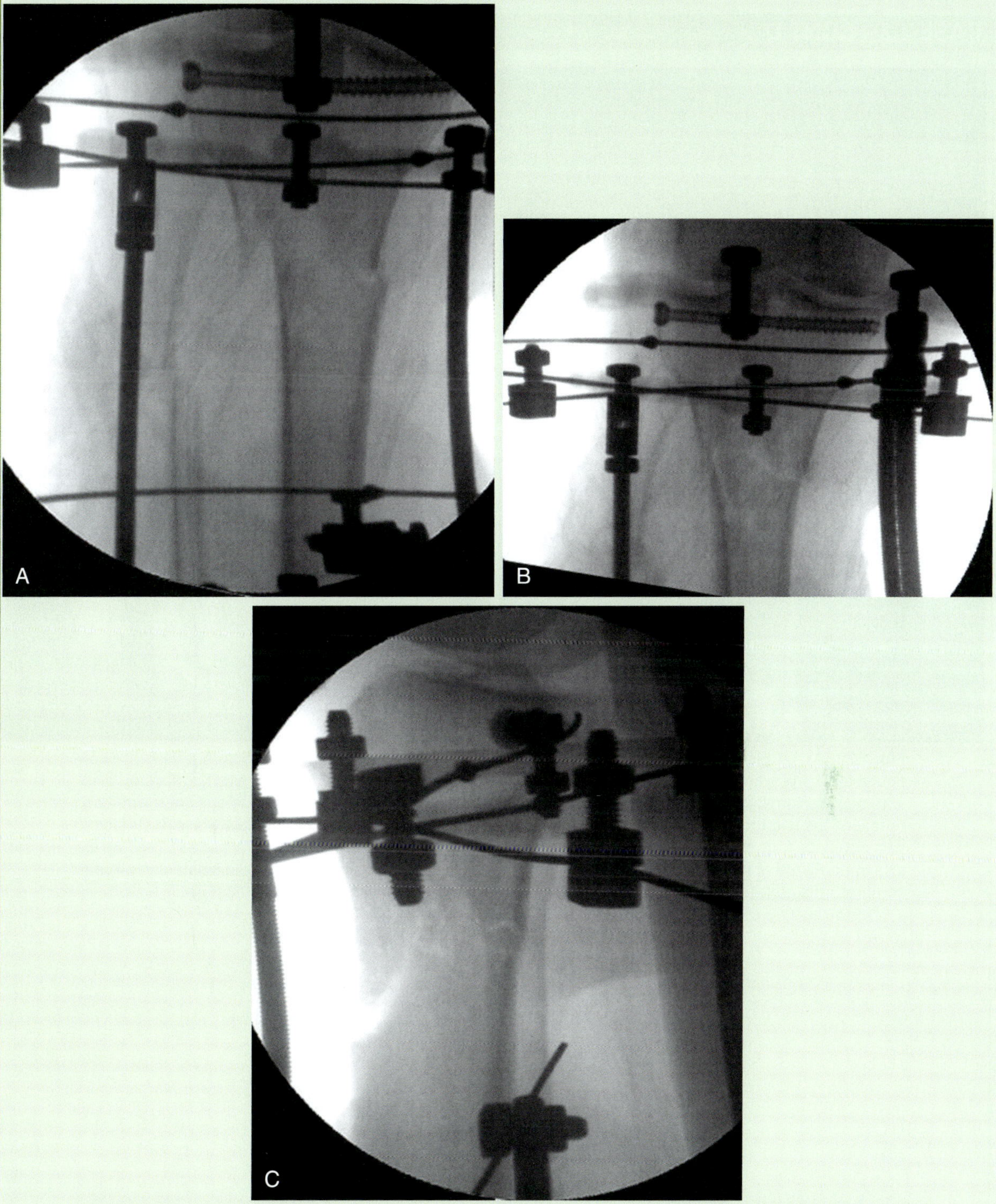

Fig. 4.28 (A) The plateau condyles are reduced with a 5.5 mm lateral to medial subcondylar lag screw and a three ring Ilizarov fixator applied to the tibia. The frame consists of a proximal tibia fracture ring and a mid-tibia two ring fixation block connected with anterior half pin on universal Rancho cube. (B) A mid tibial draw wire is manipulated to align the tibia shaft with the proximal reconstructed tibia metaphysis. (C) Three opposed tensioned wires stabilize fracture in alignment with shaft. Following the reduction and fixation a 175 sq cm meshed skin graft was placed over the proximal wound.

CASE 4.3—CONT'D

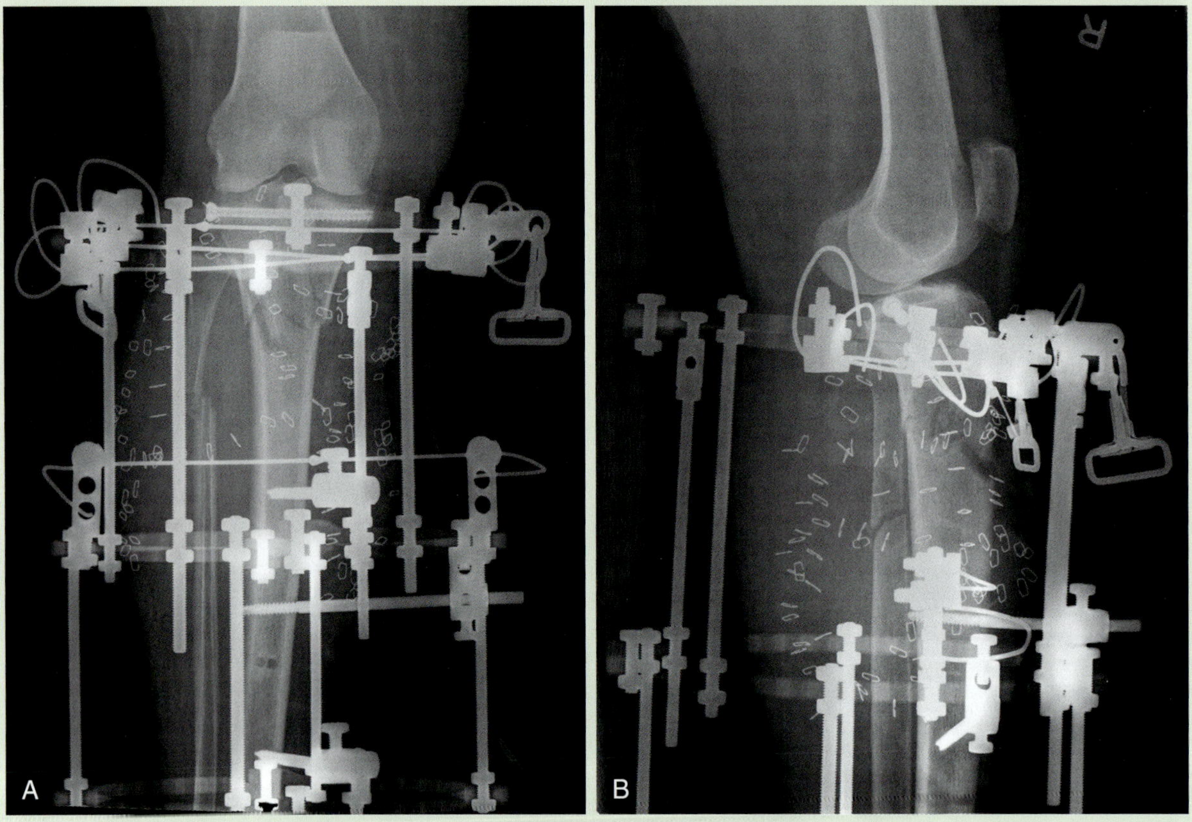

Fig. 4.29 (A) Anterior posterior x-ray of tibia plateau fracture following reduction of fracture. The frame configuration is a proximal fracture ring supported by four threaded rods connected to a two ring fixation block with two titanium hydroxyapatite AP half pins, a medial face half pin and the medial to lateral draw wire used to reduce the shaft to the condylar block. The condylar fixation screw is placed just below the joint surface to gain clearance from the horizontal reference wire. The multiple staples seen on x-ray were used to secure the skin graft. Plenty of space exists to skin graft under the frame. The frame is used to hold bolsters in place to compress the graft to the wound base. (B) Lateral x-ray shows excellent alignment of fracture.

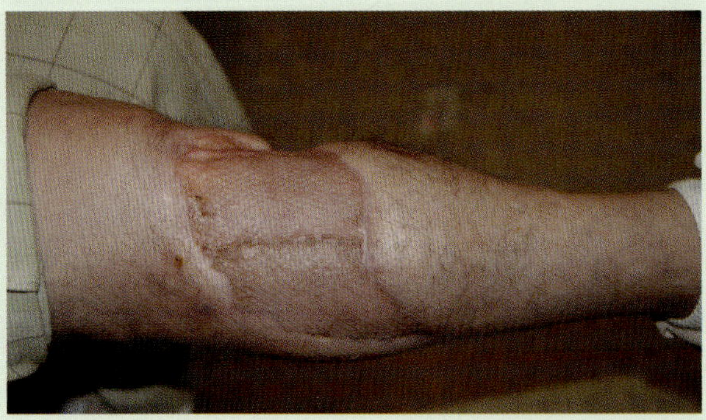

Fig. 4.30 The frame was removed under anesthesia 15 weeks following fixation. The healing pin and wire sites are observed. The patient was protected with hinged knee brace and started on 50% weight bearing. The healing skin grafts show the extent of the initial open injury.

CASE 4.3—CONT'D

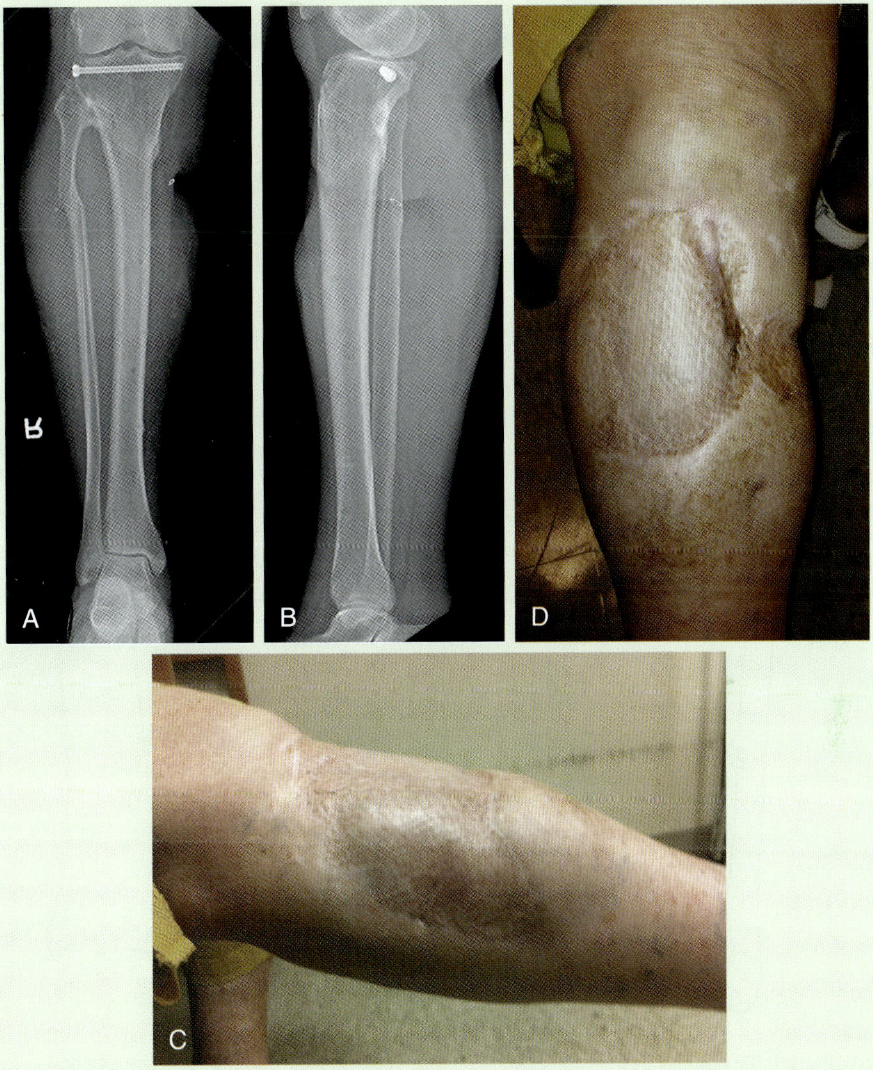

Fig. 4.31 (A and B) X-ray of tibia one year after injury with healed fracture. Notice the location of the condylar interfragmentary screw in the posterior condyle. (C and D) Clinical pictures of healed tibia fracture at one year.

Continued

CASE 4.3—CONT'D

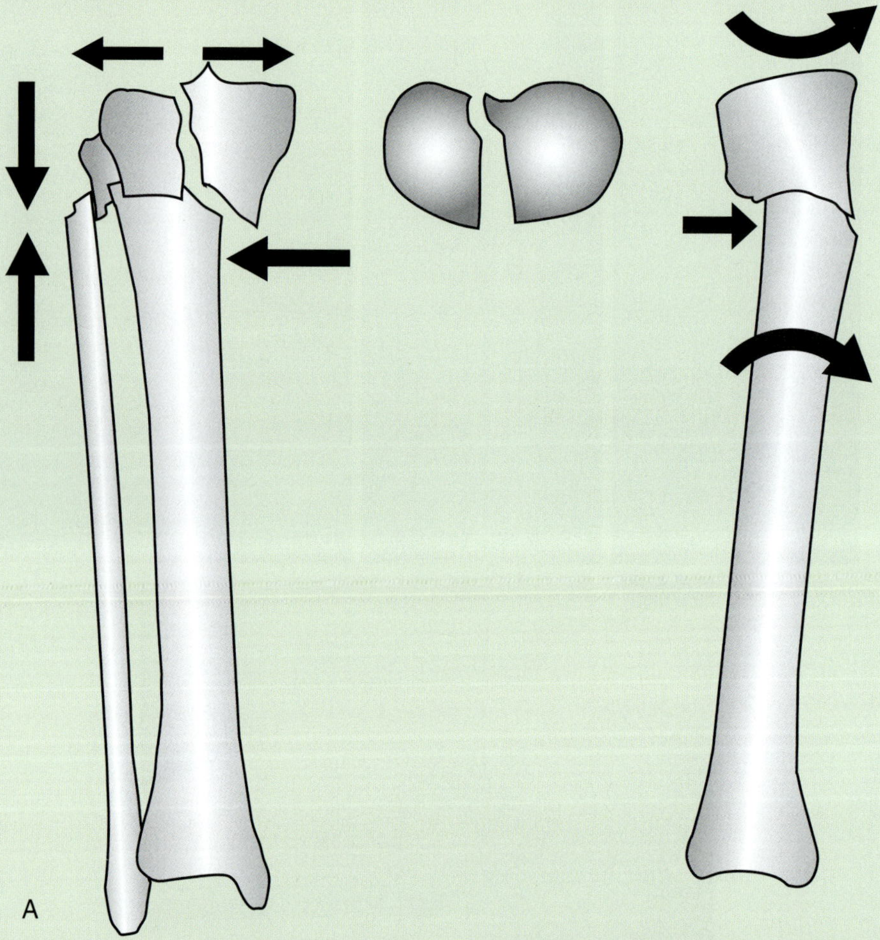

Fig. 4.32 Technique drawings. (A) C1-2 tibia plateau fractures have a split of the condyles and metaphyseal dissociation from the shaft with C2 having comminution at the metaphyseal-diaphyseal junction.

CASE 4.3—CONT'D

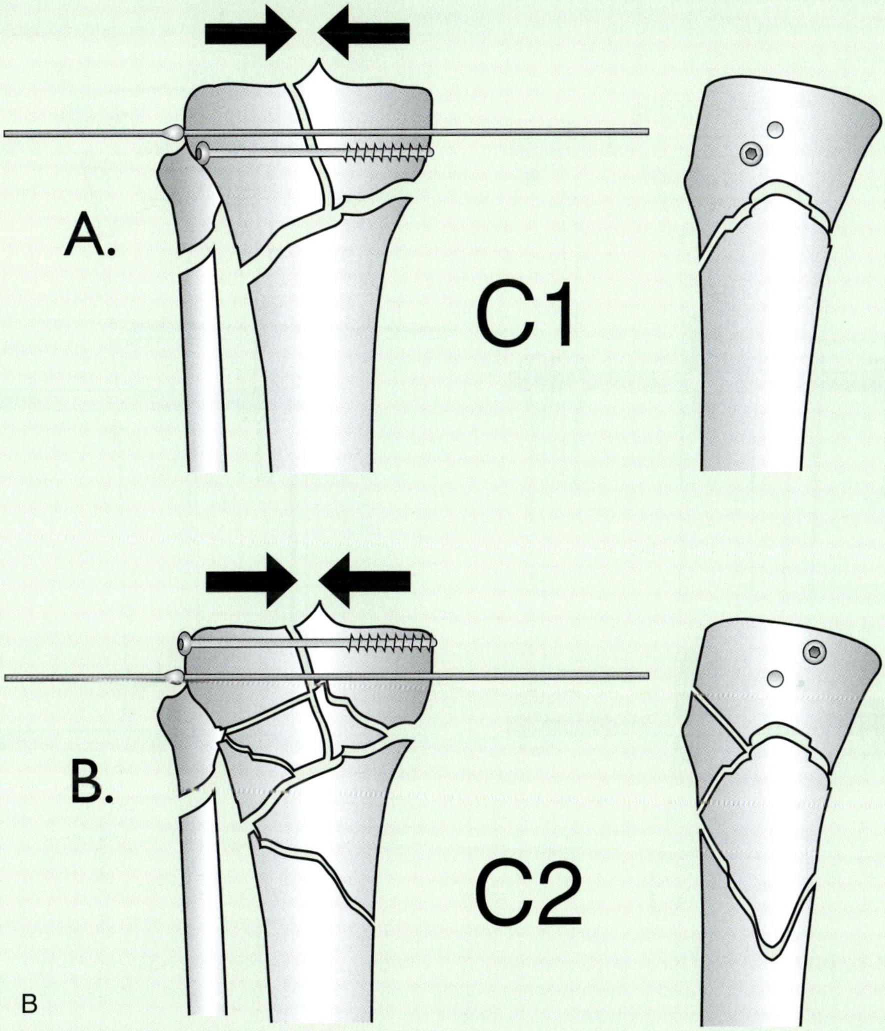

Fig. 4.32 cont'd (B) The condyles are reduced percutaneously with a large fracture reduction clamp and a 5.5mm cannulated screw placed across the fracture. Large C1 fragments can have a lag screw placed in mid condyles. C2 fractures should have a subchondral lag screw placed posteriorly in the condyles to provide clearance of the horizontal reference wire.

Continued

CASE 4.3—CONT'D

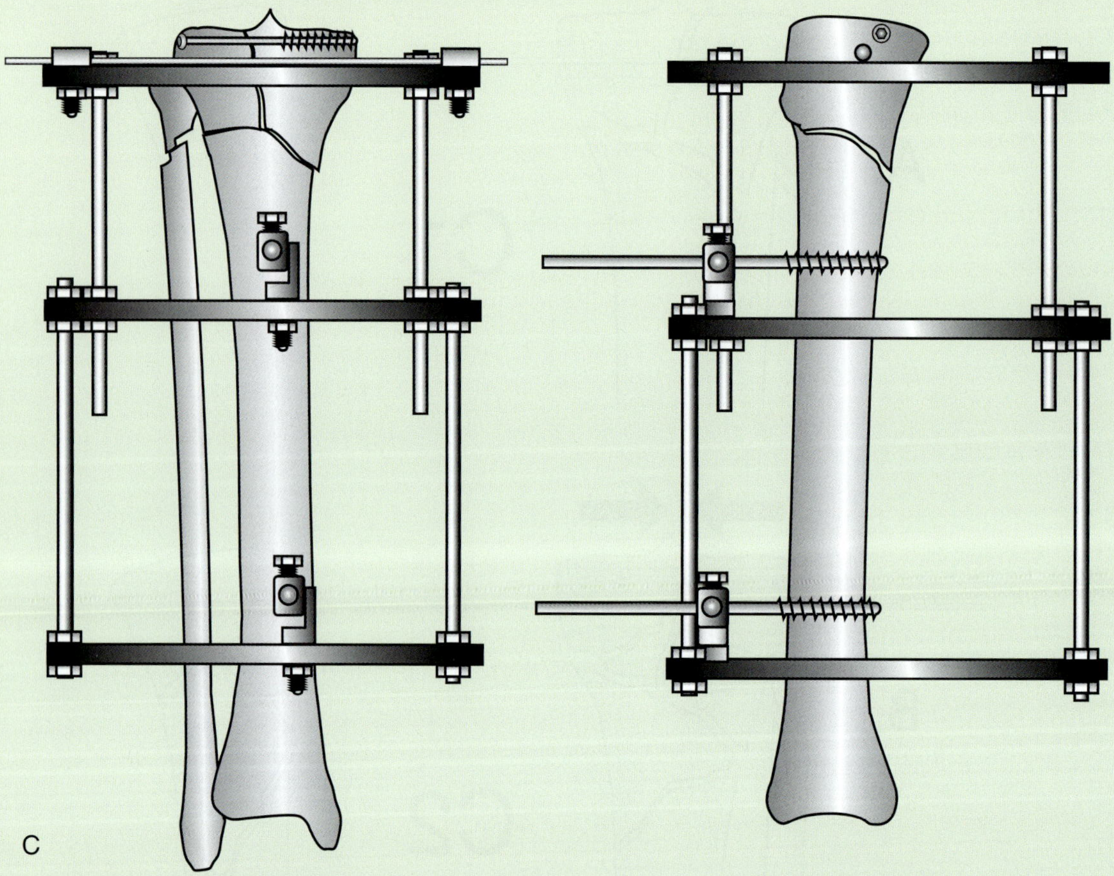

C

Fig. 4.32 cont'd (C) With the condyle reconstructed, a horizontal reference wire is placed 10-12mm below the joint. The shaft is reduced to the metaphysis using Ilizarov reduction techniques with three opposed tensioned wires in the plateau and a two ring fixation block on the shaft.

(Courtesy Dr. Hutson JJ Jr, MD, Professor Clinical Orthopedic Trauma Service, Ryder Trauma Center University of Miami Medical School, Miami, FL)

SELIGSON'S TIPS AND TRICKS

- Bolsters are used to elevate the thigh and lower leg to allow 360 degrees viewing and access to the operative limb.
- The proximal reference wire should be placed parallel to the proximal articular surface, 1 cm anterior to the midpoint of the tibia from lateral to medial.
- Crossed olive wires for a proximal ring are placed from posterior lateral and posterior medial at 60 degrees from the coronal plane and cross 1 cm posterior to the midpoint of the center of the proximal tibia.
- Construct stiffness is affected by transfixion wire spread, crossing angle, ring diameter, half-pin diameter, number of rings, and ring symmetry.
- When possible, effort should be made to place proximal pins ≥14 mm inferior to the proximal tibial joint line to avoid intra-articular pin placement.
- Half-pins placed at different angles can be used for distal ring fixation to the diaphysis.
- Three threaded rods are used to connect proximal and distal rings.

REFERENCES

1. DeCoster TA, Crawford MK, Kraut MAS. Safe extracapsular placement of proximal tibia transfixation pins. *J Orthop Trauma*. 1999;13(4):236–240.
2. Roberts CS, Dodds JC, Perry K, Beck D, Seligson D, Voor MJ. Hybrid external fixation of the proximal tibia: strategies to improve frame stability. *J Orthop Trauma*. 2003;17(6):415–420.
3. Seligson D, Mauffrey C, Roberts C. *External Fixation in Orthopedic Traumatology*. London: Springer; 2012:121–129.
4. Roberts CS, Antoci V, Antoci Jr V, Voor MJ. The effect of transfixion wire crossing angle on the stiffness of fine wire external fixation: a biomechanical study. *Injury*. 2005;36(9):1107–1112.
5. Antoci V, Raney EM, Antoci V, Voor MJ, Roberts CS. Transfixion wire positioning within the bone. *J Pediatr Orthop*. 2006;26(4):466–470.
6. Watson JT, Coufal C. Treatment of complex lateral plateau fractures using Ilizarov techniques. *Clin Orthop Relat Res*. 1998;353:97–106.
7. Geller J, Tornetta 3rd P, Tiburzi D, Kummer F, Koval K. Tension wire position for hybrid external fixation of the proximal tibia. *J Orthop Trauma*. 2000;14(7):502–504.
8. Sirkin MS, Bono CM, Reilly MC, Behrens FF. Percutaneous methods of tibial plateau fixation. *Clin Orthop Relat Res*. 2000;375:60–68.
9. Hutson Jr JJ. Chapter 2: safe wire and half pin placement in tibia fractures. *Tech Orthop*. 2002;17(1):5–11.
10. Watson MA, Mathias KJ, Maffulli N. External ring fixators: an overview. *Proc Inst Mech Eng H*. 2000;214(5):459–470.
11. Pugh KJ, Wolinsky PR, Dawson JM, Stahlman GC. The biomechanics of hybrid external fixation. *J Orthop Trauma*. 1999;13(1):20–26.
12. Pugh KJ, Wolinsky PR, Pienkowski D, Banit D, Dawson JM. Comparative biomechanics of hybrid external fixation. *J Orthop Trauma*. 1999;13(6):418–425.
13. Haidukewych GJ. Temporary external fixation for the management of complex intra- and periarticular fractures of the lower extremity. *J Orthop Trauma*. 2002;16(9):678–685.
14. Bible JE, Mir HR. External fixation: principles and applications. *J Am Acad Orthop Surg*. 2015;23(11):683–690.
15. Behrens F. A primer of fixator devices and configurations. *Clin Orthop Relat Res*. 1989;241:5–14.
16. Dendrinos GK, Kontos S, Katsenis D, Dalas A. Treatment of high-energy tibial plateau fractures by the Ilizarov circular fixator. *J Bone Joint Surg Br*. 1996;78(5):710–717.
17. Krupp RJ, Malkani AL, Roberts CS, Seligson D, Crawford 3rd CH, Smith L. Treatment of bicondylar tibia plateau fractures using locked plating versus external fixation. *Orthopedics*. 2009;32(8).
18. Debnath UK, Jha DK, Pujari PK. Results of ring (Ilizarov) fixator in high energy Schatzker type VI fractures of proximal tibia. *J Clin Orthop Trauma*. 2018;9(2):186–191.
19. Mikulak SA, Gold SM, Zinar DM. Small wire external fixation of high energy tibial plateau fractures. *Clin Orthop Relat Res*. 1998;356:230–238.
20. Keightley AJ, Nawaz SZ, Jacob JT, Unnithan A, Elliott DS, Khaleel A. Ilizarov management of Schatzker IV to VI fractures of the tibial plateau: 105 fractures at a mean follow-up of 7.8 years. *Bone Joint J*. 2015;97-B(12):1693–1697.
21. Egol KA, Tejwani NC, Capla EL, Wolinsky PL, Koval KJ. Staged management of high-energy proximal tibia fractures (OTA types 41): the results of a prospective, standardized protocol. *J Orthop Trauma*. 2005;19(7):448–456.
22. Hutson Jr JJ. The centered lateral fluoroscopic image of the knee: the key to safe tensioned wire placement in periarticular fractures of the proximal tibia. *J Orthop Trauma*. 2002;16(3):196–200.
23. Hall JA, Beuerlein MJ, McKee MD, Canadian Orthopaedic Trauma Society. Open reduction and internal fixation compared with circular fixator application for bicondylar tibial plateau fractures. Surgical technique. *J Bone Joint Surg Am*. 2009;91(suppl 2, pt 1):74–88.
24. Sales JG, Soleymaopour J, Ansari M, Afaghi F, Goldust M. Treatment results of bicondylar tibial fractures using hybrid external fixator. *Pak J Biol Sci*. 2013;16(10):491–495.

25. Bal GK, Kuo RS, Chapman JR, Henley MB, Benirschke SK, Claudi BF. The anterior T-frame external fixator for high-energy proximal tibial fractures. *Clin Orthop Relat Res*. 2000;380:234–240.
26. Kazmers NH, Fragomen AT, Rozbruch SR. Prevention of pin site infection in external fixation: a review of the literature. *Strategies Trauma Limb Reconstr*. 2016;11(2):75–85.
27. Chin TY, Bardana D, Bailey M, et al. Functional outcome of tibial plateau fractures treated with the fine-wire fixator. *Injury*. 2005;36(12):1467–1475.
28. Ramos T, Ekholm C, Eriksson BI, Karlsson J, Nistor L. The Ilizarov external fixator--a useful alternative for the treatment of proximal tibial fractures. A prospective observational study of 30 consecutive patients. *BMC Musculoskelet Disord*. 2013;14:11.
29. Mahan J, Seligson D, Henry SL, Hynes P, Dobbins J. Factors in pin tract infections. *Orthopedics*. 1991;14(3):305–308.
30. Hutson Jr JJ, Zych GA. Infections in periarticular fractures of the lower extremity treated with tensioned wire hybrid fixators. *J Orthop Trauma*. 1998;12(3):214–218.
31. Parameswaran AD, Roberts CS, Seligson D, Voor M. Pin tract infection with contemporary external fixation: how much of a problem? *J Orthop Trauma*. 2003;17(7):503–507.
32. Canadian Orthopaedic Trauma Society. Open reduction and internal fixation compared with circular fixator application for bicondylar tibial plateau fractures. Results of a multicenter, prospective, randomized clinical trial. *J Bone Joint Surg Am*. 2006;88(12):2613–2623.
33. Bertrand ML, Pascual-López FJ, Guerado E. Severe tibial plateau fractures (Schatzker V-VI): open reduction and internal fixation versus hybrid external fixation. *Injury*. 2017;48(suppl 6):S81–S85.
34. Katsenis D, Dendrinos G, Kouris A, Savas N, Schoinochoritis N, Pogiatzis K. Combination of fine wire fixation and limited internal fixation for high-energy tibial plateau fractures: functional results at minimum 5-year follow-up. *J Orthop Trauma*. 2009;23(7):493–501.

5

Internal Fixation

John T. Riehl, MD

INTERNAL FIXATION OF TIBIAL PLATEAU FRACTURES

Fixation constructs depend largely on fracture patterns and on patient factors such as associated injuries and functional status. Classification systems discussed in Chapter 2 can aid in the determination of definitive treatment for tibial plateau fractures. Many commercially available plating systems specific to the tibial plateau are available, with innovations constantly being brought to market. These provide treatment options with precontoured plates that can help secure stable fixation of difficult fracture patterns. Successful operative treatment in tibial plateau fractures begins with gaining the exposure needed to perform reduction and apply fixation (as detailed in Chapter 1). Visualization of the plateau may be obtained with fluoroscopy or arthroscopy, with minimal incisions, or with large and/or multiple incisions. It is imperative that the surgeon determines what approach can be used to reduce and adequately stabilize the fracture pattern while exposing the patient to the minimum amount of risk needed to reach those objectives. While it is recommended to perform biologically friendly fixation to the greatest degree possible, it is equally important to recognize when greater exposure is needed in order to achieve reduction and fixation goals.

INDICATIONS

Indications for the surgical treatment of tibial plateau fractures are determined primarily by fracture characteristics, such as fracture displacement and instability. These fractures involve the articular surface in the knee joint and such articular displacement leads to alterations in force transmission across the joint and accelerated degenerative changes. Articular displacement/step-off of 3 mm or more is generally cited as an indication for operative treatment. In highly active and younger patients, however, consideration may be given to reduction and fixation with any articular step-off of 1 mm or more.

Additionally, fractures that cause varus or valgus instability meet indications for operative treatment due to the risk of fracture healing with mechanical axis deformity of the tibia. Instability may be detectable by plain radiographs showing displacement on static films or alternatively determined by stress views. Examination under anesthesia in the operating room with fluoroscopy assistance can be performed if questions remain regarding fracture stability. Varus or valgus deformity of greater than 5 to 10 degrees with stress indicates instability. Metaphyseal comminution, bicondylar tibial plateau involvement, and medial tibial plateau fractures are all fracture characteristics that are often indicative of instability.

Articular surface gapping of 3 to 5 mm or more is another common indication for surgical management. This is often determined by tibial condylar widening, which can be measured by comparing contralateral tibia x-rays and/or by comparing tibial condylar width with femoral condylar width. The tibial plateau lateral margin should normally line up with the lateral margin of the femoral epicondyle.[1] The articular width of the proximal tibia should be slightly larger than the distal femoral articular width, while the total tibial condylar width should be slightly less than the overall femoral condylar width.[2]

Other potential indications for operative treatment of tibial plateau fractures may exist as well. Difficulty/inability to comply with non–weight bearing either due to cognitive deficits or injuries to multiple limbs may be a reason to proceed with surgical management in order to prevent displacement and allow early mobilization. The decision to proceed with surgical management must be individualized to the patient being treated, with consideration of both the risks and the benefits of surgery. Open fractures and compartment syndrome are indications for surgical treatment, although these do not always necessitate internal or external fixation in cases of nondisplaced and stable fractures. Indications for operative treatment of tibial plateau fractures are listed in Box 5.1.

PERCUTANEOUS FIXATION

Percutaneous fixation (PF) of tibial plateau fractures is performed in conjunction with fluoroscopy, arthroscopy, or both. PF can be used alone or as an adjunct to open fixation. PF is most applicable to situations where minimal to no displacement is present, where compression through lag screw fixation is sufficient for fracture fixation (most often in noncomminuted fracture segments), and when there is a need to avoid making large incisions to place fixation (e.g., to avoid small skin bridges, traumatic wounds).

Proper visualization of the tibial plateau is paramount to ensure an appropriate reduction and placement of hardware. Anteroposterior (AP) fluoroscopy views can be taken in a straight AP view and in a 10-degree caudad view in order to look down the slope of the plateau. This second view is helpful during placement of hardware to ensure that lag screws are placed in the subchondral bone without penetration through the joint surface. On this view, the articular surface should overlap on itself and make one solid radiographic line. Multiple angle AP views can also be taken to evaluate reduction and look for step-off deformity. Lateral views should aim to overlap the medial and lateral tibial condyles and allow the surgeon to evaluate reduction in the sagittal plane.

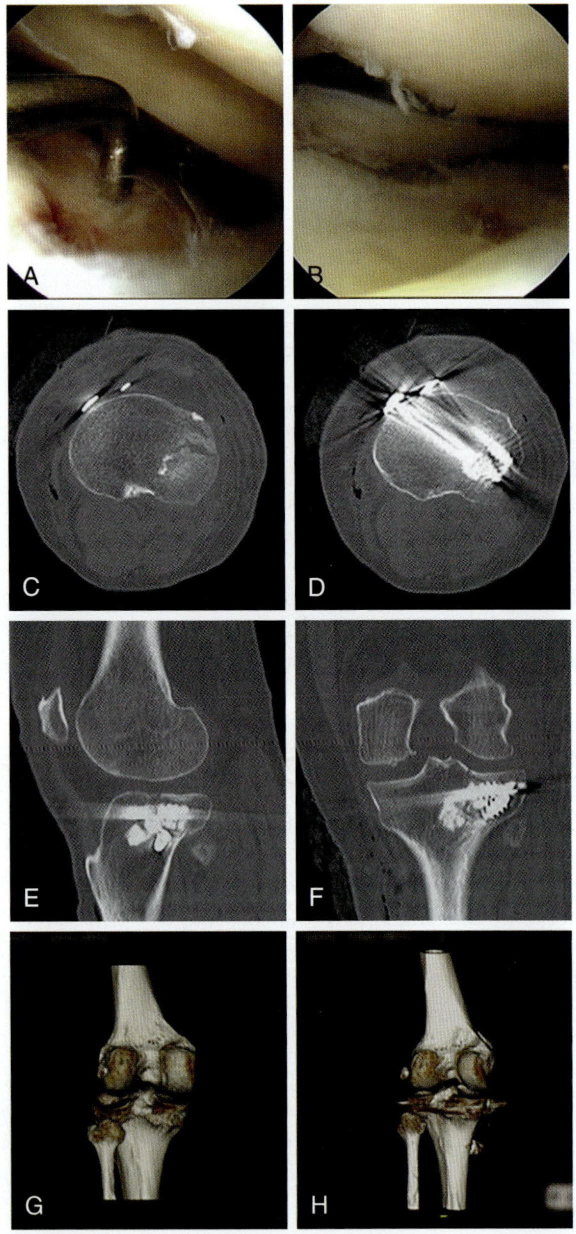

Fig. 5.1 Arthroscopic view of the lateral tibial plateau before (A) and after (B) reduction. (C–H) Postfixation computed tomography scans showing reduction and hardware placement. *Reproduced with permission, Fig. 1. Kun Chan AC, Hin Chan AP, Hung YW, Lo CK, Ho Fan JC. A novel percutaneous screw fixation of postero-lateral tibial plateau fracture using posterior cruciate ligament reconstruction femoral template: Technical note. J Orthop Trauma Rehabilitation. 2017;22:22–29.*

BOX 5.1 Indications for Operative Treatment of Tibial Plateau Fractures

- Articular step-off of ≥3 mm (1 mm in young and highly active patients)
- Varus/valgus instability of ≥5–10 degrees
- Most bicondylar fractures, medial condyle fractures, and tibial plateau fractures with metaphyseal comminution
- Articular gap of ≥3 mm (plateau widening)
- Need for early weight bearing
- Open fracture
- Compartment syndrome

Direct visualization of the tibial plateau articular surface can be achieved through the use of arthroscopy (Fig. 5.1). With arthroscopy, care must be taken not to cause extravasation into the tissues of the lower leg, which may already have some degree of damage from the initial trauma insult. Fluid extravasation into a closed compartment can induce a compartment syndrome. The operating surgeon should be aware of this if using arthroscopy to assist visualization. "Dry" scoping (using the arthroscope without water) is a technique that can be used to help avoid fluid extravasation. However, in the setting of a percutaneous approach, this can make visualization difficult (dry scoping during open approaches can be an excellent adjunct for visualization, as discussed later). An arthroscopic pump should be used with great caution or not at all in these cases. Gravity flow fluid with a separate inflow cannula may be desirable to allow for sufficient flushing of the joint. Medial and lateral portals can be established for the arthroscope and instruments (shaver, probe, etc.) and a superolateral portal for inflow. It is necessary to use a suction-shaver to remove clot in the knee and debride clot at the fracture site to provide visualization.

Several reduction instruments and techniques are available in these cases (Fig. 5.2). When slight step off or gap deformities exist, large pointed clamps (Weber, periarticular, etc.) can be used to obtain reduction. By placing both clamp tines onto bone through small stab incisions and with a force across the knee that opens up the joint space where the reduction is taking place (i.e., varus force when reducing a lateral plateau), the clamp can be twisted to elevate an inferiorly displaced fragment and then squeezed down in order to reduce and compress the fragment. In some instances, a Freer elevator may first need to be inserted into the fracture site and used to disimpact the fracture so it may be mobilized.

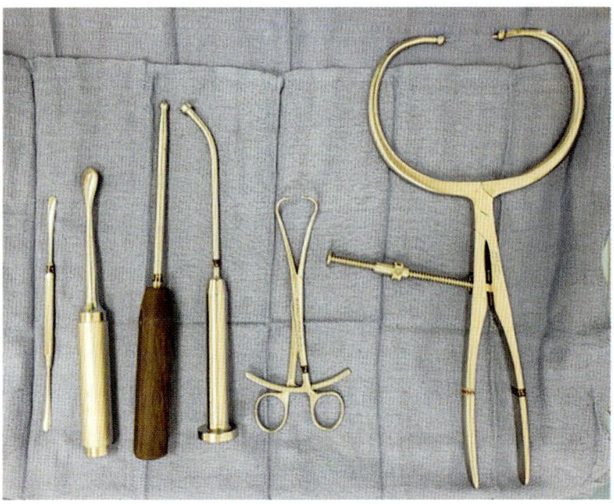

Fig. 5.2 Instruments used for reduction in tibial plateau fractures. From *left* to *right*, Freer elevator, Cobb elevator, ball spike, bone tamp, Weber clamp, and large periarticular clamp.

A ball spike (or Picador) is an invaluable tool in percutaneous (and open) reduction for tibial plateau fractures. This instrument can be placed through a small incision and used to push the fracture fragment in a desired direction (elevate, compress, etc.). A femoral distractor or external fixator can also be used to help obtain the length of the fracture and to apply varus or valgus forces across the knee joint. This concept is discussed in further detail in the Open Reduction and Internal Fixation (ORIF) section.

Articular surface depression within the central portion of the lateral condyle can be a more difficult problem to address percutaneously. This can be accomplished by making a small incision at the metaphyseal flare. If there is no break in the cortex in this region, a 4.5-mm drill bit can then be used to open the cortex. A long, curved tamp can then be inserted it into the hole created in the metaphysis and directed toward the depressed articular segment. Visualization of tamp placement using fluoroscopy can guide the tamp to the correct position on AP and lateral views. The bone can then be gently tapped back into place with a mallet, and reduction can be checked via fluoroscopy, arthroscopy, or both. An additional reduction technique that can be used here is balloon tibioplasty. This involves inserting an inflatable balloon (often a kyphoplasty balloon) into the tibial metaphysis just beneath the depressed segment and slowly inflating the balloon until the fracture has been reduced (Fig. 5.3). This technique may provide a more widespread and even pressure to the depressed fragment than a bone tamp does with less destruction to the tibia.[3,4] Once the depressed fragment has been reduced, the metaphyseal bone void can then be percutaneously filled with a bone void filler, such as a calcium phosphate cement.

Another helpful reduction technique is to use medium to large (2.0–3.2 mm) K-wires. These K-wires can be drilled into a large depressed lateral plateau fragment and stopped short of the fracture. The wires are then manipulated to elevate the tibial plateau and, once reduced, can be further inserted across the fracture site into the opposite cortex.

The use of a posterior cruciate ligament (PCL) guide has been reported as a helpful technique in localizing depressed fragments and aiming guidewires to guide tamp and screw placement.[5] The targeting portion of the PCL guide can be placed over the skin. Then, an entry point remote from the articular depression can be used for insertion of instruments in order to get accurate placement of instrumentation and the best angle possible for articular surface reduction (Fig. 5.4). This may be especially useful in percutaneous treatment of posterolateral tibial plateau fractures where instrumentation and fixation can be brought across the plateau accurately from the medial side.

After reduction has been achieved at the fracture site, provisional fixation using K-wires can be utilized to hold the reduction if necessary. Fixation is most often performed parallel to the articular surface, and often compression is desired to provide absolute stability and primary bone healing at the articular fracture site. Compression can be achieved through clamping the fracture and/or through placement of lag screws. Screws of various sizes are used for fixation in these instances (from 3.5, 4.0, 4.5, 6.5, up to 8.0). The size of the screw used may depend on fragment size, patient size, and other

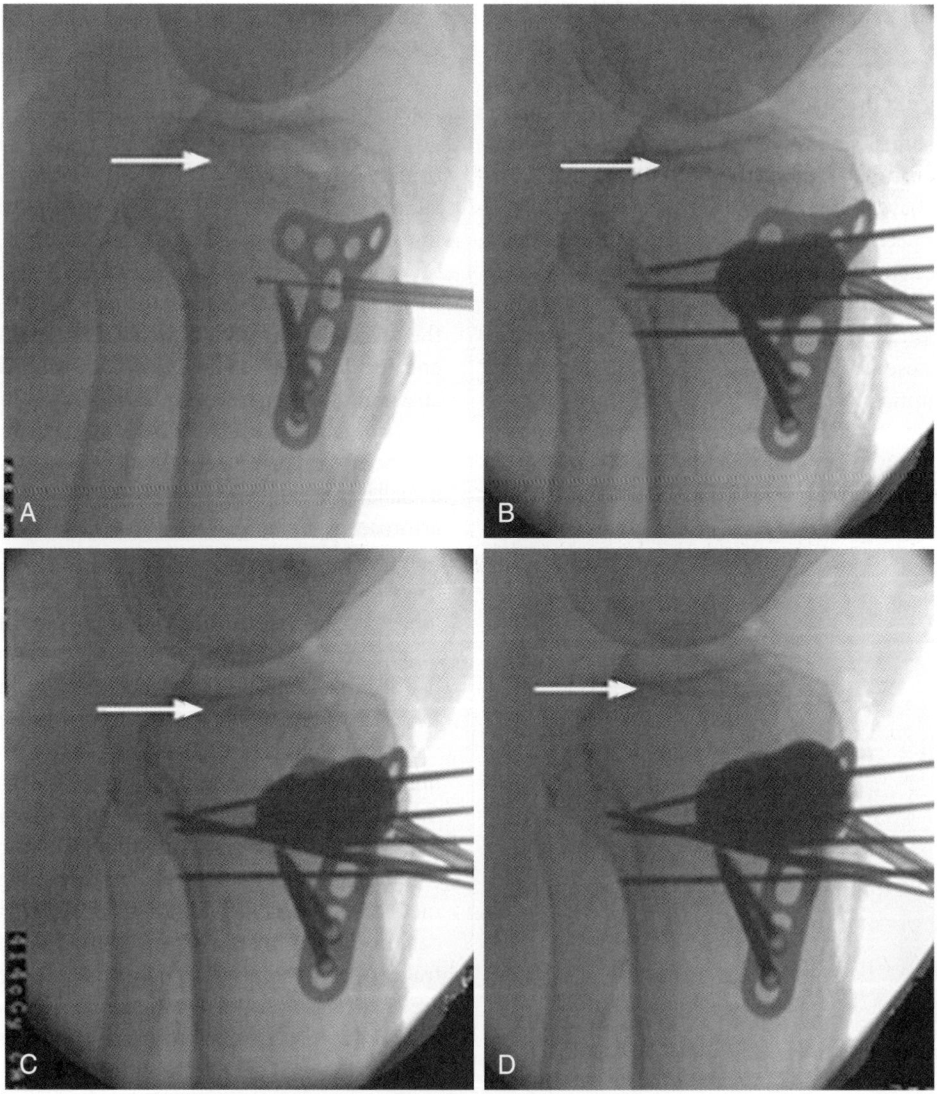

Fig. 5.3 Balloon is inserted into the tibial metaphysis (A) and slowly inflated (B–D) in order to reduce the depressed articular surface *(white arrow)*. (Skeletal Trauma, Sixth Edition, 2020).

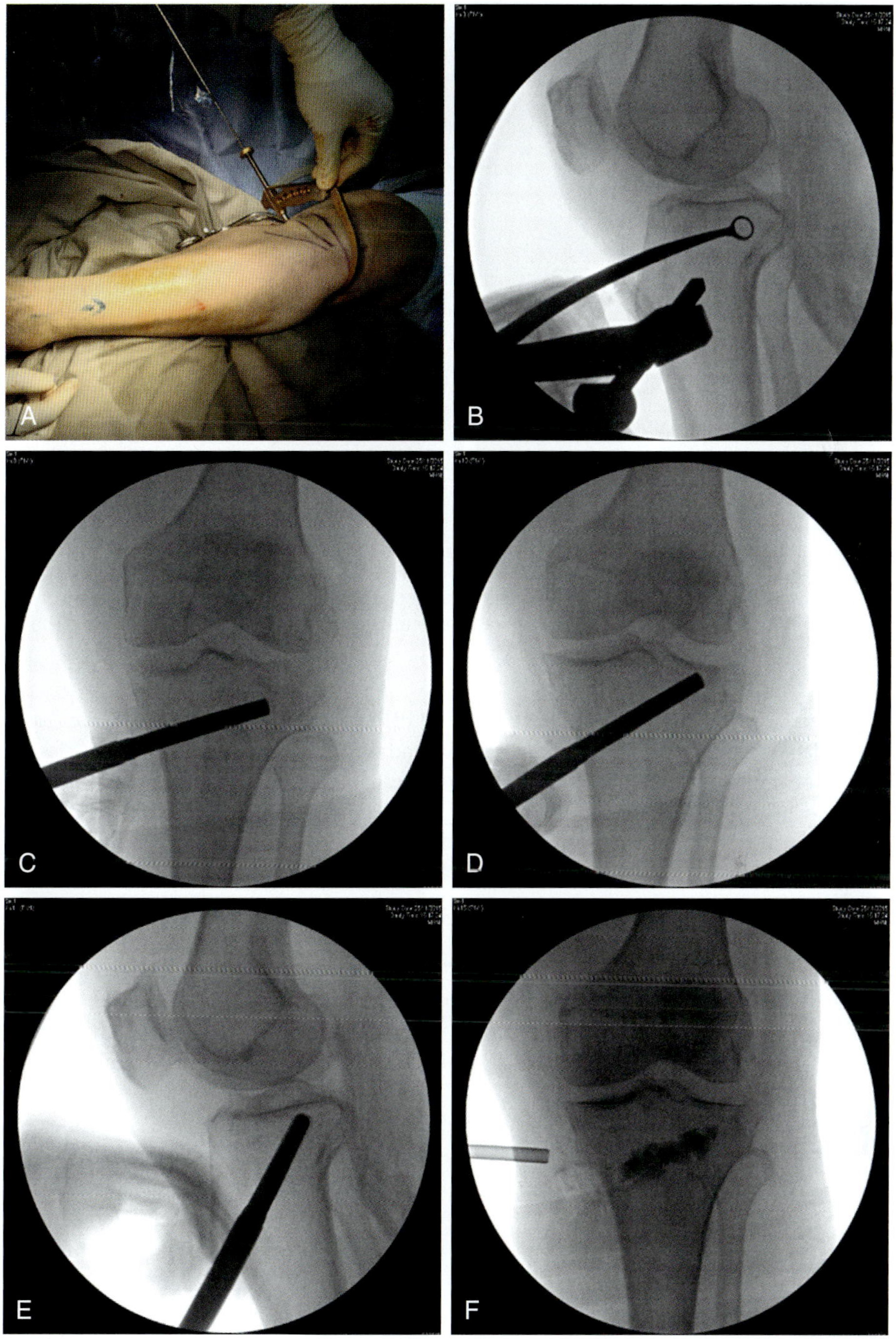

Fig. 5.4 Clinical photograph (A) and fluoroscopic picture (B) of a PCL guide being used to target the postero-lateral plateau from the medial metaphysis. A tamp is then inserted from the medial metaphysis and aimed toward the depressed posterolateral fragment (C). Reduction/elevation of the depressed plateau (D and E). Metaphyseal void can then be filled with bone void filler (F). *Reproduced with permission, Fig. 5. Kun Chan AC, Hin Chan AP, Hung YW, Lo CK, Ho Fan JC. A novel percutaneous screw fixation of postero-lateral tibial plateau fracture using posterior cruciate ligament reconstruction femoral template: Technical note. J Orthop Trauma Rehabilitation. 2017;22:22–29.*

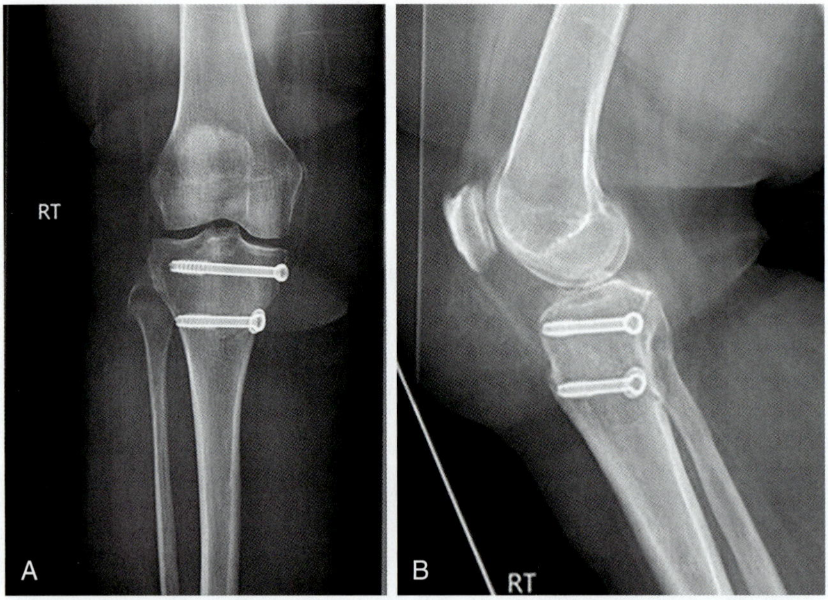

Fig. 5.5 Anteroposterior (A) and lateral (B) x-rays of a medial tibial plateau fracture treated with two large cannulated screws placed perpendicular to the fracture site. The more inferior screw has been placed at the apex of the fracture.

fixation being utilized. Lag by design (i.e., partially threaded screws) or lag by technique (i.e., overdrilling the near cortex) may be employed to compress fracture fragments. Screws may be placed with or without washers depending on bone quality and surgeon's preference. When placing screws for PF, it is helpful to ensure bicortical placement to improve construct strength. In the case of wedge fracture fragments, it is beneficial biomechanically to place a screw at the distal apex of the fracture fragment as a buttress screw to help prevent inferior displacement, in addition to subchondral screws (Fig. 5.5).

OPEN REDUCTION AND INTERNAL FIXATION

Many tibial plateau fractures, especially those resulting from a high-energy mechanism of injury, are treated with ORIF of the displaced joint surface. Large displacement and comminution of the joint surface can make percutaneous reduction and fixation less likely to result in successful radiographic outcomes. Direct visualization through an open approach allows for direct manipulation of displaced fragments. The decision of which approach or approaches to use is important and will depend on the fracture pattern present. Chapter 1 provides descriptions of several approaches to the tibial plateau.

In unicondylar lateral tibial plateau fractures, an anterolateral approach is often utilized for fixation. Once exposure is obtained and meniscus and capsule are retracted superiorly (see Chapter 1), a varus force applied across the knee will permit exposure across the lateral tibial plateau to the tibial spine. The transverse submeniscal arthrotomy can extend from the patellar tendon back to the posterolateral plateau. Varus force across the knee can be applied manually or through

CASE 5.1

A 48-year-old male presented to the emergency department after a fall from a ladder with isolated right knee pain. The patient was hemodynamically stable. His pulses were symmetric with no sign of compartment syndrome. No associated injuries were present (Fig. 5.6).

CASE 5.1—CONT'D

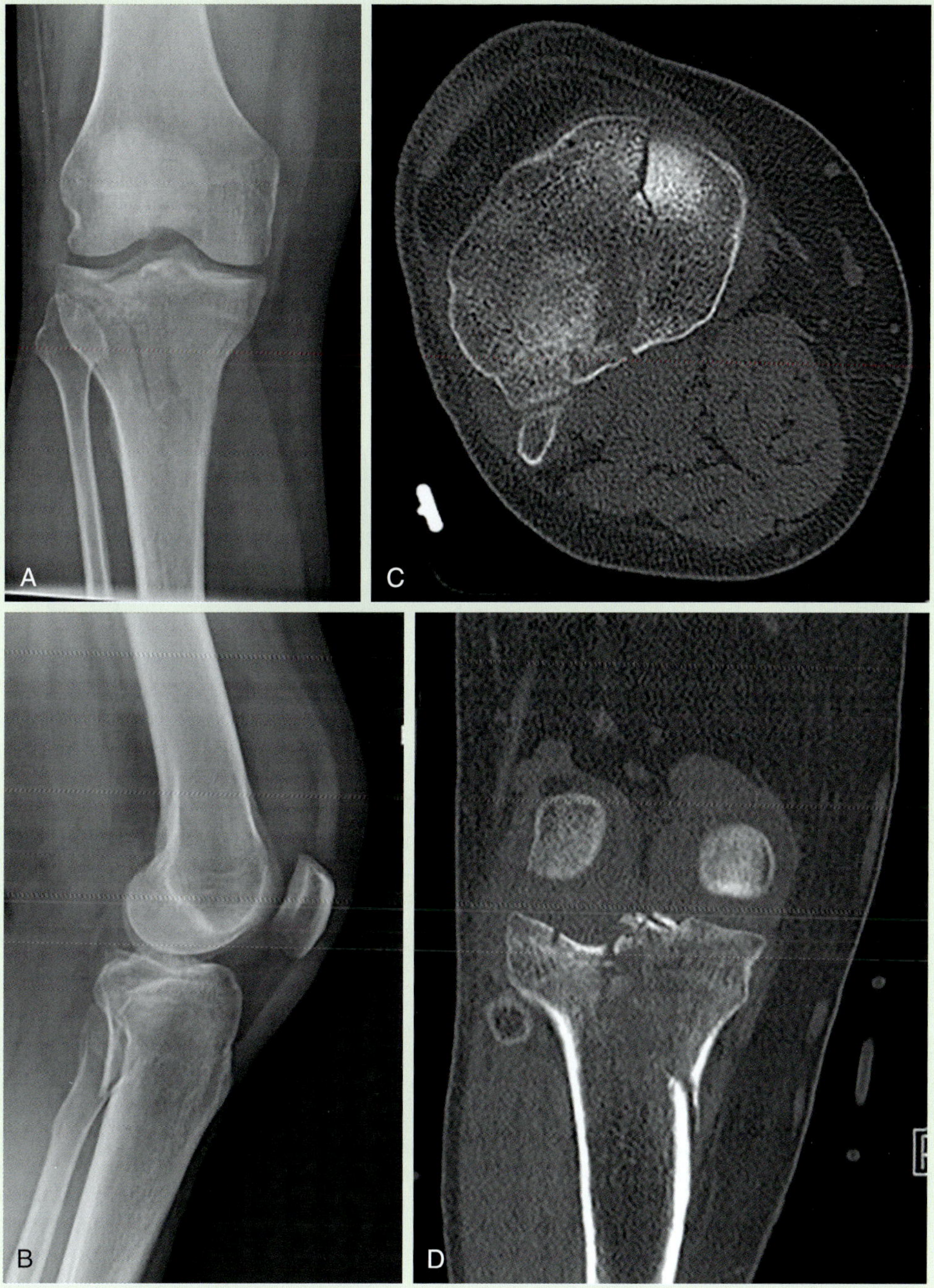

Fig. 5.6 X-rays (A and B) and computed tomography scans (C and D) showing bicondylar tibial plateau fracture (Schatzker type V) with lateral articular depression and a posteromedial fracture fragment.

Continued

CASE 5.1—CONT'D

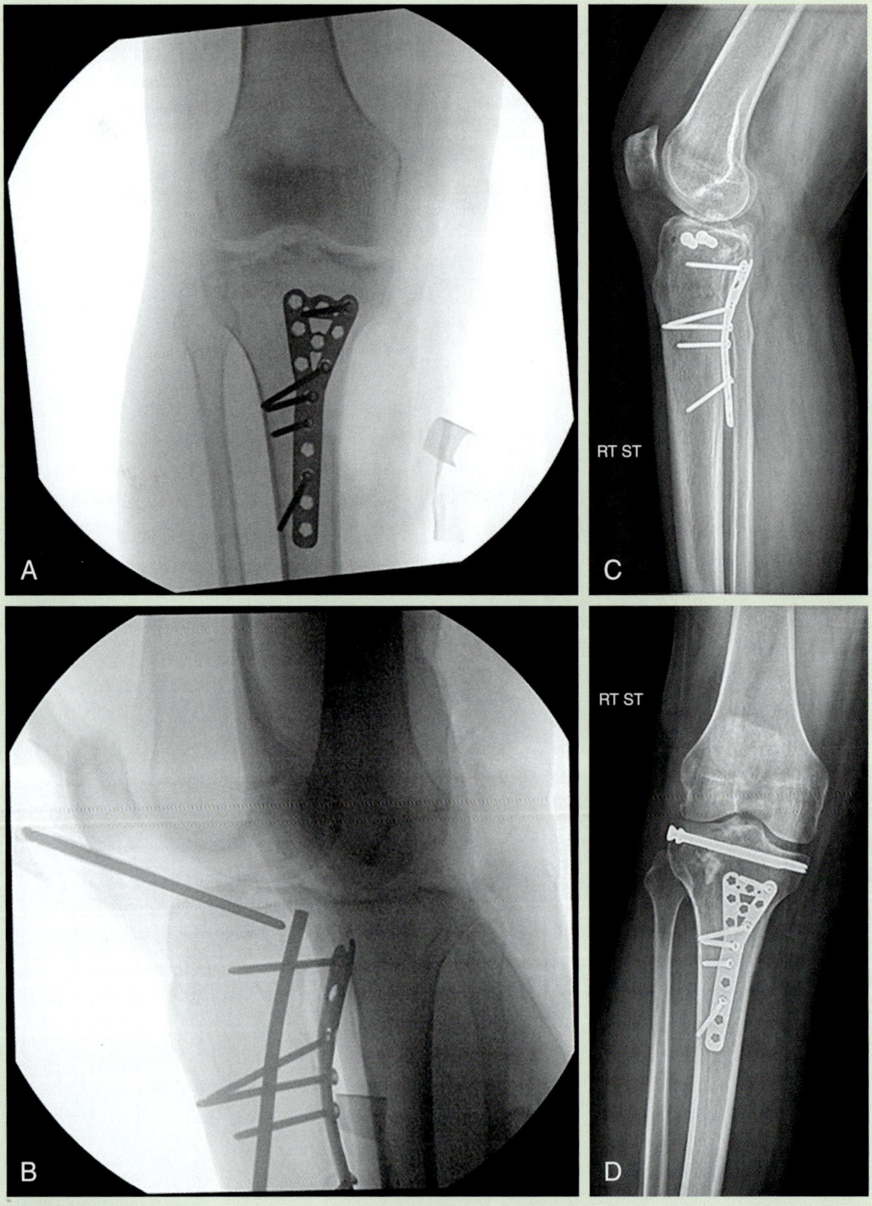

Fig. 5.7 Intraoperative x-ray showing placement of a buttress plate through a posteromedial approach (A), followed by percutaneous reduction of the lateral plateau using a bone tamp (B). The tamp was introduced through a corticotomy made in the lateral tibial metaphysis. Definitive fixation of the lateral plateau (C and D) was performed by placing two 6.5-mm partially threaded cannulated screws, and the metaphyseal void was filled with calcium phosphate.

A knee immobilizer was placed, ice was applied, and elevation was performed overnight. The patient was taken to the operating room the following morning. Intraoperative examination under anesthesia showed greater than 10 degrees of instability with varus stress testing. Open medial buttress plating was performed with percutaneous treatment of the lateral plateau (Fig. 5.7).

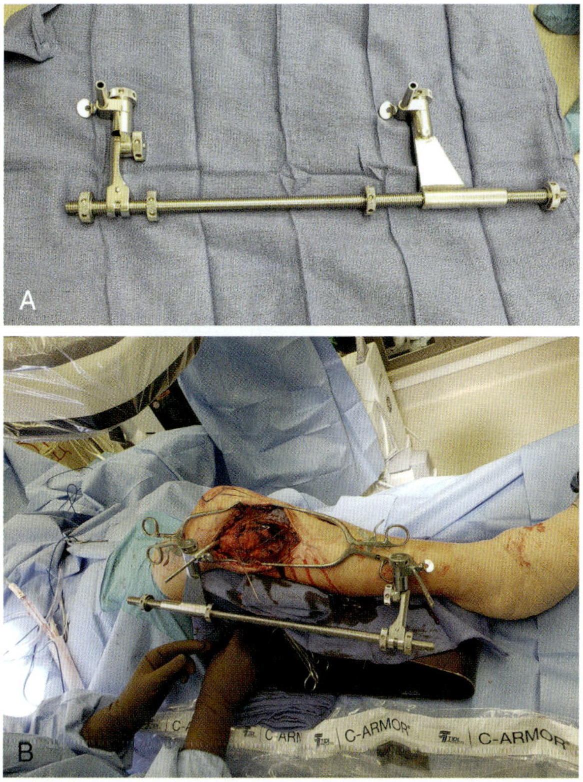

Fig. 5.8 Femoral distractor assembled (A). The femoral distractor is applied in such a way that it does not block access to the surgical field or to C-arm visualization, pins are out of the way of planned hardware placement, and knee motion is allowed for (B).

use of a distraction device. When available, a femoral distractor is a helpful tool that provides a steady force across the knee and allows for greater visualization of the lateral tibial plateau. To apply the femoral distractor, a half-pin is placed in the femur from lateral to medial in the lateral epicondyle (or just distal and posterior to the lateral epicondyle[6]). This location for the femoral pin allows for flexion and extension of the knee if needed, while the distractor is in place. A second pin is placed from lateral to medial in the tibia well distal to the most distal aspect of any anticipated fixation. Care should be exercised in placement of this pin to avoid injury to the superficial peroneal nerve. The distractor can be assembled on the sterile back table, and the holding sleeves are placed over the half-pins. Wing screws are then tightened to hold the sleeves in place on the pins. The distractor should be assembled and applied such that the bar comes off parallel and posterior to the tibia (Fig. 5.8) so that it remains out of the surgical field to improve access to the surgical site and to remain out of the way of x-ray. The far spindle nut in the mobile segment is loosened to the end of the bar. Distraction can then be performed by first applying manual traction and varus to the leg, followed by tightening the near spindle nut (moving the nut away from the fracture site). After familiarizing yourself with this device, its application takes only a few minutes and ultimately saves operative time due to the increased exposure.

As an alternative to a femoral distractor, an external fixator may be used. Half-pins are placed as mentioned earlier, and clamps and carbon fiber rods are then added to the pins, manual distraction applied, and clamps tightened. A third clamp can then be placed on the carbon fiber rod just proximal to the distal pin and tightened to the bar. A large lamina spreader is placed between the two distal clamps, and the most distal clamp is loosened. The lamina spreader is used to move the distal pin and clamp more distal on the carbon fiber rod, providing further distraction. The distal clamp is then retightened, and the lamina spreader can be removed (Fig. 5.9).

Another technique that can be used to gain visualization within the joint is by using an arthroscope without fluid (dry scope). After the submeniscal arthrotomy has been performed, an arthroscope can be placed beneath the meniscus to visualize across the plateau. If necessary, the scope can also be placed through anterolateral or anteromedial portals.

With the arthrotomy performed and direct visualization of the joint, the lateral meniscus can be inspected. Tears in the periphery can often be repaired, whereas more central tears will be debrided. Despite having an open approach with the arthrotomy, an arthroscopic backbiter is a helpful tool to easily reach in and debride the meniscus back to a smooth and stable edge (Fig. 5.10).

In order to gain access to the more depressed medial segments of the lateral plateau, the lateral cortical fragment will often need to be "booked" open. A Cobb elevator or an osteotome can be placed within the sagittal fracture line and is used to lever open the lateral plateau (Fig. 5.11). This can be held open with a lamina spreader or with a self-retaining retractor. Reduction then proceeds from medial to lateral on the tibial plateau (Box 5.2).

Depressed articular fragments are often impacted into the metaphyseal bone and must be first disimpacted with an osteotome or elevator. The osteotome should be placed at least 1 cm below the articular surface to elevate a sufficiently large osteochondral fragment.

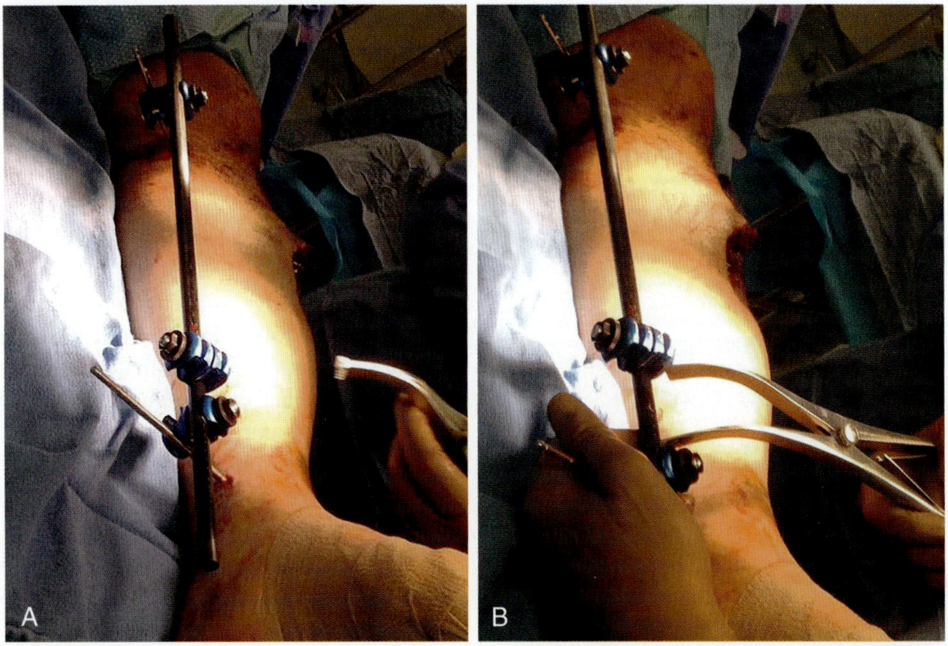

Fig. 5.9 Distraction obtained with an external fixator and lamina spreader. A third bar clamp is tightened to the carbon fiber rod just proximal to the distal clamp (A). A lamina spreader is used to increase the distance between the two clamps after loosening the most distal clamp (B), which is then retightened after further distraction has been achieved (Arthro FX external fixator system pictured, Arthrex Inc., Naples, FL).

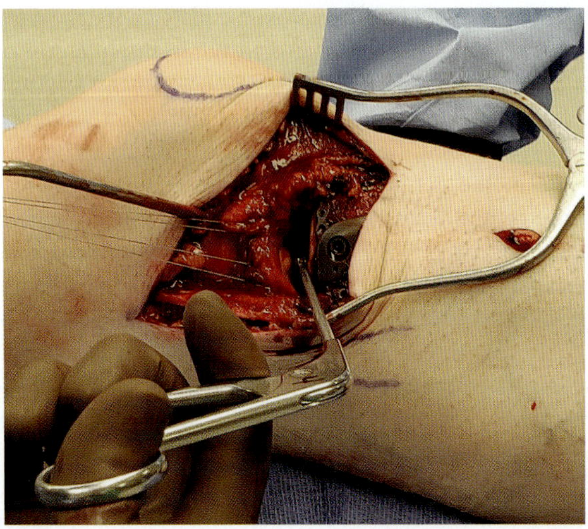

Fig. 5.10 Arthroscopic backbiter used to debride central tear of the lateral meniscus through a submeniscal arthrotomy.

Once the osteotome is placed, it can be used to elevate the fragment with superiorly directed force on the osteotome directly. As an alternative, a second osteotome can be placed just beneath the first, and the osteotomes can be spread apart to lever the articular fragment back into place (Fig. 5.12). Cobb elevators, Freer elevators, or a tamp with or without the simultaneous use of an osteotome can also be used to elevate fragments (Fig. 5.13).

Once the articular fragment has been reduced, a Kirschner wire (K-wire) can be placed for provisional fixation. This K-wire can be driven through the medial plateau and skin and advanced by pulling the medial side of the pin until the lateral end of the pin is flush with the articular fragment it is holding in place (Fig. 5.14). This allows the fragment to be held by a K-wire without interfering and getting in the way of further reduction of more lateral fragments. Additionally, bioabsorbable pins can be placed in these more medial fragments that will stay in place as definitive fixation (Fig. 5.15). K-wires can also be used to help reduce varus deformity to the lateral plateau by insertion into fragments with a slight superior aim (parallel to the displaced joint surface). The K-wire can then be used to manipulate the fragments into a reduced (or slightly over-reduced) position, and an additional K-wire can be inserted to secure the reduction. Once the more medially positioned fragments have been

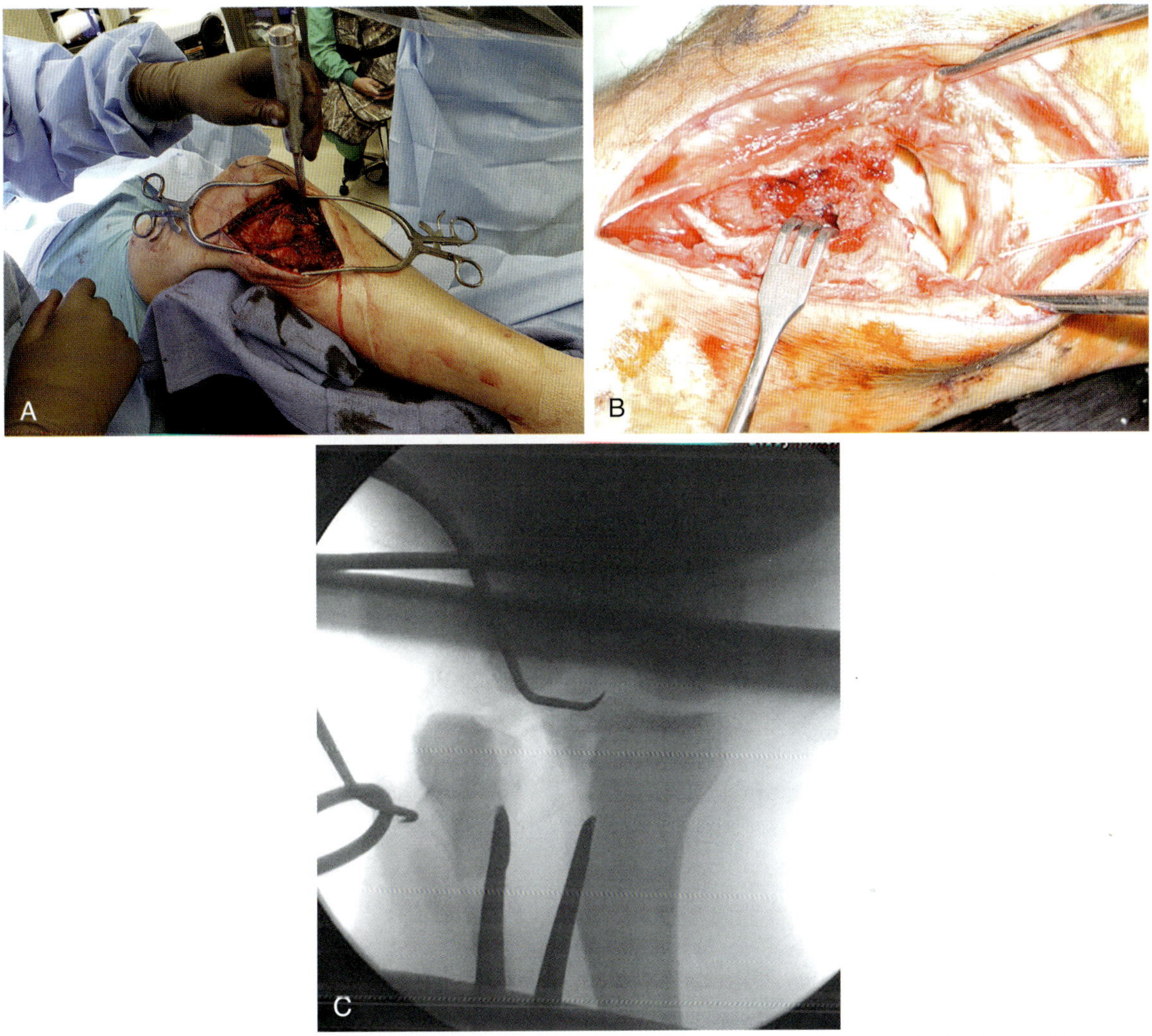

Fig. 5.11 A Cobb elevator being used to develop the sagittal plane fracture line of the lateral tibial plateau (A). Retractor used to "book" open the lateral tibial fracture fragment (B). X-ray showing lamina spreader being used to book open lateral fracture in order to obtain visualization of more medial comminuted fragments (C).

BOX 5.2 Reduction Techniques/Aides for Tibial Plateau Fractures

- Double osteotomes used to disimpact and lever depressed fragments into place
- Pointed clamps
- K-wire joystick
- Tamp and mallet
- Distractor
- Ball spike
- Push/pull device

reduced, the lateral cortical segment can be reduced and compressed. Depending on the bone graft/graft substitute used to fill the metaphyseal void, it may be placed (packed) prior to reduction of the lateral cortical fragment or can be injected after fixation. Compression can be achieved via a ball spike or a reduction clamp. Reduction can be checked both by direct visualization and by using a Freer elevator to "feel" the articular surface and note any step-off deformity. Radiographic confirmation of reduction is performed with standard AP view and AP view aimed 10 degrees caudad (in line with the tibial

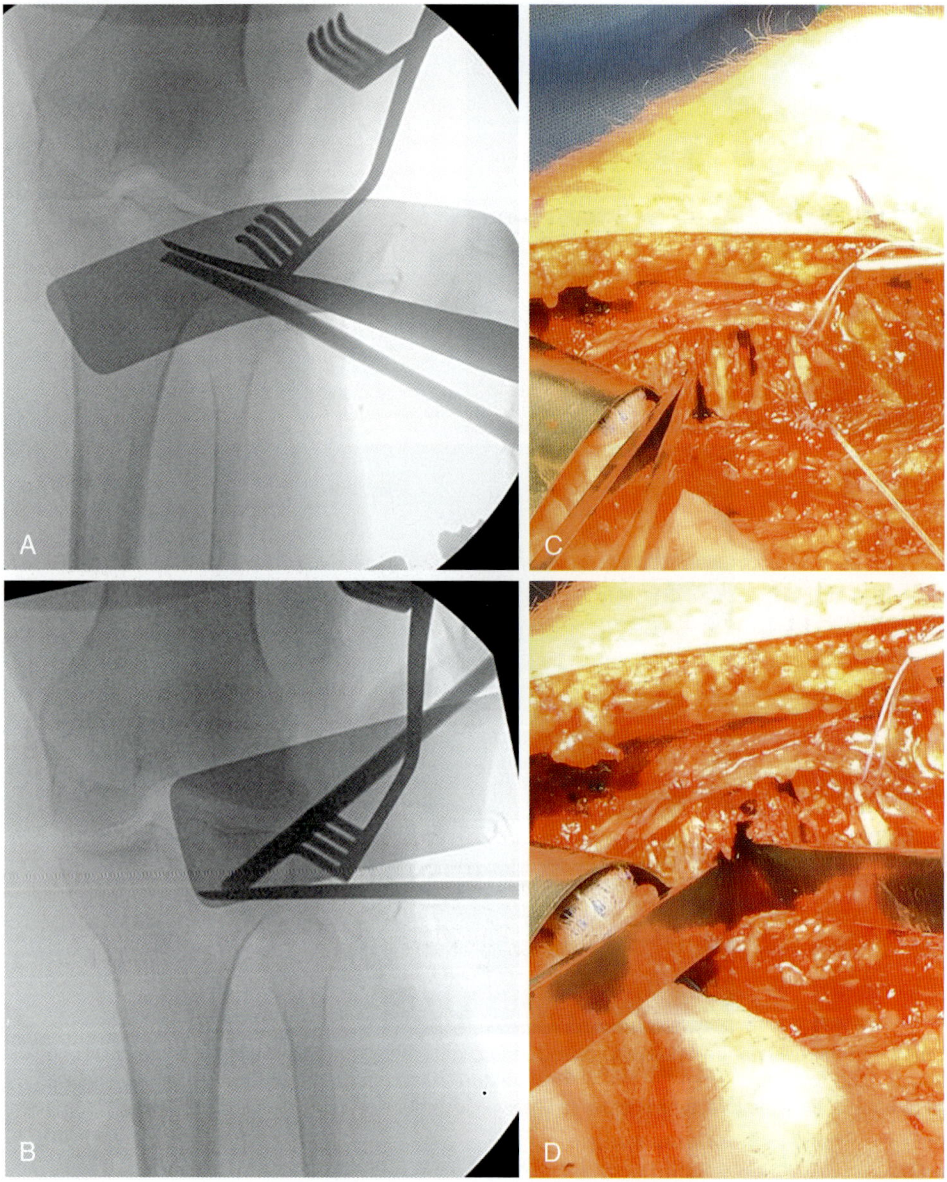

Fig. 5.12 Osteotomes placed underneath a depressed lateral articular fragment. The osteotomes are placed parallel to the depressed joint surface and stacked on each other (A). By holding the more distal osteotome in place and spreading the handles apart, the depressed fragment is reduced (B). Clinical pictures showing reduction of depressed fragments using two osteotomes (C and D).

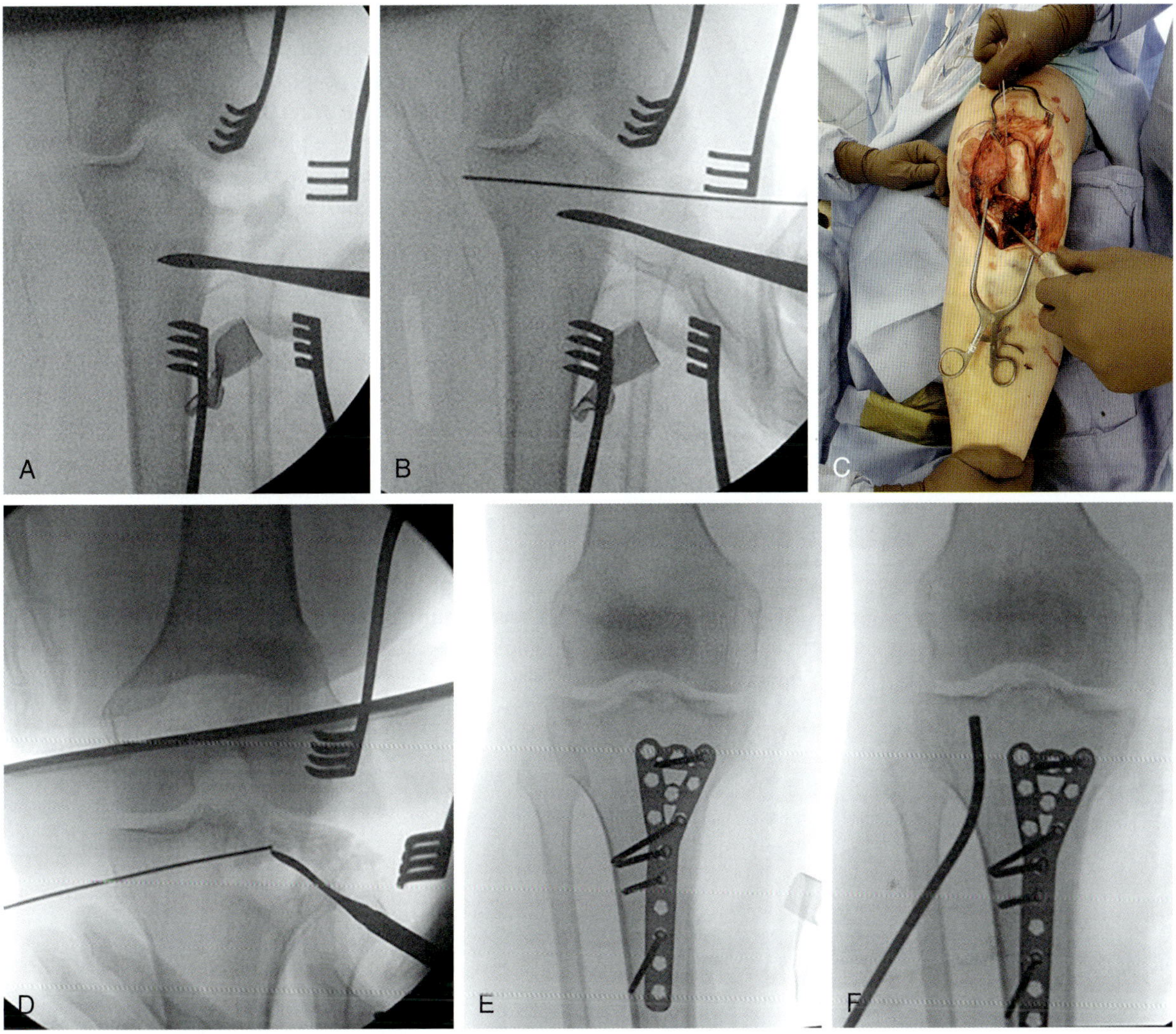

Fig. 5.13 A Cobb elevator provides a large flat surface that can be used to reduce depressed articular fragments with underlying subchondral bone and, once reduced, fragments can be pinned in place (A–C). Freer elevators may also be used to elevate small fragments (C). Alternatively, a tamp may be used to reduce depressed fragments (E and F).

plateau posterior slope) as well as on lateral x-ray with medial and lateral femoral condyles aligned.

With reduction accomplished and K-wires flush to the lateral cortex, placement of definitive fixation can begin to be placed. If independent lag screws are to be used, they can be placed at this point from lateral to medial in the subchondral bone and parallel to the articular surface. Lag by design may be utilized by placing a partially threaded screw, or lag by technique may be employed by first drilling a gliding hole to the fracture site and then drilling for the core diameter of the screw across the remainder of the plateau. Lag screw placement will provide further compression at the articular surface (Fig. 5.16).

A lateral plate can then be placed along the lateral tibial cortex. Site-specific plates are available and are most often used for fixation of lateral tibial plateau fractures. The plate should be placed as a buttress plate and will ideally be slightly undercontoured in order to obtain an intimate fit to the lateral cortex and apply pressure, especially at the articular surface and at the apex of the fracture site (Fig. 5.17). A periarticular clamp may

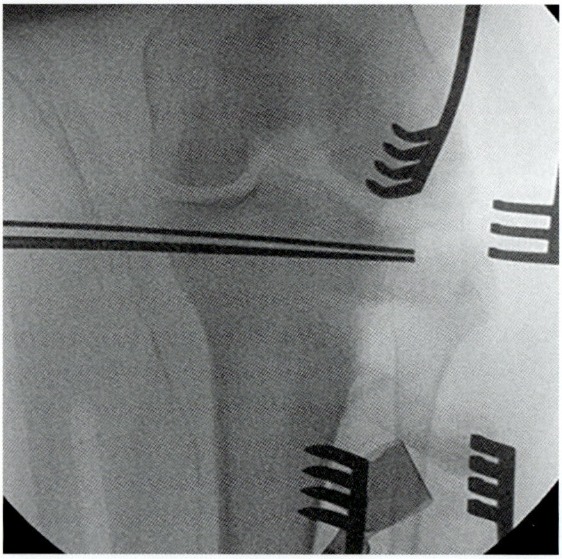

Fig. 5.14 K-wires holding reduction of more medial fragments of the lateral tibial plateau, driven through the medial skin until flush with the reduced fragments to prevent interference with more lateral reduction and hardware placement.

be used to help compress the plate to bone if needed. Once the plate is aligned in the desired position, a nonlocking screw may be placed near the metaphyseal/diaphyseal junction to bring the plate intimately down to bone. Lag screws may be placed in the proximal portion of the plate to further compress the articular surface. Once compression has been achieved, locking screws may be placed in the additional proximal screw holes if desired to provide a fixed angle construct. This is especially desirable in cases with poor bone quality, in cases with a sagittal split in the medial plateau that has already been compressed, or in cases where subchondral support is needed for small fragments. Distally, nonlocking or locking screws can be placed in the shaft portion of the plate, again based on patient's bone quality or other factors that would provide an indication for the use of locking screws. Finally, a "kickstand" screw can be placed to obtain additional proximal fixation (Fig. 5.18).

If graft has not been placed previously, injectable graft such as calcium phosphate[7] may now be injected into the metaphyseal void. The joint is then irrigated. Sutures that

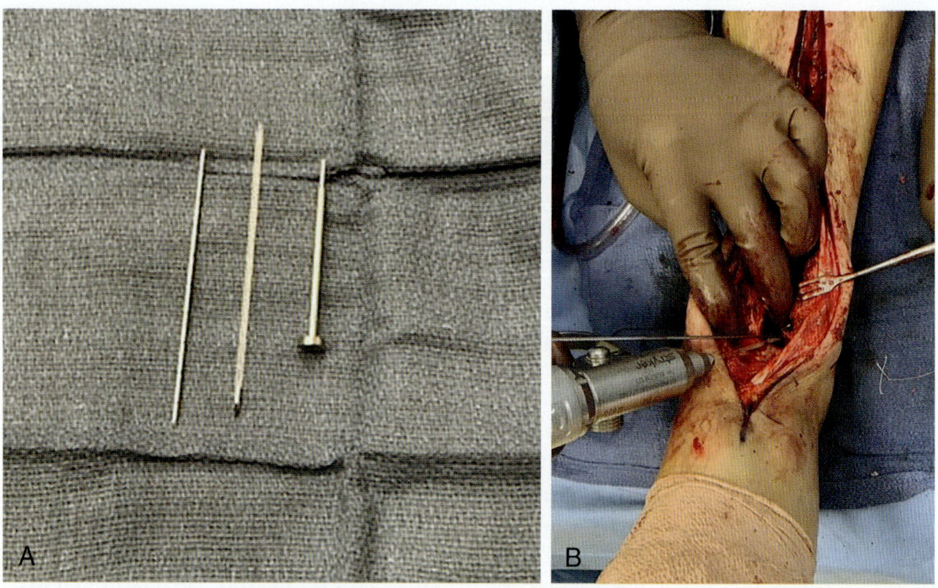

Fig. 5.15 Bioabsorbable pins can be used to provide fixation of central fragments (A). With some systems, these pins can be drilled in place similar to using a K-wire, as seen here in this pilon fracture (B). The pin can then be cut flush with the fragment using a pin cutter or a battery powered cautery.

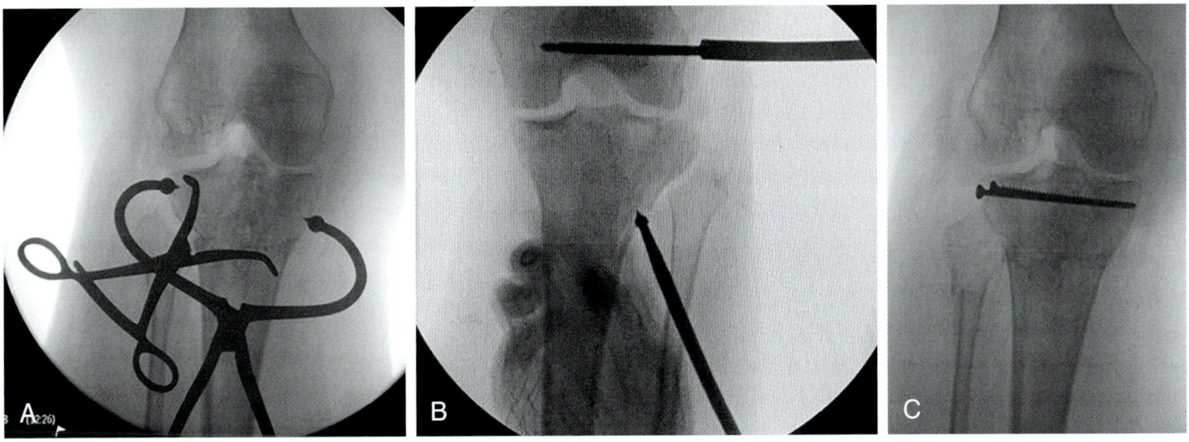

Fig. 5.16 Compression at the articular fracture site achieved through clamp placement (A), ball spike (B), and independent lag screws (C).

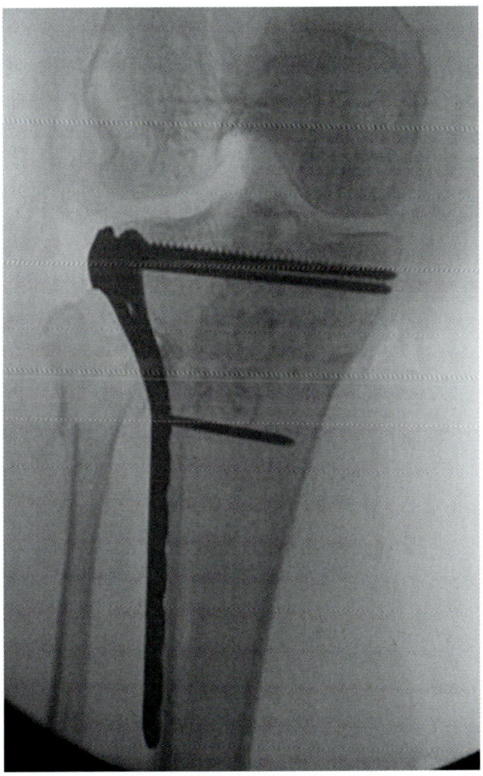

Fig. 5.17 Lateral buttress plating of a tibial plateau fracture.

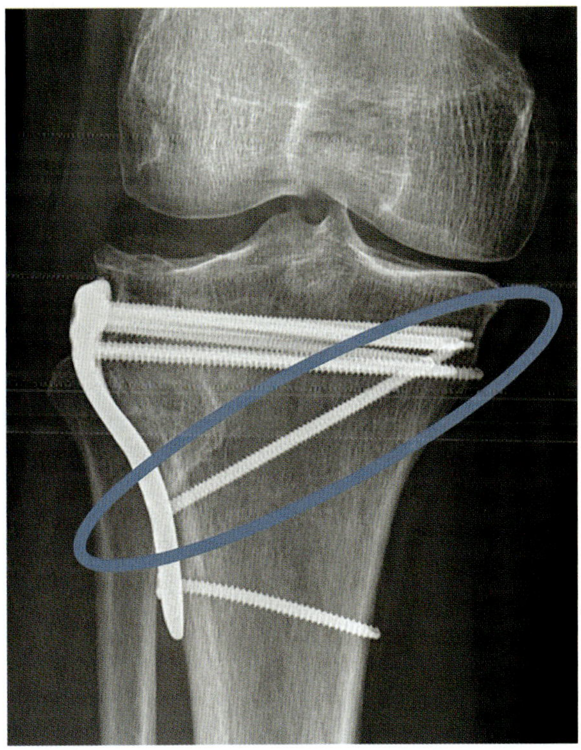

Fig. 5.18 Lateral buttress plating of a Schatzker type II tibial plateau fracture with the "kickstand" screw circled.

have been placed into the periphery of the lateral meniscus can then be tied down into the plate or into a cuff of tissue on the lateral plateau. Anterior compartment muscle and fascia can then be repaired back over the plate, but care should be taken to avoid overtightening. Knee retinaculum is also repaired, followed by subcutaneous tissue and staples in the skin. Irrigation is performed at each layer of closure. With stable fixation, a soft dressing is applied, and the patient is allowed full range of motion and is made non–weight bearing on the operative extremity for 6 weeks. An extension brace may be used at night during the first 6 weeks to prevent flexion contracture.

When a medial condyle fracture is present in isolation (Schatzker type IV injury), a posteromedial approach (Chapter 1) is performed to access fracture reduction and placement of fixation. This approach is also utilized for many bicondylar fracture patterns in combination with the anterolateral or direct anterior approach. In cases of bicondylar fracture patterns, the medial approach is usually made first and the medial fracture reduced, followed by reduction and fixation of the lateral tibial plateau. Commonly, the medial fragment can be reduced by applying a valgus force across the knee, and a ball spike can be used to push the medial plateau back into place. A Hohmann retractor can also be placed within the fracture site and used to lever the medial fragment superiorly and back into place, especially in instances when an inferiorly displaced fragment is difficult to reduce. A plate can then be placed to buttress the medial or posteromedial fragment. Nonlocking screws are placed into the plate just below the apex of the fracture to bring the plate down to bone. Additional screws are placed distal to that in the shaft. Proximal screw holes are either left empty at this point or short screws are placed so they do not inhibit the reduction of the lateral plateau. The medial wound is left open while an anterolateral (or direct anterior) approach is made, and the lateral plateau is reduced and fixed as described earlier. Additional screws can then be placed across the plateau from the medial side, if desired (see Case 5.2). Medial fascia, subcutaneous tissue, and skin are closed, and irrigation is performed at each layer of closure.

Some medial fractures can be treated with lateral locked plating alone. This may be especially appropriate when soft-tissue injuries and comorbid medical conditions raise concerns for medial wound healing problems. However, caution and careful attention should be utilized before deciding to treat a bicolumnar plateau fracture with lateral locked plating alone. Fractures with a sagittally oriented medial fracture line may be amenable to treatment with lateral plating alone, as lateral to medial screws will travel perpendicular to the fracture line, and multiple screws can obtain purchase in the medial fragment. On the other hand, medial fracture lines that are oriented in a posteromedial plane are generally not amenable to treatment from lateral plating (Fig. 5.19). Fixation obtained from lateral plating is poor

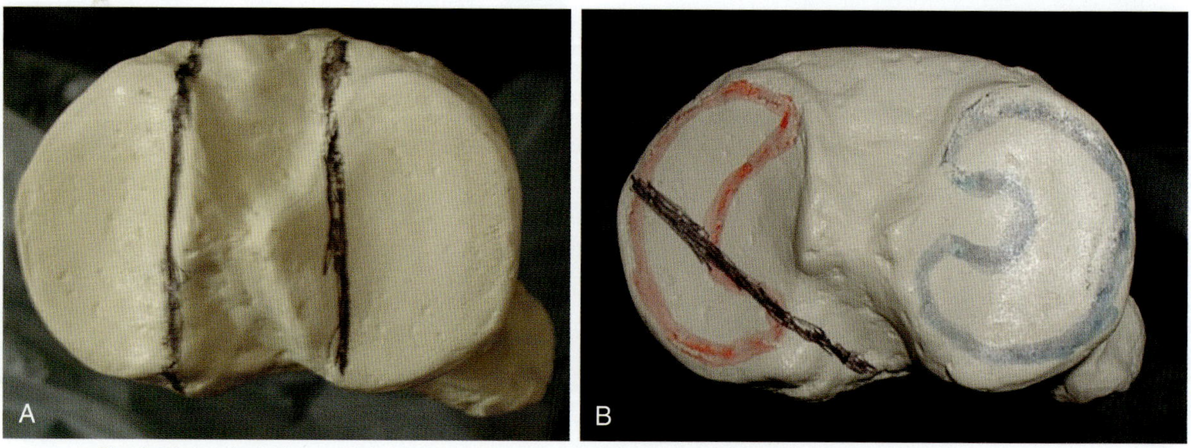

Fig. 5.19 Synthetic bone models with medial fracture lines depicted. Fracture lines oriented in a more anterior to posterior direction (A) may be amenable to treatment without medial based fixation in some cases. Medial fracture lines that run more closely to the coronal plane (B), however, often require a medial approach for fixation. (Pictures courtesy Jim Widmaier, MD.)

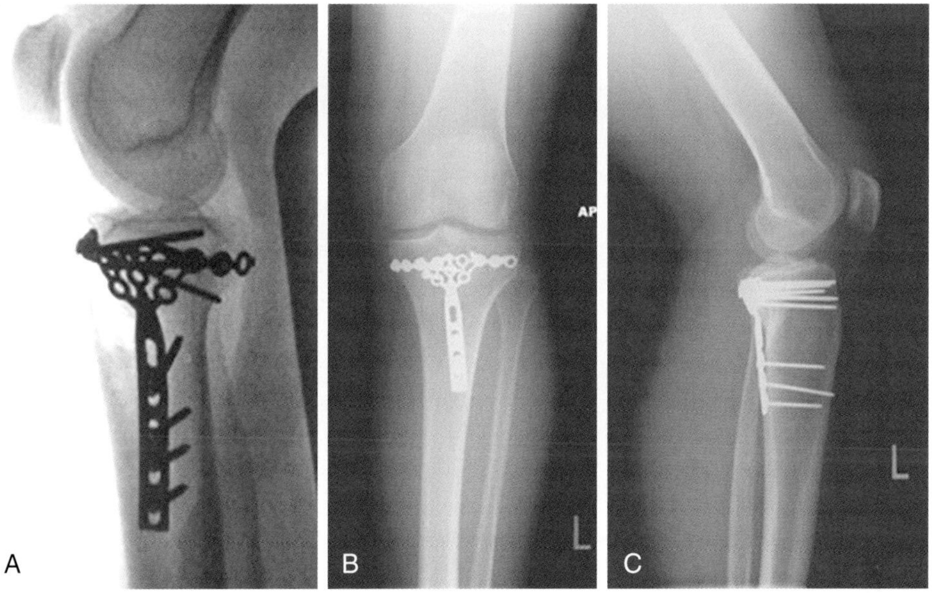

Fig. 5.20 Buttress plating through a posterior medial incision reaching anterior and posterior around the tibial articular surface to stabilize comminution (A). Through flexion at the knee and external rotation of the tibia, plates can be placed posterior with the patient supine using a posteromedial approach as seen on these anteroposterior and lateral views (B and C).

in posteromedial fractures and may result in displacement prior to healing.

Posterior fracture fragments can often be captured through a posteromedial approach. A malleable retractor can be used to retract the gastrocnemius laterally. Through flexion at the knee and external rotation of the tibia, greater access to the posterior plateau can be reached through the posteromedial approach. Utilizing implants that can wrap around the posterior plateau proximally, posterior fragments can be effectively buttressed without the need to place the patient prone and perform a direct posterior approach (Fig. 5.20).

Posterolateral fracture fragments are approached through extension of the anterolateral approach, direct posterior approach, or direct posterolateral approach (Chapter 1). These fragments are often comminuted and/or depressed and are reduced back into place utilizing the techniques described earlier. Small plates can then be contoured and placed along the posterolateral rim to support the reduced fracture (Fig. 5.21).

MINIMALLY INVASIVE PLATE OSTEOSYNTHESIS

Minimally invasive plating of tibial plateau fractures can take different forms. In cases of nondisplaced articular surfaces or in extraarticular proximal tibia fractures, direct joint visualization may not be necessary, and small incisions for plate insertion may be desirable (especially in the cases of patients with comorbidities and concurrent soft-tissue injuries that may put them at higher risk of wound complications). Additionally, in cases where articular displacement is present with metaphyseal comminution, a combined technique whereby direct joint visualization can be performed through an open approach proximally and submuscular plate insertion with percutaneous screw fixation can be performed distally is useful.

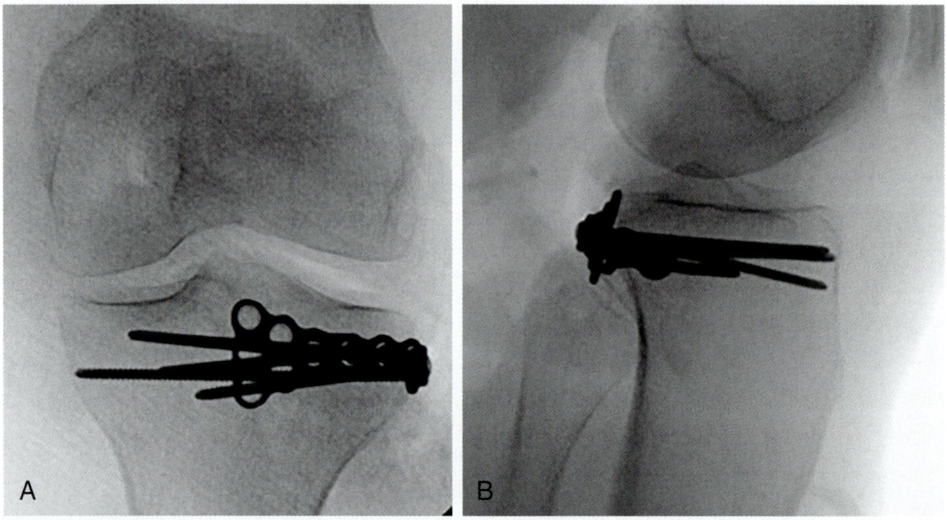

Fig. 5.21 A 2.7-mm locking plate used to buttress a posterolateral tibial plateau fracture placed through a direct posterolateral approach with the patient in a lateral position (A and B).

CASE 5.2

A 41-year-old male was cleaning his boat in his driveway and jumped approximately 5 feet off the back developing pain in the left knee. The patient presented to the emergency department with left knee pain and mild swelling. The patient was hemodynamically stable and neurovascularly intact without signs of compartment syndrome. There were no other injuries (Fig. 5.22).

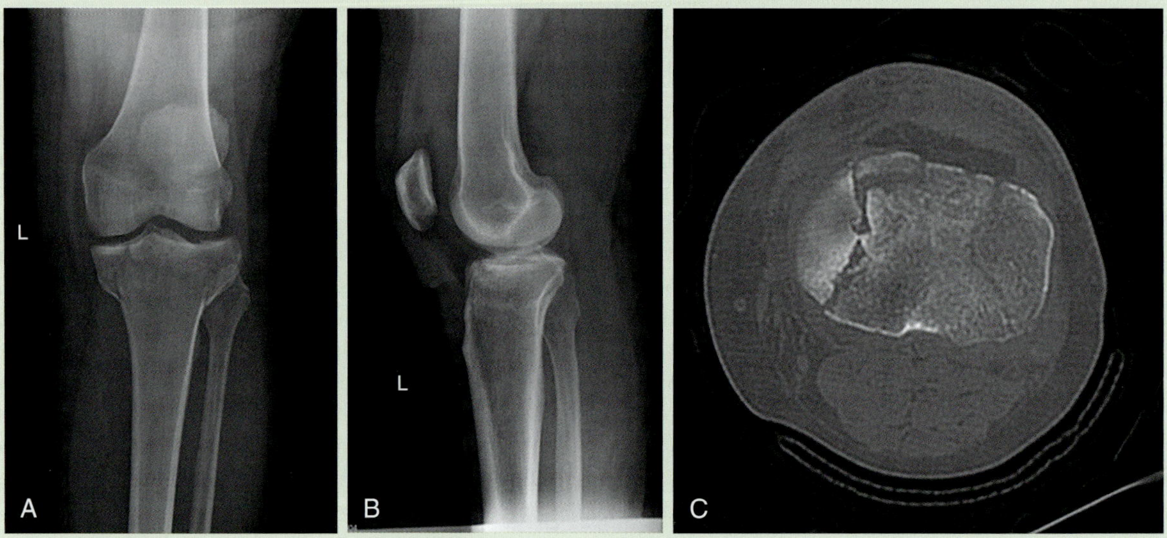

Fig. 5.22 X-rays (A and B) and computed tomographic scan (C) showing a bicondylar (Schatzker type V) tibial plateau fracture with minimal displacement.

CASE 5.2—CONT'D

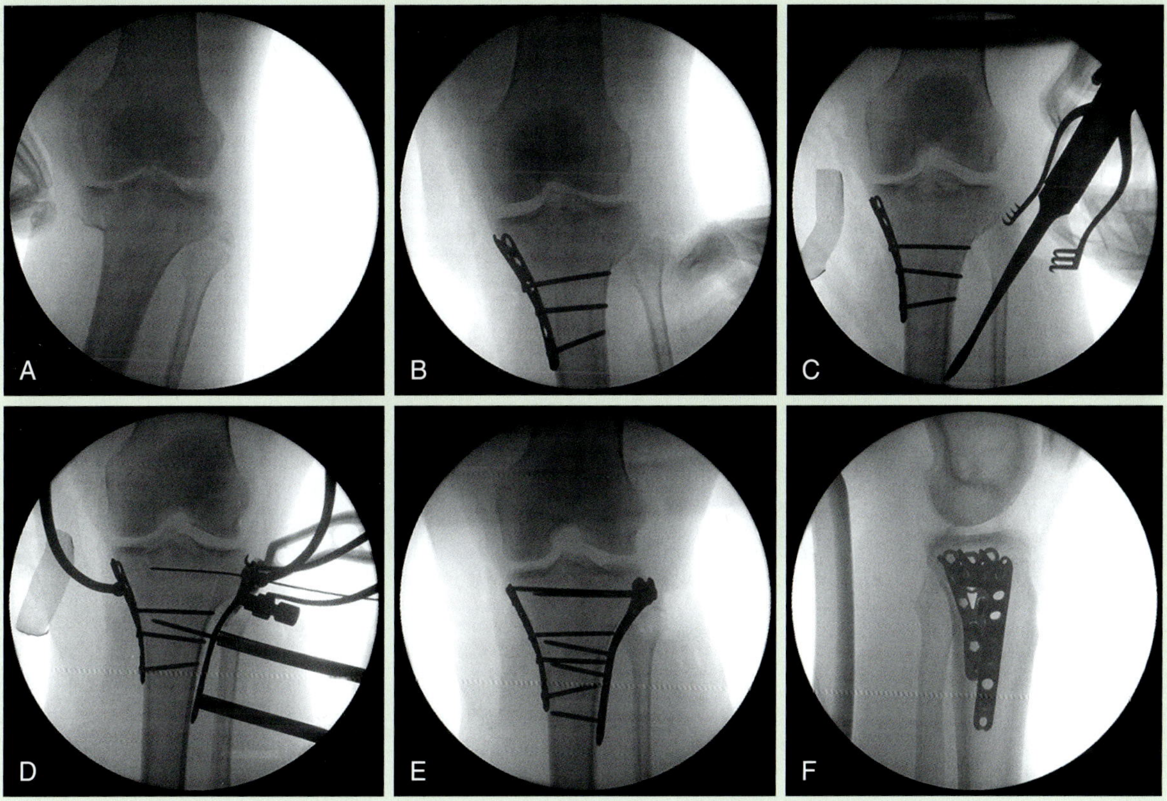

Fig. 5.23 Intraoperative x-rays. Varus stress examination under anesthesia demonstrates significant coronal plane instability (A). Medial buttress plating performed first through a medial incision (B). Note proximal screw holes left empty to avoid interfering with lateral reduction and fixation. A Cobb elevator placed laterally to elevate anterior musculature in preparation for placement of lateral plate using minimally invasive plate osteosynthesis technique (C). Lateral plate applied with compression clamp proximally and push-pull device at the apex of the fracture (D). Anteroposterior (E) and lateral (F) views of the final construct.

The patient was taken to the operating room the following day (Fig. 5.23). Coronal plane instability was seen on stress examination. Open medial buttress plating was performed, followed by lateral plating through a minimally invasive approach.

The patient healed his fractures uneventfully and returned to his preinjury functional status (Fig. 5.24).

Continued

CASE 5.2—CONT'D

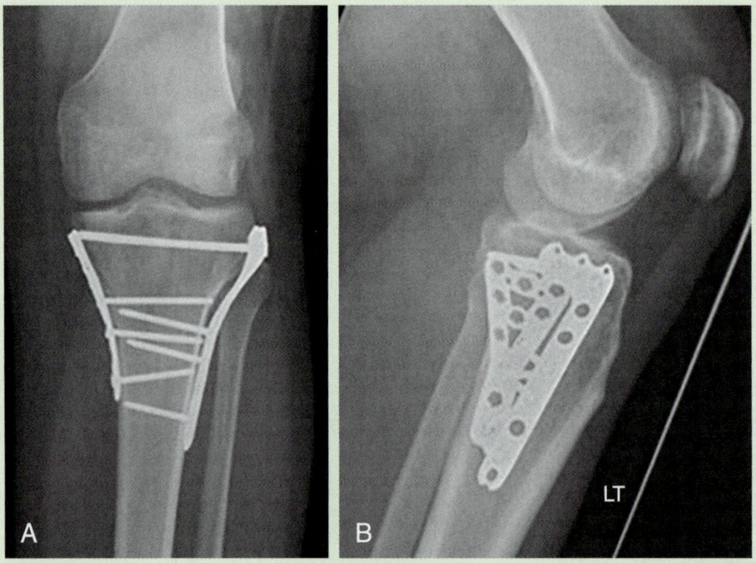

Fig. 5.24 Anteroposterior (A) and lateral (B) views at 6 months postoperatively.

CASE 5.3

A 28-year-old male restrained passenger in a motor vehicle collision (MVC) was brought to the emergency department by ambulance with right knee pain and mild swelling, but no breaks in the overlying skin. The patient also presented with chest pain and left shoulder pain (shoulder x-rays negative for fracture). The patient was hemodynamically stable. The patient's Glasgow Coma Scale (GCS) score was 15 and serum lactate was elevated. Computed tomography (CT) scan of the chest showed pulmonary contusions. Bilateral upper and lower extremities were neurovascularly intact, calf was soft and compressible without compartment syndrome (Fig. 5.25).

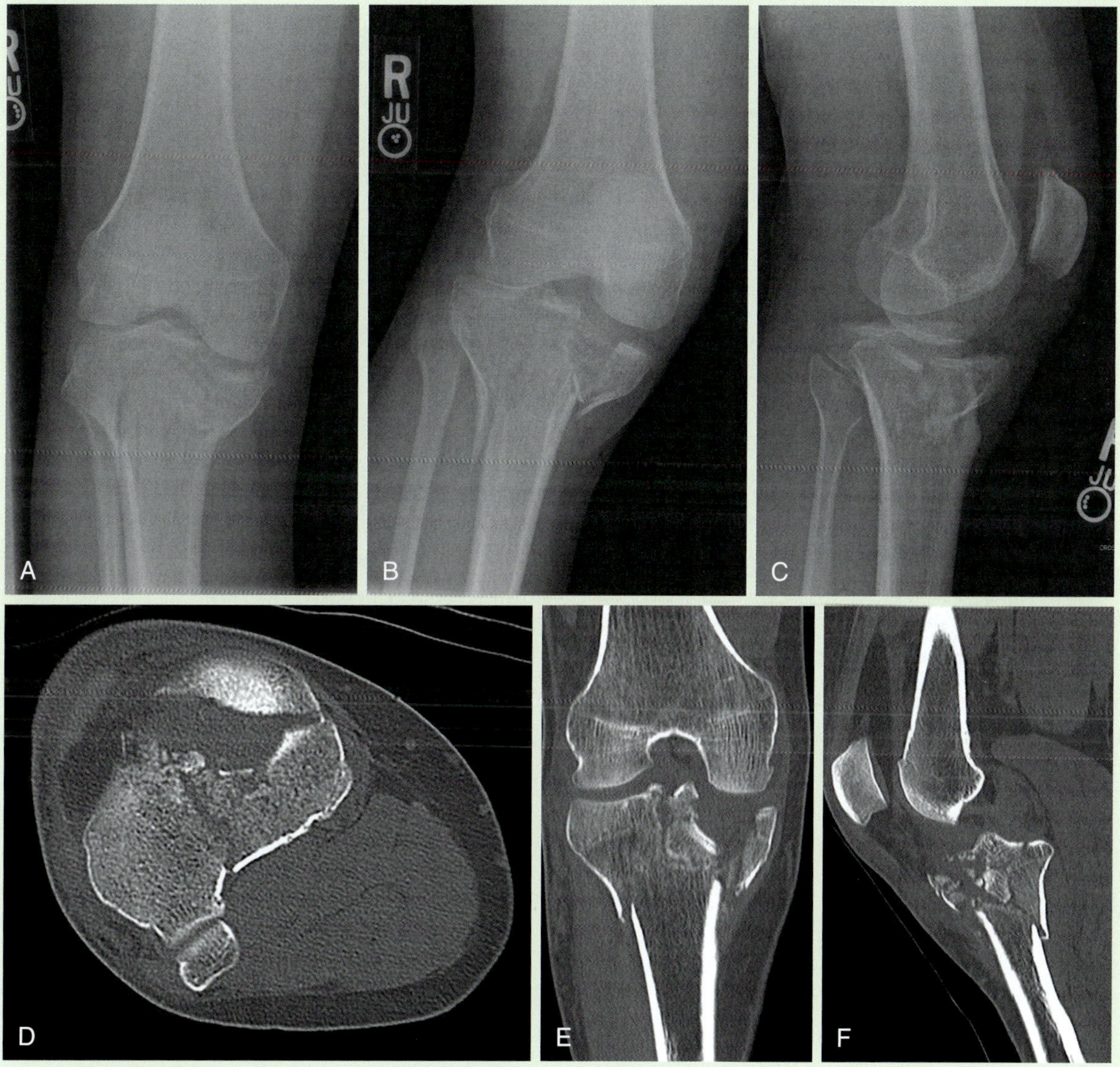

Fig. 5.25 Preoperative x-rays (A–C) and computed tomography (CT) scan (D–F) demonstrating a bicolumnar (Schatzker type VI) tibial plateau fracture. A posteromedial fracture fragment can be readily appreciated on CT scan axial view (D). This is a length unstable fracture with shortening and deformity.

Continued

CASE 5.3—CONT'D

The leg was initially splinted, and the patients taken to the operating room for external fixation (Fig. 5.26) employing damage control orthopedic techniques to assist with ongoing resuscitation, allow the patient's lung function to improve, and for local soft-tissue swelling to subside prior to proceeding with the added surgical insult from definitive fixation. Nine days after external fixation, the patient returned to the operating room for external fixator removal and definitive fixation utilizing a dual approach and medial and lateral plates to provide stable fixation. Given the high degree of medial comminution and the separate posteromedial fracture fragment (seen most reliably on axial CT views), this injury was best treated with medial and lateral plates (Fig. 5.27).

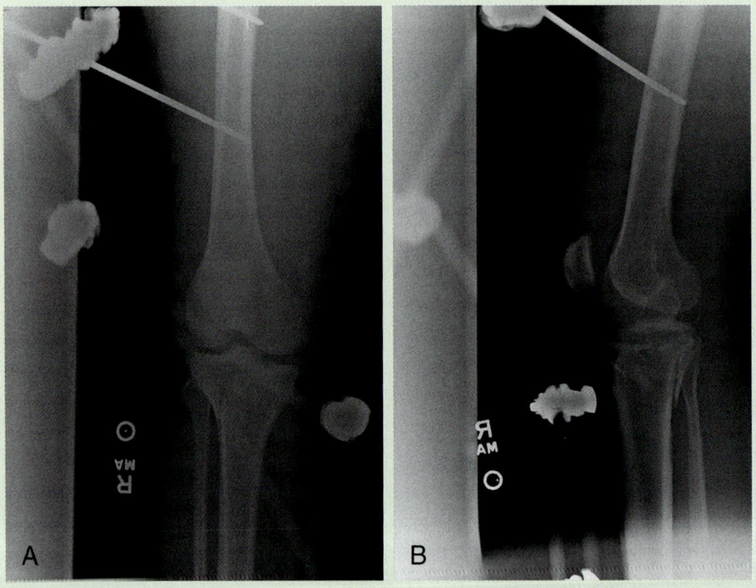

Fig. 5.26 X-rays following external fixation spanning the knee (A and B). Length has been restored, and stability was provided by external fixation while awaiting definitive treatment.

CASE 5.3—CONT'D

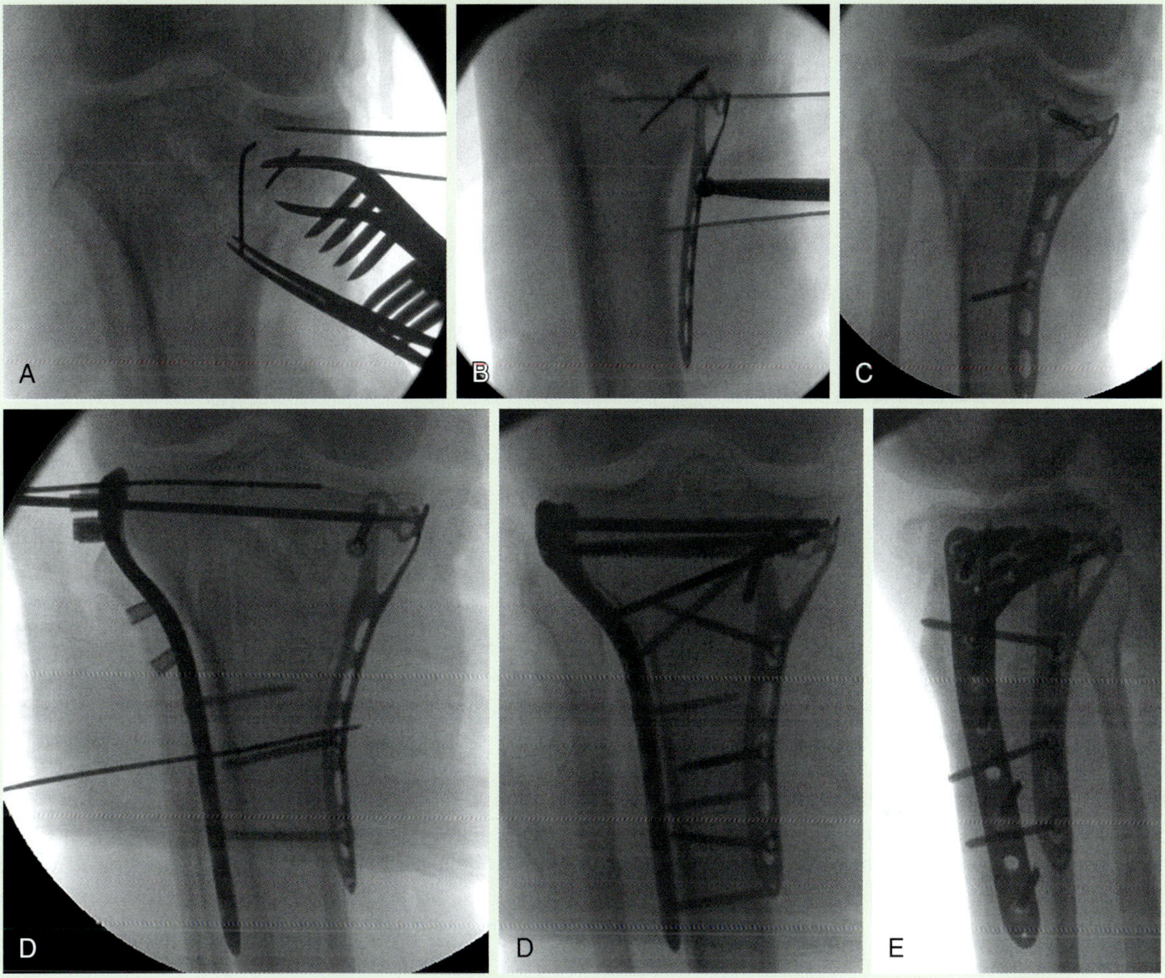

Fig. 5.27 Intraoperative imaging. Reduction/elevation of medial articular fragments (A). Application of undercontoured medial plate held in place with ball spike (B). Nonlocking screw first placed in the shaft portion of the plate to compress to bone (C). Application of lateral plate with nonlocking screw placed at the apex of the fracture to compress plate to bone (D). Note that at this point, fixation has been left out of the proximal portion of the medial plate to avoid blocking lateral reduction. Final anteroposterior (E) and lateral (F) views.

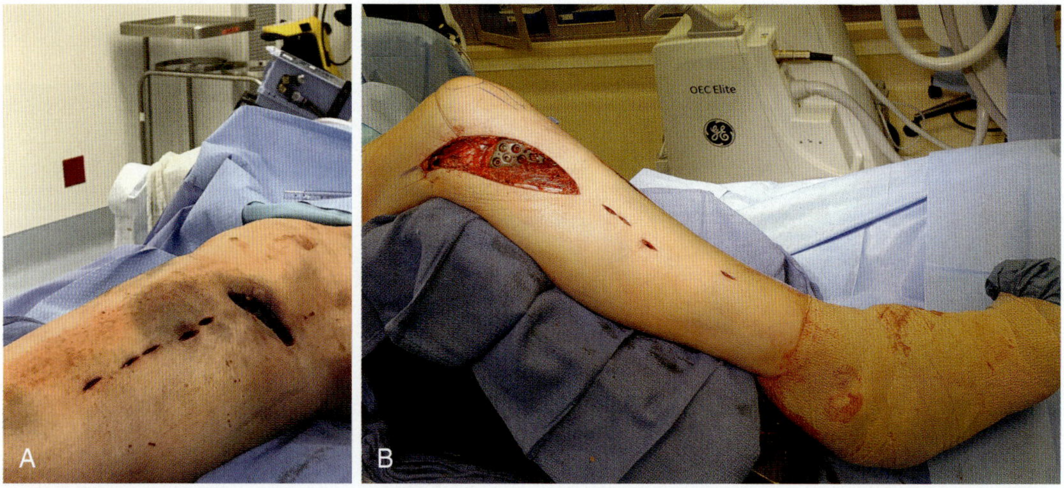

Fig. 5.28 Minimally invasive approaches for tibial plateau fracture plating (A and B). Note that a submeniscal arthrotomy was performed in (B) providing direct visualization of the joint.

Minimally invasive plate osteosynthesis (MIPO) techniques in tibial plateau fracture treatment most often involve lateral locked plating. Often, it is possible to make an angled incision directly overlying the lateral plateau that is just large enough to accommodate the proximal attachments to a plateau plate–aiming arm or, if an insertion jig is not being used and the incision large enough, to perform a submeniscal arthrotomy and to directly visualize the proximal row(s) of the plate being used (Fig. 5.28). Through this proximal incision, direct joint visualization, reduction, and provisional fixation can be performed through the techniques for the anterolateral approach described earlier. A plate can then be inserted submuscularly along the lateral surface of the tibia. Once the plate is placed and determined radiographically to be centered on the tibia on the lateral view and placed at the appropriate superior to inferior location, K-wires are placed proximally and distally through the plate to hold it in place. If difficulty is encountered in centering the plate, K-wires can be placed percutaneously to "block" the plate into the proper position (Fig. 5.29). Direct manipulation of the leg and traction can help to realign the mechanical axis of the tibia in the coronal and sagittal planes. Bumps can also be placed under the leg to help reduce sagittal deformity. Nonlocking screws and/or push/pull devices can be used to bring the plate down to bone when desired and to help perform additional reduction when necessary (Fig. 5.30).

Locking or nonlocking screws can be placed in the proximal portion of the plate as indicated. Screws can also be placed in the shaft portion of the plate either using insertion instruments/cannulas or by using x-ray and "feel." Several commercially available insertion guides exist that attach to tibial plateau locking plates and line up with screw holes in the plate to aid in screw insertion. Cannulas are used to place K-wires, drill bits, and screws (Fig. 5.31). Care should be taken in placing distal screws in long plates that extend down the leg into close proximity to the superficial peroneal nerve. Outer cannulas should be placed with inner trocars in place followed by placement of an inner drill bit cannula. Once the tibia has been drilled and measured off of the drill bit, the drill sleeve is removed, and the screw can be placed down the outer cannula and into the plate. Some surgeons prefer percutaneous insertion without the use of a guide. In those instances, or when a guide is not available, insertion can be performed using x-ray to localize incision, drill bit placement, and screw placement. AP and lateral views can be used to ensure that the incision is made at the

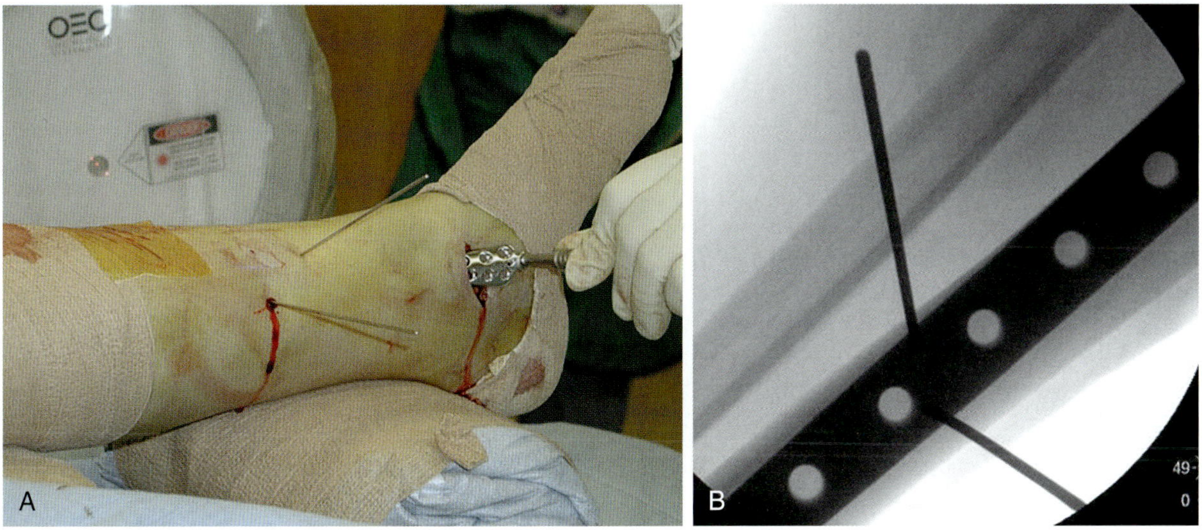

Fig. 5.29 "Blocking wire" technique used for minimally invasive plate placement. Clinical photograph (A) and x-ray (B). In this case, the technique was used for a medial distal tibia plate but is applicable to tibial plateau plating as well. Wires can be placed anterior and/or posterior to direct the path of the plate to sit in the middle of the bone. This technique is especially useful when placing longer plates percutaneously.

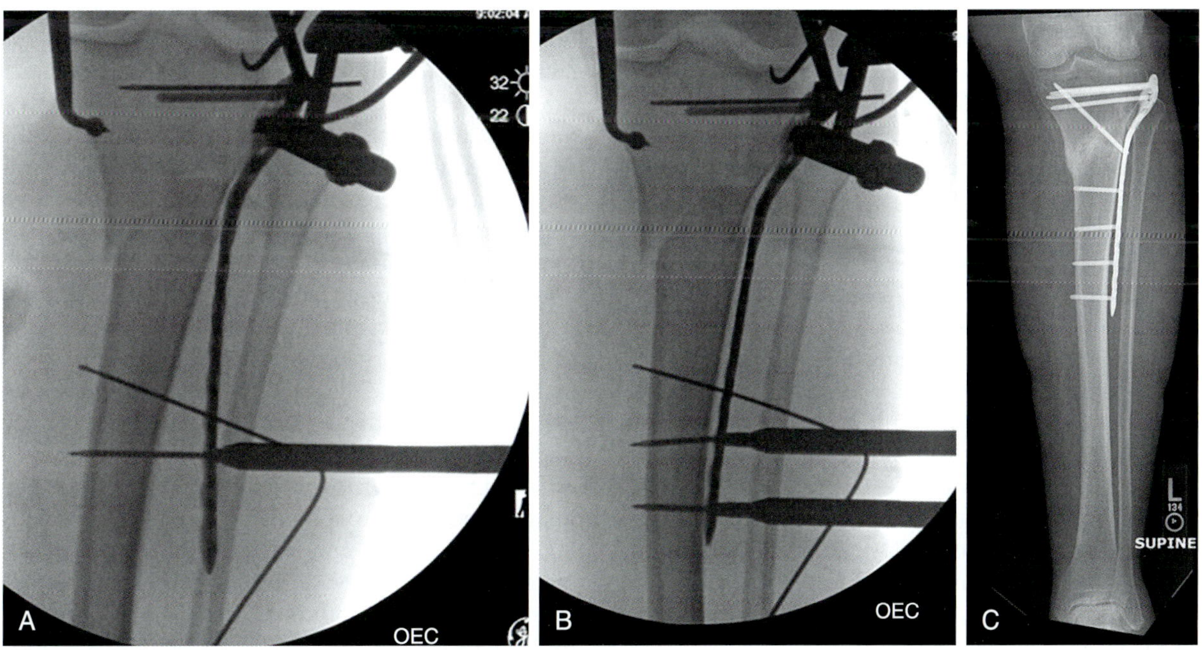

Fig. 5.30 After minimally invasive plate osteosynthesis application of the plate and insertion of one proximal locking screw, varus deformity remains (A). Push/pull devices are applied through the insertion jig and cannulas and used to pull the distal fragment to the plate, reducing the coronal plane deformity (B). Final anteroposterior x-ray (C).

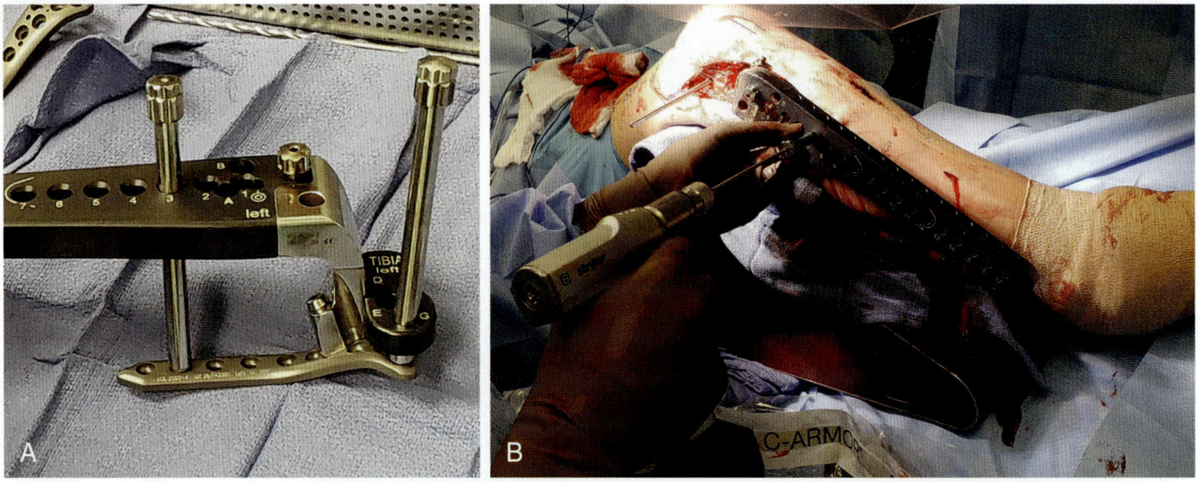

Fig. 5.31 Insertion guide and cannulas used for percutaneous placement of lateral tibial plateau plates (A and B). Two important features of these aiming systems are that they consistently hit their targets and that the attachment to the plate takes up a small footprint proximally (to allow for small insertion incisions). When reduction forces are applied with long plates, deforming forces can occur on the plate causing aiming arms to miss. It is important, therefore, with longer plates to form connections proximally and distally at the beginning of screw insertion. Distal K-wires (or drills, or push/pull devices) can be left in place through cannulas, increasing the accuracy of the more proximal shaft screw insertion. Finally, after placing more proximal screws, the most distal screws can be placed.

proper location. The incision is made through skin only, and a hemostat is used to spread the soft tissues down to the plate. The drill bit can then be inserted into the wound and can be used to feel the outline of the plate hole, and x-ray can be used to confirm drill bit placement. After drilling, the screw can be inserted, again through feel and by utilizing x-ray if needed.

With nearly all orthopedic applications of plates, all plate holes need not (and perhaps should not) be filled with screws. This is especially true when utilizing MIPO techniques. While the exact best ratio of screw holes left empty to those filled is unknown (biomechanical and clinical studies have produced conflicting results), the author recommends one-half to two-thirds density for screws in the shaft of a tibial plateau plate when performing MIPO. With four screws spread out and placed in the distal segment, this ensures that a long enough plate will be used to allow for a sufficient working length that will spread forces out over a greater plate area.

NAILING

Intramedullary nail treatment of proximal tibia fractures may be with nail alone (as in the case of extra-articular proximal tibia fractures) or in combination with plates and/or screws. Proximal tibia metaphyseal fractures (such as AO/OTA type A fractures) may be amenable to intramedullary nail treatment as a minimally invasive and biomechanically advantageous treatment.[8] Proximal fragment extension (or apex anterior fracture deformity) and valgus angulation are commonly encountered deformities in these fractures. Although nailing can be performed in a hyperflexed position, semiextended nailing (suprapatellar or semiextended extra-articular) approaches can be helpful in such cases in order to help prevent flexion deformity at the fracture site. These approaches are performed with the patient supine with a bump under the hip and the operative extremity elevated on a radiolucent platform (in order to obtain lateral images without the contralateral extremity obscuring a lateral view), and the knee is flexed approximately 15 to 20 degrees. The suprapatellar approach is made with a longitudinal incision just proximal to the patella, and the quadriceps tendon is sharply incised in line with its fibers. Specialized instrumentation is then required to traverse the patellofemoral joint down to the tibial starting point. With the

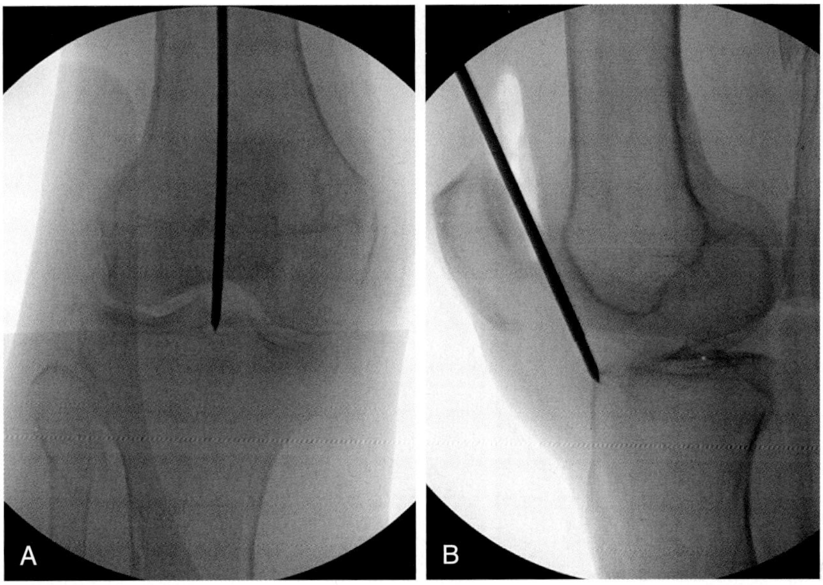

Fig. 5.32 Correct starting point for tibial nailing with the wire at the medial aspect of the lateral tibial spine on anteroposterior view (A) and at the anterior edge of the articular margin on perfect lateral view of the tibial plateau (B).

semiextended extra-articular approach, an incision is made lateral to the patella. The retinacular layer of the knee is incised, and the synovial layer is left intact. Working distally within this plane, the starting point can be accessed (posterior to the patellar tendon and anterior to the knee fat pad).

The starting point for nailing in proximal tibia fractures should be obtained with care, as a starting point too medial may cause accentuation of valgus deformity. The correct starting point is the medial aspect of the lateral tibial spine on the AP view and the anterior edge of the articular margin on the perfect lateral view.[9] With rotation of the tibia, an incorrect starting point can look correct, so careful attention must be given to limb positioning. On the AP view, correct positioning is confirmed with either a "fibular bisector radiograph" (lateral tibial plateau lines up with a point that bisects the fibula into halves)[10] or a "twin peaks AP view" (AP view with the sharpest profile of the tibial spines)[11] (Fig. 5.32). On the lateral view, the medial and lateral tibial plateaus should overlap. A slightly more lateral starting point may be appropriate in some cases to help avoid valgus deformity.[12]

As with many nailing procedures, it is extremely important when nailing proximal tibia fractures that reduction is achieved prior to nailing (Box 5.3).

BOX 5.3 Reduction Techniques for Proximal Tibial Nailing

- Poller screws
- Pointed clamps
- Joysticks
- Distractor
- Ringed external fixator
- Unicortical plating

One very useful and minimally invasive technique to aid in reduction of deformity in proximal tibia fractures is the use of "poller" or "blocking" screws, first described by Dr. David Seligson in 1983 and later by others.[13,14] These screws decrease the effective intramedullary space, "forcing" the nail along a certain path within the bone and preventing the nail from taking a line that will allow deformity to persist. As a general rule, these screws are placed first in the shorter bone segment on the concave side of the deformity (i.e., lateral on a valgus deformity, posterior on a flexion deformity) (Figs. 5.33 and 5.34). If additional screws are needed to increase stability or improve reduction, they can be placed as well

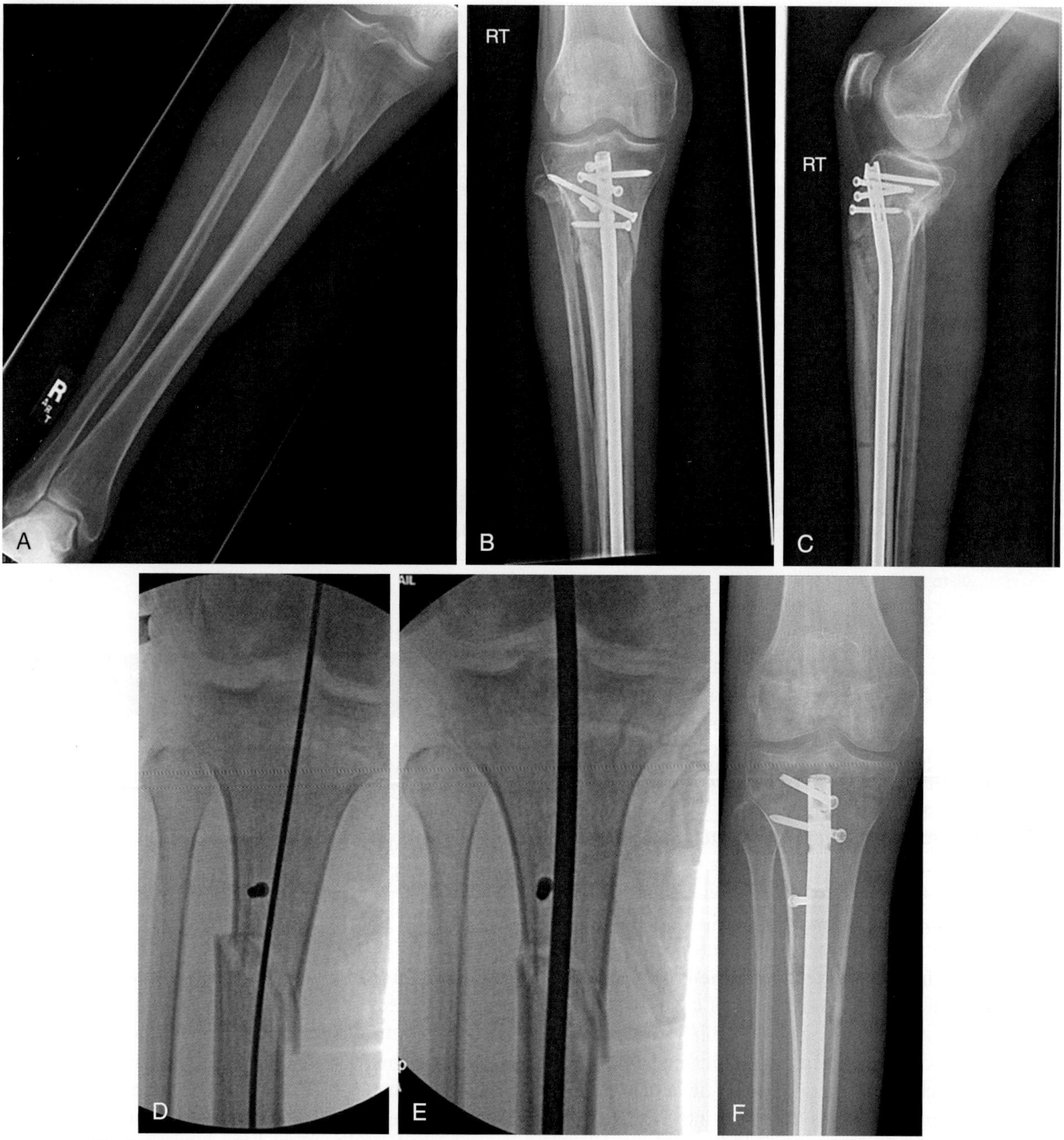

Fig. 5.33 Blocking screws used to correct coronal plane deformity. Valgus deformity is seen in this proximal tibia fracture (A). Final x-rays with a blocking screw having been placed lateral (concave side) to the expected path of the nail in the proximal (short) segment (B and C). The tibia fracture depicted in (D) shows a translational deformity rather than an angular deformity. In this case, the screw is placed lateral in the canal to force the nail more medially, allowing the proximal segment to line up with the shaft (E and F).

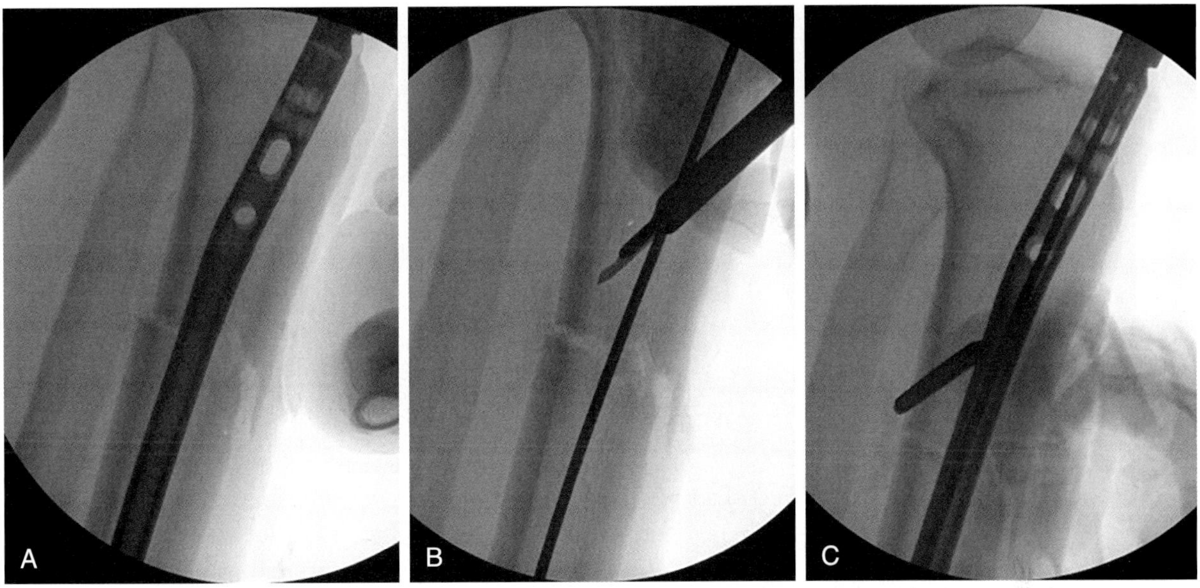

Fig. 5.34 Blocking screws used to correct sagittal plane deformity. In this case, the proximal segment shows a slight anterior translational and extension deformity with nail passage (A). The nail is removed, and location for blocking screw placement is determined using C-arm (B). Deformity correction following blocking screw and nail placement (C).

(place screws in the location where you do not want the nail to go). While ideally these screws are placed prior to reaming and reaming is done with the fracture reduced, there are instances where nail passage results in deformity prior to placing blocking screws. In this instance, removing the nail, placing blocking screws, and passing reamers again followed by nail insertion can result in successful reduction.

Placement of clamps (periarticular clamps, Weber clamps) through small percutaneous incisions can be helpful in reducing proximal tibia fractures. Using a Schanz pin as a "joystick" to manipulate fracture fragments is another technique that can be employed. Use of a distractor and that of a half-ringed external fixator connected to skinny wires are other techniques that can be used to help maintain reduction.[15,16] Olive wires or cerclage wires can be used to adjust translational deformities after length has been reestablished with threaded rods. When using skinny wires and a ringed frame, it is important to place wires parallel to the proximal and distal tibial articular surfaces prior to attachment to the rings, so when traction is applied, angular deformities will be corrected. Staples can be used as low-profile extramedullary implants that can help reduce fracture fragments. Finally, unicortical plate placement is another strategy that can be helpful in reduction of proximal tibia fractures (Fig. 5.35). After exposure of the fracture site, a low-profile plate can be placed to hold fracture reduction while nailing. While the plate can be placed at various points around the tibia, posteromedial plate placement may be advantageous as this location is readily accessible yet allows for greater soft-tissue coverage over the plate and may provide a biomechanical advantage as well. Cortical screws may be placed initially to aid in reduction, but unicortical locking screws are often utilized to avoid getting in the way of eventual nail placement. Bicortical screws may be desired at times to serve the dual purpose of holding the plate in place and acting as blocking screws.

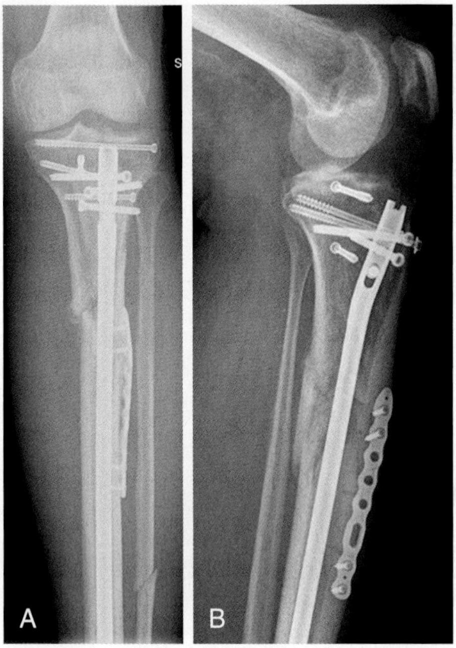

Fig. 5.35 Anteroposterior (A) and lateral (B) views of unicortical plate used as a reduction aid in proximal tibial nailing.

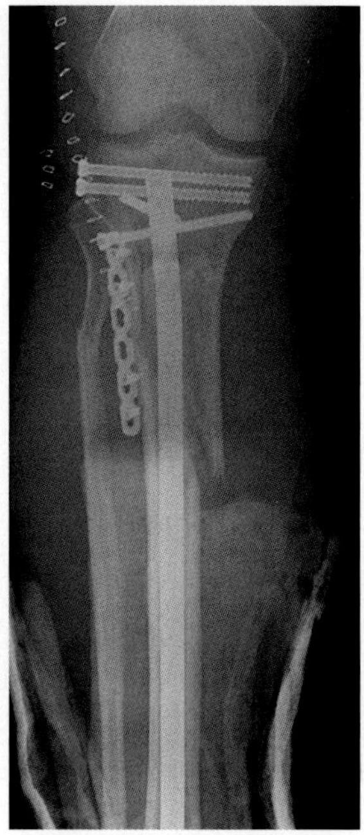

Fig. 5.36 Tibial plateau fracture treated with large cannulated lag screws providing joint compression and a tibial nail.

Proximal tibial fractures involving the articular surface (AO/OTA type C fractures) may be amenable to nail treatment as well, especially when high degrees of metaphyseal comminution or shaft extension is present. These fractures require additional implants to address the articular surface portion of the fracture. With nondisplaced articular fractures, this can often be accomplished with partially threaded cannulated screws with or without a washer (Fig. 5.36). In such instances, treatment can often be performed in a minimally invasive manner. Large cannulated screws are placed prior to nailing and are placed outside of the projected path of the nail (posteriorly). Percutaneous clamping of the tibial plateau may be desirable prior to placement of the screws. Screws are placed from the side (medial or lateral) where the plateau split is present.

Proximal tibiofibular joint disruption is an occasionally overlooked injury that can be present with proximal tibia fractures. Failure to recognize dislocation can result in long-term deformity and pain. Treatment may consist of open reduction and fixation with screws (Fig. 5.37) or with suture fixation similar to that used for the distal tibiofibular joint (i.e., Arthrex Tightrope or Internal Brace, Arthrex Inc., Naples, FL).

With more complex articular fractures involving displacement and associated metaphyseal/diaphyseal comminution, an open approach may be necessary. As described in Chapter 1 and earlier in this chapter, a direct anterior midline approach or a mini-lateral approach with arthrotomy can be made to expose the fracture for reduction and to expose the lateral tibia for plating. The articular fracture is reduced as previously described, and a lateral plate is placed. Often, avoiding the use of the most anterior screw holes in the proximal rows of a plate will avoid the nail insertion point. If screws have been placed that will interfere with the path of the nail, then after articular reduction and plate placement, these screws can be removed or replaced with unicortical screws (Fig. 5.38).

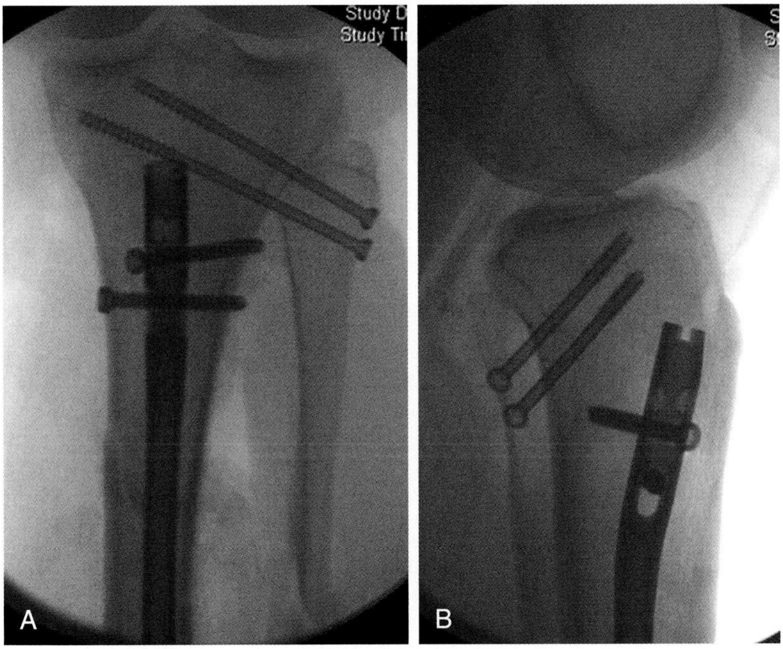

Fig. 5.37 Treatment of proximal tibiofibular joint dislocation with two cannulated screws (A and B). The peroneal nerve was visualized and protected prior to joint reduction and hardware placement.

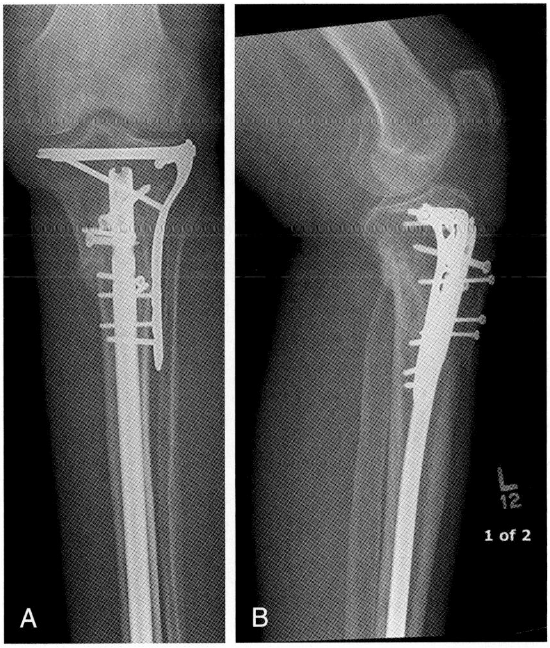

Fig. 5.38 Tibial plateau fracture treated with proximal tibia locking plate and tibial nail. The articular surface is first reduced, and the plate is applied. One shaft screw is placed (aimed posteriorly) along with the more posterior proximal row screws. With the articular surface stabilized, the nail is then placed. Additional screws can then be placed through the plate around the nail. Anteroposterior (A) and lateral (B) x-rays after healing.

CASE 5.4

A 39-year-old male involved in a motorcycle collision was brought to the emergency department via ambulance. The patient was hemodynamically stable. Closed injury to the left tibia was present along with multiple abrasions on all four extremities. There were no additional fractures, closed head injury was present (Fig. 5.39).

The patient was resuscitated in the emergency department, and the leg was initially splinted. The patient was taken to the operating room the following day for tibial fixation (Fig. 5.40). Given the high degree of both intraarticular and metaphyseal comminution, it was felt that this case would best be definitively treated through a direct anterior approach and nail/plate combination fixation (Fig. 5.41). Cancellous bone allograft was used to fill the metaphyseal void after articular surface reduction. In this case, an incisional negative pressure wound therapy dressing was placed to increase perfusion to the soft tissues around the incision.

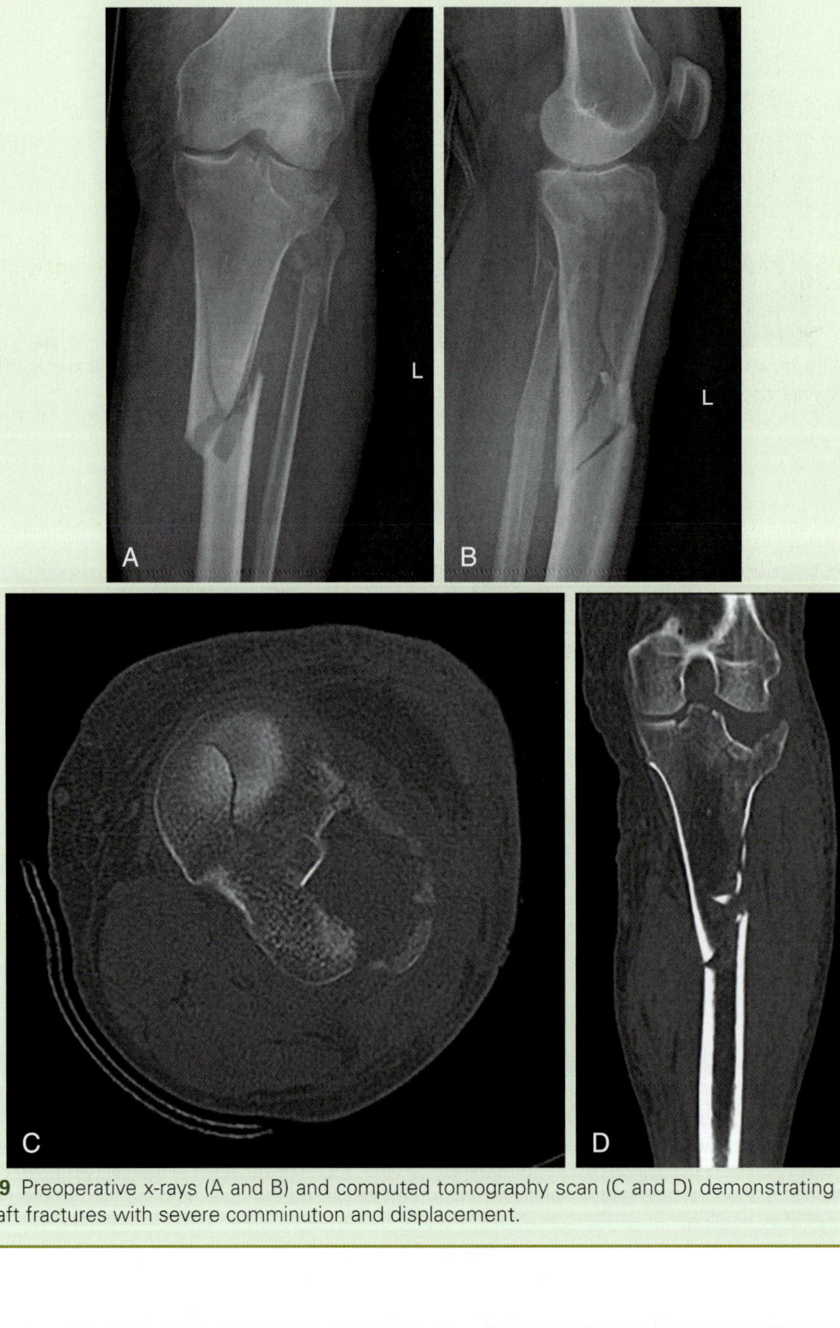

Fig. 5.39 Preoperative x-rays (A and B) and computed tomography scan (C and D) demonstrating tibial plateau/shaft fractures with severe comminution and displacement.

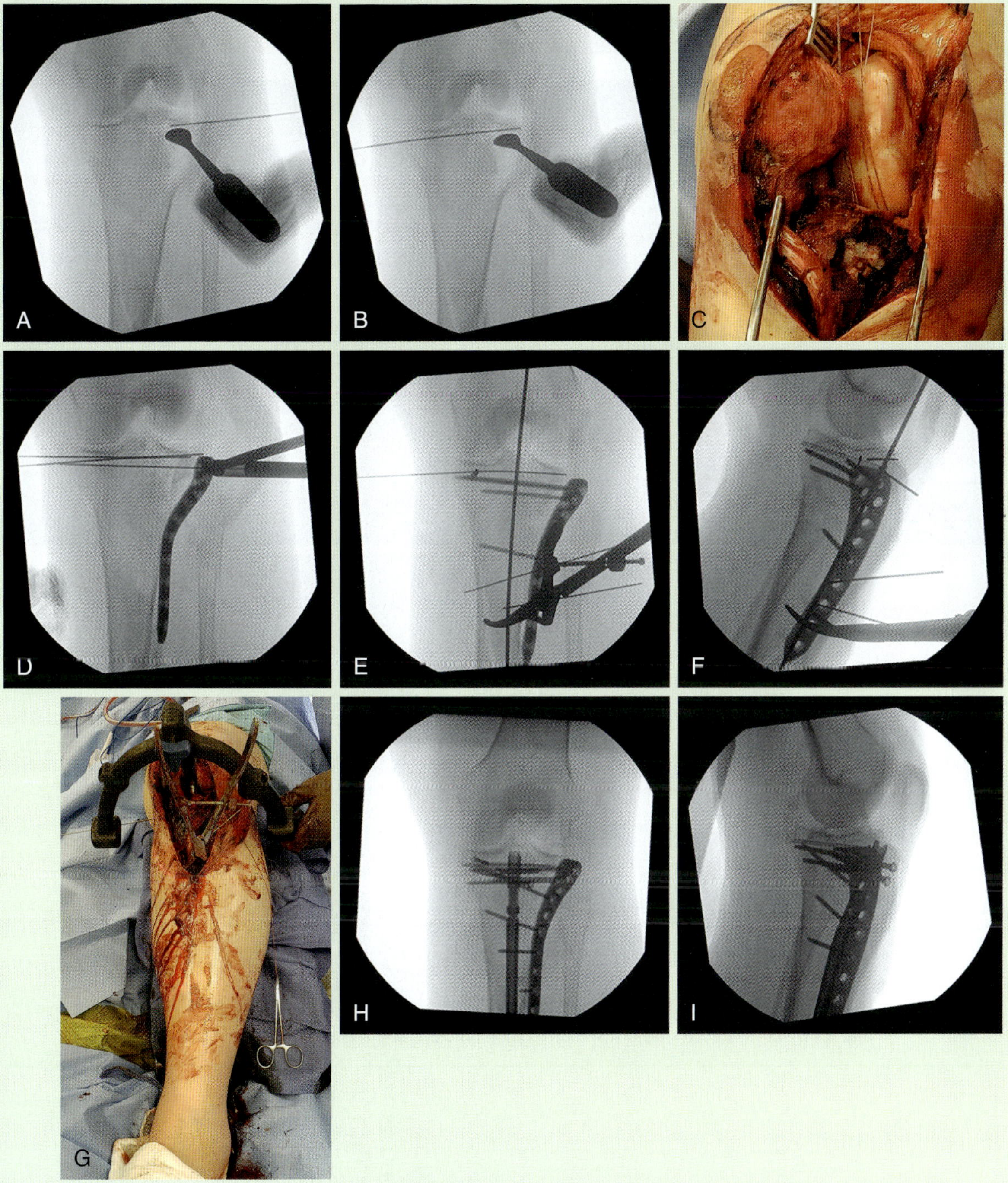

Fig. 5.40 Intraoperative x-rays and clinical images. Reduction of lateral tibial plateau comminution using a Cobb elevator to elevate the articular surface with underlying metaphyseal bone (A). K-wire then driven across fracture until the tip of the K-wire rests at the edge of the fragment, allowing reduction of additional lateral fracture fragments (B). Metaphyseal bone void packed with cancellous allograft (C). Lateral plate applied (D) and screws placed outside of expected path of the nail. Guidewire placed for tibial reaming anteroposterior (E) and lateral (F) views. Clinical photograph showing tibial nail insertion (G). (H and I) X-rays with nail and plate in place. A negative pressure dressing was utilized to help promote blood flow to injured soft tissues around the incision.

Continued

CASE 5.4—CONT'D

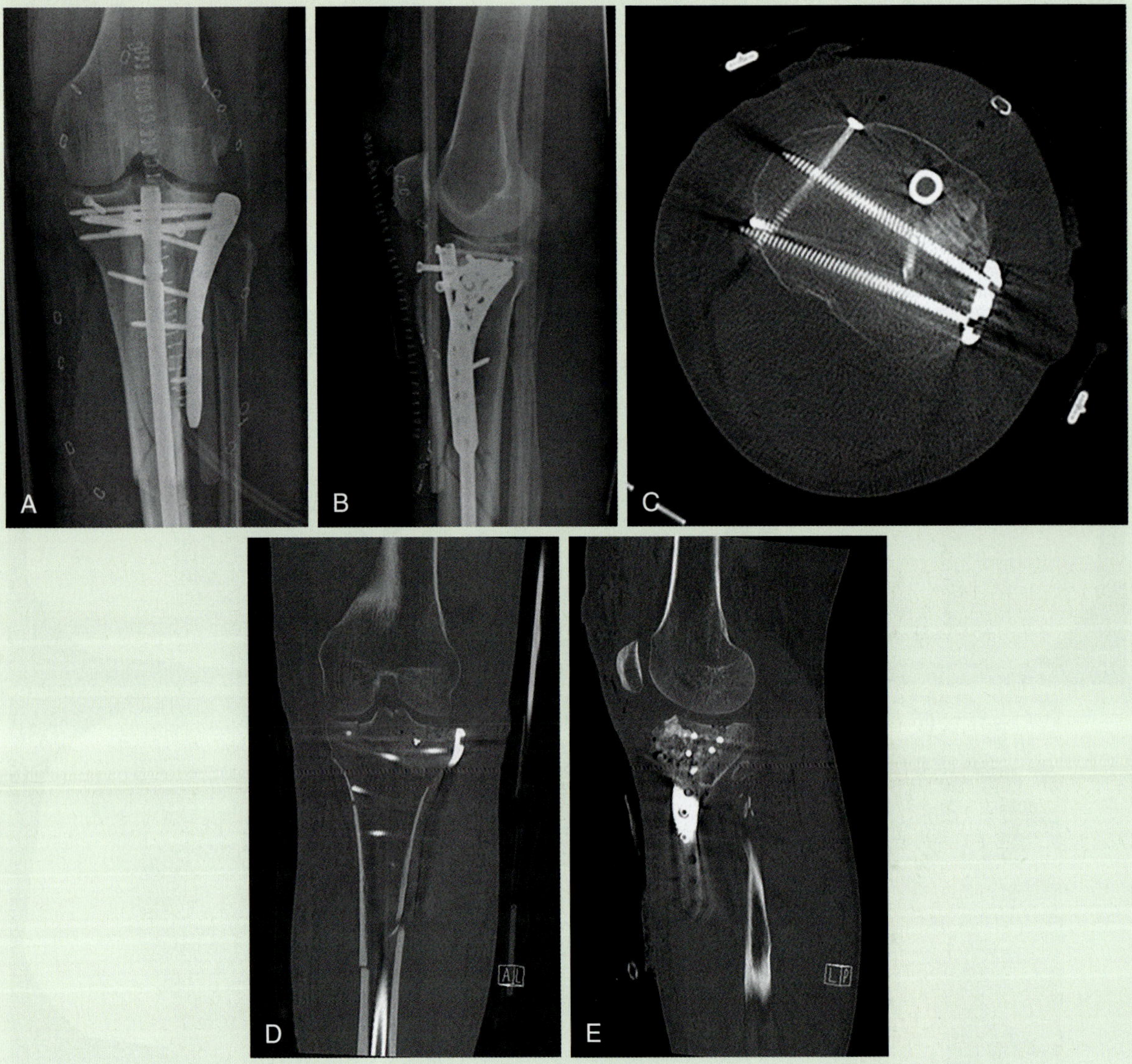

Fig. 5.41 Postoperative x-rays (A and B) and computed tomography scan (C–E) after fixation.

RIEHL'S TIPS AND TRICKS

- When there is difficulty with reducing a fracture, first assess exposure and consider increasing the exposure.
- A femoral distractor or external fixator can be an extremely helpful aid in exposure.
- Drive temporary K-wires through the opposite cortex and skin to prevent them getting in the way of reduction of additional articular fragments, lateral cortex, or plate placement.
- Bioabsorbable pins can help maintain reduction of central plateau fragments without interfering with reduction or fixation of more peripheral plateau fragments.
- Malleable plates with long extensions proximally can help significantly in capturing direct posterior and anteromedial fracture fragments through a posteromedial approach.
- Semiextended positioning can help reduce fracture deformity in proximal tibial fractures treated with intramedullary nails.
- Nail/plate combinations are an effective treatment for tibial plateau fractures with metaphyseal comminution.

REFERENCES

1. Johannsen AM, Cook AM, Gardner MJ, Bishop JA. Defining the width of the normal tibial plateau relative to the distal femur: Critical normative data for identifying pathologic widening in tibial plateau fractures. *Clinical Anatomy*. 2018;31(5):688–692.
2. Thamyongkit S, Fayad LM, Jones LC, Hasenboehler EA, Sirisreetreerux N, Shafiq B. The distal femur is a reliable guide for tibial plateau fracture reduction: A study of measurements on 3D CT scans in 84 healthy knees. *Journal of Orthopaedic Surgery and Research*. 2018;13(1):224.
3. Pizanis A, Garcia P, Pohlemann T, Burkhardt M. Balloon tibioplasty: a useful tool for reduction of tibial plateau depression fractures. *J Orthop Trauma*. 2012;26(7):e88–e93.
4. Vendeuvre T, Grunberg M, Germaneau A, et al. Contribution of minimally invasive bone augmentation to primary stabilization of the osteosynthesis of Schatzker type II tibial plateau fractures: Balloon vs bone tamp. *Clin Biomech (Bristol, Avon)*. 2018;59:27–33.
5. Kun Chan AC, Hin Chan AP, Hung YW, Lo CK, Ho Fan JC. A novel percutaneous screw fixation of posterolateral tibial plateau fracture using posterior cruciate ligament reconstruction femoral template: Technical note. *J Orthop Trauma Rehabilitation*. 2017;22:22–29.
6. Yin L, Chen K, Guo L, Cheng L, Wang F, et al. Identifying the functional flexion-extension axis of the knee: an in-vivo kinematics study. PLOS ONE. 10(6):e0128877. https://doi.org/10.1371/journal.pone.0128877
7. Welch RD, Zhang H, Bronson DG. Experimental tibial plateau fractures augmented with calcium phosphate cement or autologous bone graft. *J Bone Joint Surg Am*. 2003;85(2):222–231.
8. Chen HW, Liu GD, Ou S, Jiang XY, Fei J, Wu LJ. Comparison of three fixations for tibial plateau fractures by biomechanical study and radiographic observation. *Int J Surg*. 2015;13:292–296.
9. McConnell T, Tornetta 3rd P, Tilzey J, Casey D. Tibial portal placement: the radiographic correlate of the anatomic safe zone. *J Orthop Trauma*. 2001;15(3):207–209.
10. Walker RM, Zdero R, McKee MD, Waddell JP, Schemitsch EH. Ideal tibial intramedullary nail insertion point varies with tibial rotation. *J Orthop Trauma*. 2011;25(12):726–730.
11. Bible JE, Choxi AA, Dhulipala SC, Evans JM, Mir HR. Tibia-based referencing for standard proximal tibial radiographs during intramedullary nailing. *Am J Orthop (Belle Mead NJ)*. 2013;42(11):E95–E98.
12. Weninger P, Tschabitscher M, Traxler H, Pfafl V, Hertz H. Intramedullary nailing of proximal tibia fractures--an anatomical study comparing three lateral starting points for nail insertion. *Injury*. 2010;41(2):220–225.
13. Ricci WM, O'Boyle M, Borrelli J, Bellabarba C, Sanders R. Fractures of the proximal third of the tibial shaft treated with intramedullary nails and blocking screws. *J Orthop Trauma*. 2001;15(4):264–270.
14. Donald G, Seligson D. Treatment of tibial shaft fractures by percutaneous Küntscher nailing. Technical difficulties and a review of 50 consecutive cases. *Clin Orthop Relat Res*. 1983 Sep;(178):64–73.
15. Jackson M, Topliss CJ, Atkins RM. Fine wire frame-assisted intramedullary nailing of the tibia. *J Orthop Trauma*. 2003;17(3):222–224.
16. Belangero WD, Santos Pires RE, Livani B, Rossi FL, de Andrade ALL. Clothesline technique" for proximal tibial shaft fracture fixation using conventional intramedullary nail: a simple, useful, and inexpensive technique to prevent fracture malalignment. *Eur J Orthop Surg Traumatol*. 2018 May;28(4):721–725.

6

Treatment of Associated Soft-Tissue Injuries

John D. (JD) Adams Jr., MD

INTRODUCTION

Historically, restoring the bony architecture in tibial plateau fractures has been the focus of surgical management. While this remains the primary objective in treatment algorithms, management of the soft-tissue structures around the knee has become a secondary objective. Failure to address soft-tissue compromise can lead to continued pain or instability to the knee. This chapter focuses on the nature of the soft-tissue problem, recognizing the entire extent of injury, and surgical techniques to address specific ligament or meniscal pathology.

NOT JUST A BONE INJURY

The bones provide very little stability to the knee joint, in comparison to other highly constrained joints like the hip. Instead, the knee relies on a variety of soft-tissue structures to provide stability of this hinge joint. Ligaments, capsule, and the menisci provide important static stabilizers, and injury can result in instability and poor long-term outcomes. As a result, treatment plans that focus only on the bone, without addressing soft tissues, can fail to restore stability and may lead to a less than functional knee. Despite our best efforts in the treatment of tibial plateau fractures, patients continue to have pain, instability, deformity, wound complications, and stiffness.[1–4]

In the past, management of the soft tissues primarily focused on the skin and handling of the soft tissues during surgical management. The routine use of temporary external fixation and delaying definitive internal fixation until the inflammatory response of the soft tissues has resolved have led to lower wound complications.[1,3,5,6] While this tactic has certainly helped in managing the soft tissue, it only addresses part of the problem. More recently, an increased focus on the ligaments and menisci has been the topic of more clinical research.

While high-energy mechanisms are more commonly associated with soft-tissue injuries, low-energy injuries can also affect the ligaments and menisci. When angular, rotational, and axial loads are applied to the knee, both static and dynamic stabilizing structures can be injured. A large axial load is not as common in lower-energy mechanisms, but patients can certainly be exposed to rotational or angular loads.[1,6–9]

INCIDENCE OF SOFT-TISSUE INJURY IN TIBIAL PLATEAU FRACTURES

Bennett and Browner began to shed light on the associated injuries in tibial plateau fractures in 1994. By using a combination of diagnostic tools, soft-tissue injury was described in 30 patients with tibial plateau fractures. Overall, the incidence of soft-tissue injury was 56%. The most common pathology described was injury to the meniscus and medial collateral ligament (MCL), reported in 20% of patients. In addition, injury to the anterior cruciate ligament (ACL) was noted in 10% and 3% had injury to the lateral collateral ligament (LCL).[5,10] Specific soft-tissue injuries were also correlated with certain bony injuries. Injury to the MCL was commonly associated with Schatzker type II injuries, while injury to the meniscus was more common in type IV injuries.[5,11] A couple of years later, Colletti et al. highlighted the high incidence of soft-tissue injuries in these fractures.[12] Some form of soft-tissue injury was noted in 28 of 29 patients with acute tibial plateau fractures. The MCL was the most commonly injured ligament (55%), and the lateral meniscus was torn in 45% of patients. Most likely due to the sample size, they were not able to correlate certain soft-tissue injuries with fracture type or degree of articular depression. Interestingly, complete ligament disruptions and meniscal tears have been described even in minimally displaced plateau fractures.[13]

In 2005 and 2010, two large studies highlighted the incidence of soft-tissue injuries in tibial plateau fractures. Using magnetic resonance imaging (MRI), Gardner et al. evaluated 103 patients who underwent operative repair of a tibial plateau fracture.[14] Confirming Colleti's findings, 99% of patients had some form of soft-tissue pathology, with the most common injury being a tear of the lateral meniscus (91%). In addition to meniscal injury, complete tear or avulsion of at least one ligament was found in 77% of patients. The ACL was the most common ligament injured, followed by the LCL, MCL, and posterior cruciate ligament (PCL). Table 6.1 describes the specific incidences of injury to the ligaments and menisci. In addition to the larger sample size, Gardner et al. also highlighted other soft-tissue structures that may be injured in plateau fractures by specifically addressing the structures of the posterolateral corner (PLC). Of the 103 patients, tears of the popliteofibular ligament and/or the popliteus were found in 68%. Stannard et al. published a similar article in 2010. They also evaluated 103 tibial plateau fractures with MRI.[2] In their case series, 71% of patients had at least one major injured ligament and half of the patients had more than one torn ligament. In addition to describing the high incidence of soft-tissue injury, this report was the first to correlate a higher incidence of soft-tissue injury with severity of the bony injury. The authors concluded that higher energy fracture types (Schatzker types IV–VI) had a higher incidence of soft-tissue pathology compared with lower energy fractures (Schatzker types I–III) (Table 6.2).

TABLE 6.1 Incidence of Soft-Tissue Structures Injured.[14]

Structure	% (Absolute Number)
ACL	57 (59)
PCL	28 (29)
MCL	32 (33)
LCL	29 (30)
Medial meniscus	44 (45)
Lateral meniscus	91 (94)
PLC	68 (70)

ACL, Anterior cruciate ligament; *LCL*, lateral collateral ligament; *MCL*, medial collateral ligament; *PCL*, posterior cruciate ligament; *PLC*, posterolateral corner.

TABLE 6.2 Incidence of Ligament Injury by Schatzker Type.[2]

Schatzker Type	% With Ligament Injury
I	46
II	45
IV	69
V	85
VI	79

Note: Schatzker III fractures were not identified in the study.

EVALUATION OF SOFT-TISSUE INJURIES

Identification of associated soft-tissue injuries in the setting of tibial plateau fractures can be challenging. A traditional examination of the knee with a ligamentous injury is usually not possible in the acute setting. Therefore, examination under anesthesia and advanced imaging play an important role in diagnosis.

Obtaining the correct diagnosis begins with understanding the mechanism of injury. As discussed previously, the suspicion for soft-tissue injury should heighten with increasing energy mechanisms. For example, an axial load from a motor vehicle accident may have a variety of ligamentous and meniscal injuries, while a low-energy valgus load to the knee may only have injury to the lateral meniscus and MCL. As with most fractures, diagnostic imaging usually begins with radiographs. Using a combination of anteroposterior (AP), lateral, and oblique views can usually provide a clear understanding of the primary fracture lines. A modified AP view in which the beam shoots down the normal posterior slope of the tibia can also be helpful to assess differences between the slopes of the medial and lateral aspects of the plateau.[1,6,15] Contralateral radiographs can also be helpful in assessing bony alignment and subtle discrepancies of the medial and lateral joint spaces.[1] As with the bony injury, soft-tissue evaluation starts with initial radiographs. Joint subluxation in either the coronal or sagittal plane can be an indicator of ligamentous injury. Fracture of the fibular head or dislocation of the proximal tibiofibular joint can be a sign of lateral sided compromise.

Preoperative stress imaging has primarily now been replaced by advanced imaging techniques, such as MRI or computed tomography (CT).[16] However, intraoperative stress imaging, particularly after bony stabilization, continues to play an important role. Because of the excellent bony detail provided, CT remains the most commonly used advanced imaging technique, but it lacks soft-tissue detail.[1,6,17,18] In fact, a study that compared CT with MRI in the diagnosis of soft-tissue injury found that CT only had a sensitivity of 80% for ligamentous tears.[19] Therefore, MRI has remained the gold standard for evaluating ligamentous and meniscal injuries, but its role in the setting of tibial plateau fractures remains controversial.[1,2,20] As MRI techniques have improved, the author has found that MRI provides appropriate evaluation of the soft tissues, while not sacrificing bony detail.

Several studies have attempted to correlate bony findings with concomitant soft-tissue injuries in hopes to negate the need for MRI. Sixty-two patients with Schatzker type II fractures were evaluated by Gardner et al. They found that articular depression of greater than 6 mm and condylar widening of greater than 5 mm were associated with a lateral meniscus tear 83% of the time.[21] In addition to correlation with lateral meniscus tears, a later study showed that condylar widening of greater than 8 mm and articular depression of greater than 6 mm were found to have a high incidence of concomitant cruciate and collateral ligament injuries.[22] A definitive amount of articular depression or condylar widening that correlates with soft-tissue injury has yet to be fully accepted, but it is generally understood that with increasing depression or condylar widening, the incidence of soft-tissue pathology increases.[18,23,24]

In addition to obtaining the correct diagnosis, it also appears that MRI alters treatment plans. Holt et al. found that by adding MRI, the treatment plan changed in nearly 20% of patients.[25] In addition, MRI has been shown to have a higher interobserver agreement in fracture classification. Comparing plain radiographs, CT, and MRI, Yacoubian et al. showed that surgeons agreed 85% of the time with MRI and 73% of the time with CT. In addition, treatment plan agreement was greatest with MRI, 86% compared to 77%.[20]

The routine use of MRI for tibial plateau fractures remains controversial, likely due to cost and availability. Unfortunately, there has been little success correlating reliable radiographic parameters to predict soft-tissue injuries. Therefore, many authors who have evaluated the different advanced imaging modalities recommend MRI.[19,20,23,25–27] Currently, MRI is the advanced imaging technique of choice at the author's institution. While there may be a small initial learning curve for those that traditionally used CT, anecdotally the transition to MRI from CT seems to be quite easy.

THERAPEUTIC OPTIONS/SURGICAL TECHNIQUES

The surgical techniques of external fixation and open reduction internal fixation (ORIF) of tibial plateau fractures are well established and discussed in previous chapters. A foundational principle in the surgical management of these fractures is respect of the soft tissues. This concept was reinforced in a study by Egol et al. in which 57 high-energy plateau fractures underwent initial external fixation followed by staged ORIF. Compared with previously published data, a 5% wound infection rate was reported, in contrast to 13% to 88% in prior studies performing acute ORIF.[28] In general, the following algorithm exists at the author's institution. Length-stable, low-energy unicondylar plateau fractures usually undergo ORIF within 5 to 7 days as long as the soft-tissue envelope is amenable to an incision. Bicondylar, length-unstable fractures, especially those that are higher energy, undergo initial external fixation followed by eventual ORIF in 7 to 21 days. As mentioned previously, MRI is used in both cases for preoperative planning purposes.

Currently, scant literature exists to guide the management of soft-tissue injuries in combination with plateau fractures. Therefore, most of the treatment algorithm is built on experience and the principle of obtaining a stable knee through full range of motion. It is also believed that the meniscus is an important protector against posttraumatic arthritis, and therefore meniscal pathology should be addressed whenever possible.

In general, ORIF is performed through anterolateral and medial approaches to the proximal tibia and knee, both of which can be used to address the soft tissues. Lateral approaches should be performed in conjunction with a submeniscal arthrotomy.[1,6,29,30] This provides direct visualization of the plateau and also allows the surgeon to evaluate the lateral meniscus. In most cases of lateral meniscus tears in combination with plateau fractures, the meniscus tear is peripheral and amenable to repair. If a tear is present, an outside-in repair is performed using nonabsorbable sutures (author usually uses 2-0 FiberWire). The suture is passed through the capsule, into the meniscus, and then back through the meniscus and capsule in either a horizontal or vertical orientation. The suture is then tied on the outside of the capsule to secure the repair. In most cases, 3 to 4 sutures are used. Medial meniscal tears are usually addressed by arthroscopy, either acutely or later in the recovery. For example, a bucket-handle tear would be addressed at the time of ORIF, but a horizontal tear may be followed clinically and only addressed if symptomatic. Arthroscopic repair in the acute setting can be quite challenging, and positioning the knee in an optimal position may not be possible with an acute fracture. Therefore, only significantly displaced medial meniscal tears are addressed acutely.

Based on the preoperative MRI, if there is suspicion of a PLC injury, the incision should be adjusted slightly to allow access to the fibular head and provide access for dissection of the peroneal nerve. For the medial side of the knee, the standard medial approach allows easy access for repair or reconstruction of the collateral.

The choice between repair and reconstruction of the collateral ligaments can usually be made preoperatively by findings on the MRI. For example, mid-substance tears are usually reconstructed, while footprint avulsions are repaired. In addition, stress views after ORIF are used to assure appropriate stability. If coronal plane instability is present, collateral ligament repair or reconstruction is important to obtain appropriate stability to the knee. If the instability is recognized at a later stage, reconstruction is usually warranted instead of repair.

Cruciate injuries can be quite challenging due to the fact that reconstructions require sockets that are passed through areas of fixation for the plateau fracture. For large tibial avulsions, the fractures are usually addressed at the time of ORIF with either screw fixation or suture repair. PCL avulsions can usually be visualized through the posteromedial approach and can be secured with fixation of posteromedial fracture fragments. Mid-substance tears are usually treated using a staged approach. For example, the tibial plateau undergoes ORIF and the cruciates are not addressed. Once adequate bone healing has occurred, instability is assessed with physical examination of the ACL and/or PCL. If instability is noted, partial removal of implants is performed to allow for reconstruction. Surprisingly, this is seldomly needed. Anecdotally, these patients do not seem to complain of instability symptoms later. It may be that the fracture healing response allows for healing of the cruciates, similar to the increased healing rates of meniscal injuries in the setting of ACL reconstruction.[31]

SURGICAL MANAGEMENT OF COLLATERAL INJURIES

As described earlier, most cruciate injuries are managed nonoperatively initially, and detailed techniques for cruciate reconstruction are outside the scope of this chapter. However, collateral injuries are often addressed at the time of ORIF, so it is prudent for the treating surgeon to be able to perform repair or reconstruction if indicated.

A thorough understanding of anatomy is paramount to the success of either a repair or a reconstruction. The MCL originates at the isometric point of the femur. The most reliable method to find this isometric point is using a lateral radiograph. The isometric point is found at the intersection of a line drawn down the posterior femoral cortex and Blumensaat's line (Fig. 6.1), approximately 3 mm proximal and 5 mm posterior to the medial epicondyle. If repairing an MCL avulsion off the femur, the ligament should be repaired down to that point. If performing a reconstruction, a tibialis anterior allograft is used and should be at least 150 mm in length. The femoral limb of the reconstruction begins at the isometric point. Several options exist for fixation of the graft at both the origin and insertion points. The insertion of the MCL is on the posteromedial aspect of the tibia, just distal to the semitendinosus. It is on average approximately 6 cm from the joint line.[32] The new ligament should pass underneath the pes anserinus tendons prior to docking at the tibial insertion site. The graft is usually tensioned with the knee at 30 degrees of flexion with slight varus stress. In more severe injuries, the entire posteromedial corner (PMC) may need to be reconstructed. The primary ligaments reconstructed in this setting are the MCL and the posterior oblique ligament (POL). An option for reconstruction is to use a double-ended graft that is docked at the isometric point on the femur. The MCL

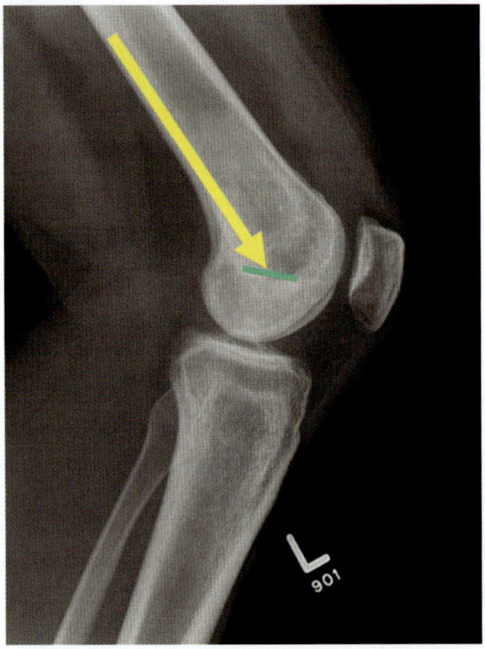

Fig. 6.1 A lateral radiograph depicting the isometric point of the femur. This is identified by the intersection of a line drawn down the posterior femoral cortex and blumensaat's line.

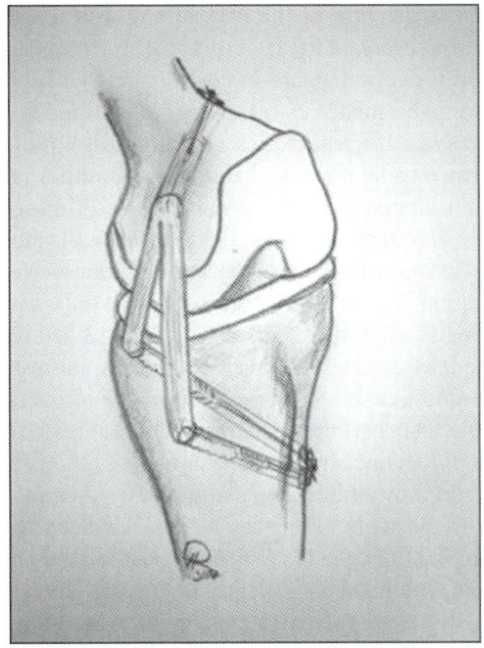

Fig. 6.2 Drawing of a reconstruction of medial collateral ligament and posterior oblique ligament with double-ended semitendinosus graft. (From Weimann A, Schatka I, Herbort M, et al. Reconstruction of the posterior oblique ligament and the posterior cruciate ligament in knees with posteromedial instability. *Arthroscopy*. 2012;(9):1283-1289.)

is then reconstructed in a similar manner as described earlier, and the graft for the POL is passed behind the semimembranosus tendon and then anchored into the posteromedial tibia (Fig. 6.2). With the graft in place, a posteromedial capsular shift/imbrication can be performed, as a capsular stretch injury and redundant capsule will often be present.

The PLC is slightly more complex than the medial side of the knee. The LCL originates at the same isometric point as the MCL, but on the lateral femur, and can be found using the lateral radiograph as described earlier. This point correlates with approximately 3 mm posterior and 1 to 2 mm proximal to the lateral epicondyle. The popliteus inserts approximately 18 mm distal and anterior to the LCL origin and passes underneath the LCL.[33] There are many options for reconstruction of the PLC, but the author's preferred technique is based on the one described by Grimm et al.[34] In this case, a single allograft is used to reconstruct the LCL and popliteus. In most cases, a tibialis anterior or posterior graft, at least 25 cm in length, is utilized. While traditional tenodesis screws can be used, the author prefers to use a double suspensory construct, which utilizes the Arthrex GraftLink technique and TightRope buttons (Arthrex, Naples, FL). Two sockets are drilled, one at the isometric point on the femur and the other 18 mm anterior and distal for the popliteus. Each socket is drilled to a depth of approximately 40 to 50 mm to provide ample room for tensioning. A tunnel equal to the size of the graft is then drilled in the fibular head, from anterior-lateral to posterior-medial. The allograft is first brought into the popliteus tunnel on the femur by flipping the TightRope button on the medial cortex of the femur and using the adjustable loop to pull the graft into the tunnel. Once approximately 15 mm of graft is secured into the socket, the graft is then tunneled underneath the iliotibial (IT) band and directed toward the posterior-medial aspect of the fibular head. The graft is then brought through the fibular head from posteromedial to anterolateral, passed back up under the IT band (and over the popliteus limb of the graft), and then into

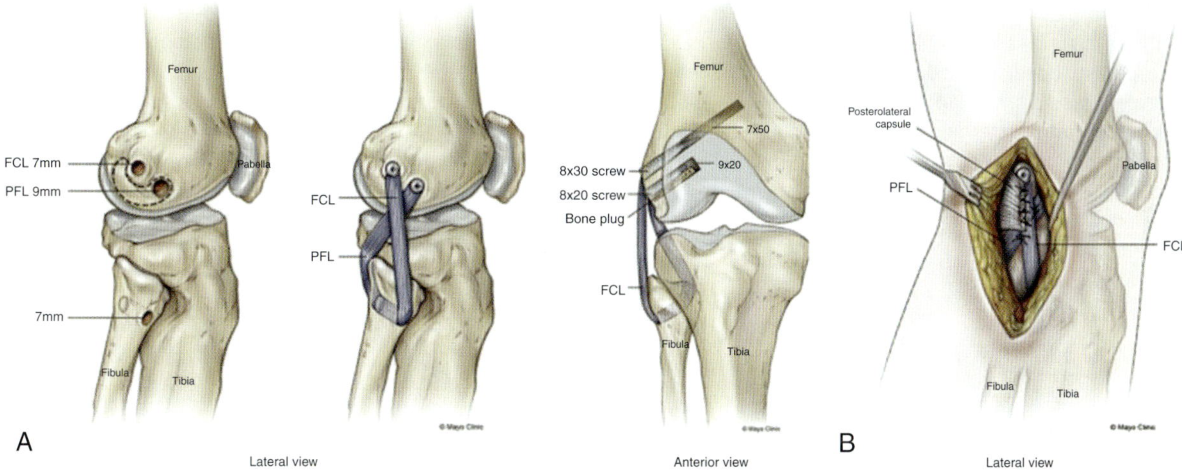

Fig. 6.3 Drawing of single tendon allograft posterolateral corner reconstruction technique showing femoral and transfibular tunnel placement and final construct, in this case utilizing interference screws in the femoral tunnels (A) and posterolateral capsular shift and imbrication (B). (From Kuzma S, Chow R, Engasser, W et al. Reconstruction of the posterolateral corner of the knee with achilles tendon allograft. *Arthrosc. Tech.* 2014;(3)3:e393-e398.)

the socket at the isometric point. The other button is flipped on the medial femoral cortex, and the graft is brought into the socket using the adjustable loop. The graft is then tensioned at 30 degrees of knee flexion and slight valgus using both of the adjustable loops (Fig. 6.3). A posterolateral capsular shift can then be performed as well.

As mentioned earlier, reconstructions are preferred when intrasubstance tears are present. If the ligamentous injury is better characterized as an avulsion, repair can be an option. The origins and insertions are the same for a repair, as with a reconstruction. The author's preferred method of repair consists of #5 FiberWire (Arthrex, Naples, FL) placed into the ligament using a locking Krackow stitch. The ligament is then repaired back to the bone using a SwiveLock anchor (Arthrex, Naples, FL).

CLINICAL OUTCOMES

Despite the high incidence of soft-tissue injuries in the setting of tibial plateau fractures, there has been little correlation with clinical outcomes. In fact, a recent study in 2018 attempted to correlate findings on MRI with patient-reported outcomes, but was unable to show that a soft-tissue injury affected outcomes. However, criticism of the study was that it did not specifically address the PLC and had lower cruciate injury rates than previously reported.[2,5,35,36] This may have been due to the large number of low-energy fractures included in the study (67% were Schatzker type I or II). In addition, only 82 patients were evaluated in this retrospective study. This sample size is severely underpowered to identify a causal relationship with certain injuries and outcomes. Despite not being able to correlate soft-tissue injuries with outcomes, there were valuable points that can be taken from the study. While there was no control group, patients with lateral meniscus tears repaired at the time of ORIF should expect good results. Also, if instability exists after ORIF, the collaterals should be addressed in order to have a good outcome. Therefore, the paper did show that the soft tissues cannot be ignored if good results are to be expected.

Currently, we know that there is a high incidence of meniscal and ligamentous injury in the setting of plateau fractures, but we do not specifically know if and when we should be addressing these injuries surgically. Due to the wide spectrum of injury, randomized controlled trials may not be feasible. Therefore, further prospective studies evaluating injuries, outcomes, and treatment algorithms are warranted.

CASE 6.1

A 31-year-old female injured her right knee in an all-terrain vehicle accident. Initial injury radiographs (Fig. 6.4A,B) show a bicondylar tibial plateau fracture. Unfortunately, the patient developed compartment syndrome and underwent fasciotomies and spanning external fixation. An MRI scan after external fixation highlights a lateral meniscal injury with a posterior root injury (Fig. 6.4C). In addition, the MCL was avulsed off the tibia, which was not easily seen on the MRI. She later underwent ORIF. After stabilizing the medial plateau, the posterior lateral tibial plateau was elevated under direct visualization along with the use of a femoral distractor (Fig. 6.4D). The posterior root of the lateral meniscus was avulsed off the fragment and had to be repaired. This was done by drilling a hole in

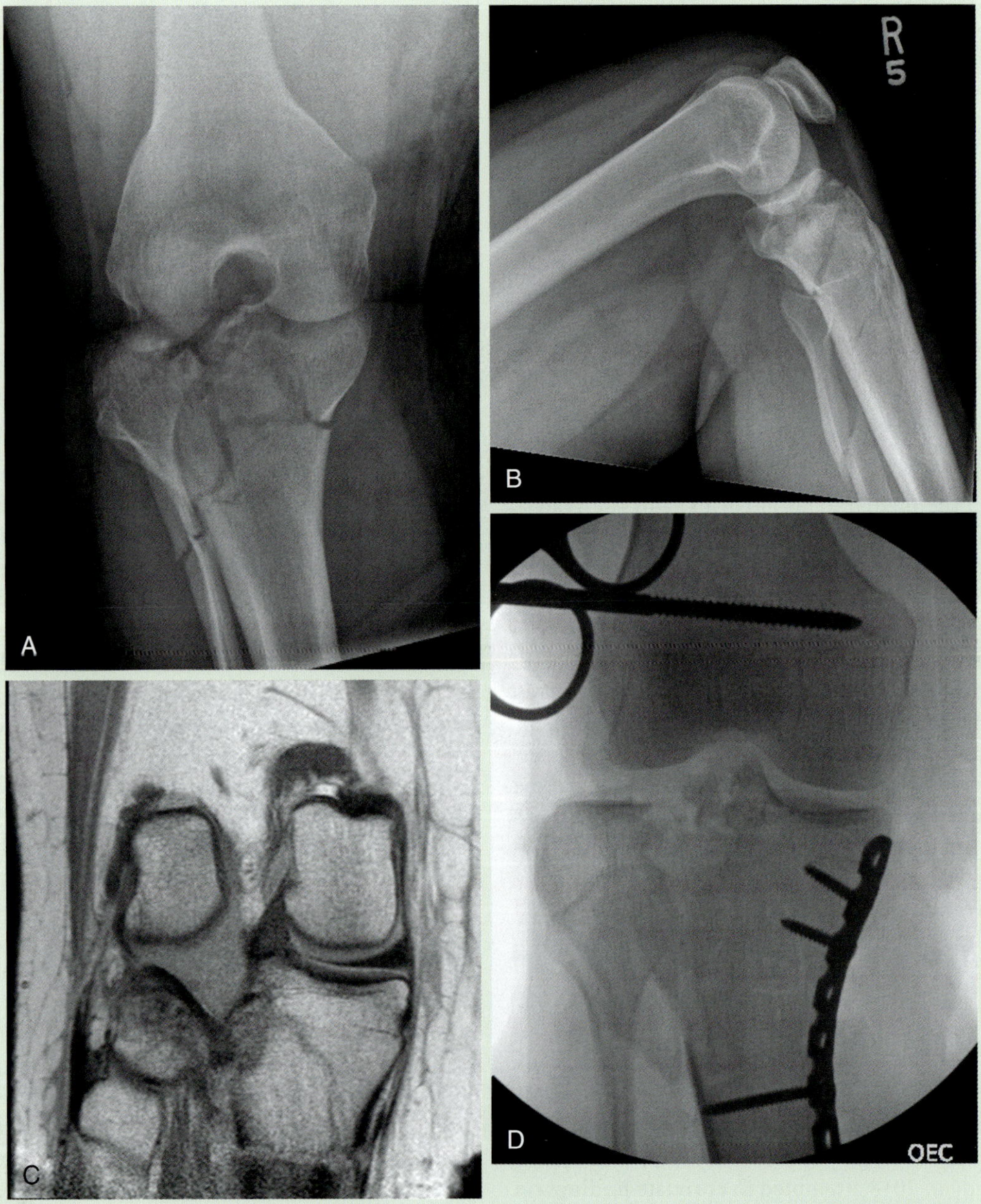

Fig. 6.4 (A and B) Injury radiographs demonstrating a bicondylar tibial plateau fracture. (C) Magnetic resonance imaging showing a lateral meniscal injury, specifically the posterior root. (D) Use of a laterally based femoral distractor and submeniscal arthrotomy to visualize and reduce the lateral plateau. (E and F) The lateral plateau is elevated using a tamp and then supported with the use of calcium phosphate. (G) The meniscal root is repaired by suture repair over a button (highlighted by the arrow). (H and I) Case 1 final radiographs.

CASE 6.1—CONT'D

the fracture fragment and passing FiberWire suture into the root, through the suture hole in the posterior plateau. The remainder of the lateral tibial plateau was reduced and stabilized with a lateral plate. To support the posterior plateau, calcium phosphate cement was injected under the fragment (Fig. 6.4E, F). After final fixation, the sutures from the lateral meniscal root were tied over a button to secure the root repair (Fig. 6.4G, button highlighted by the arrow). The MCL was repaired using a suture anchor in the tibia. At the 6-month follow-up, the patient was ambulating without pain and had full range of motion of the knee. Final radiographs are seen in Figs. 6.4H and I.

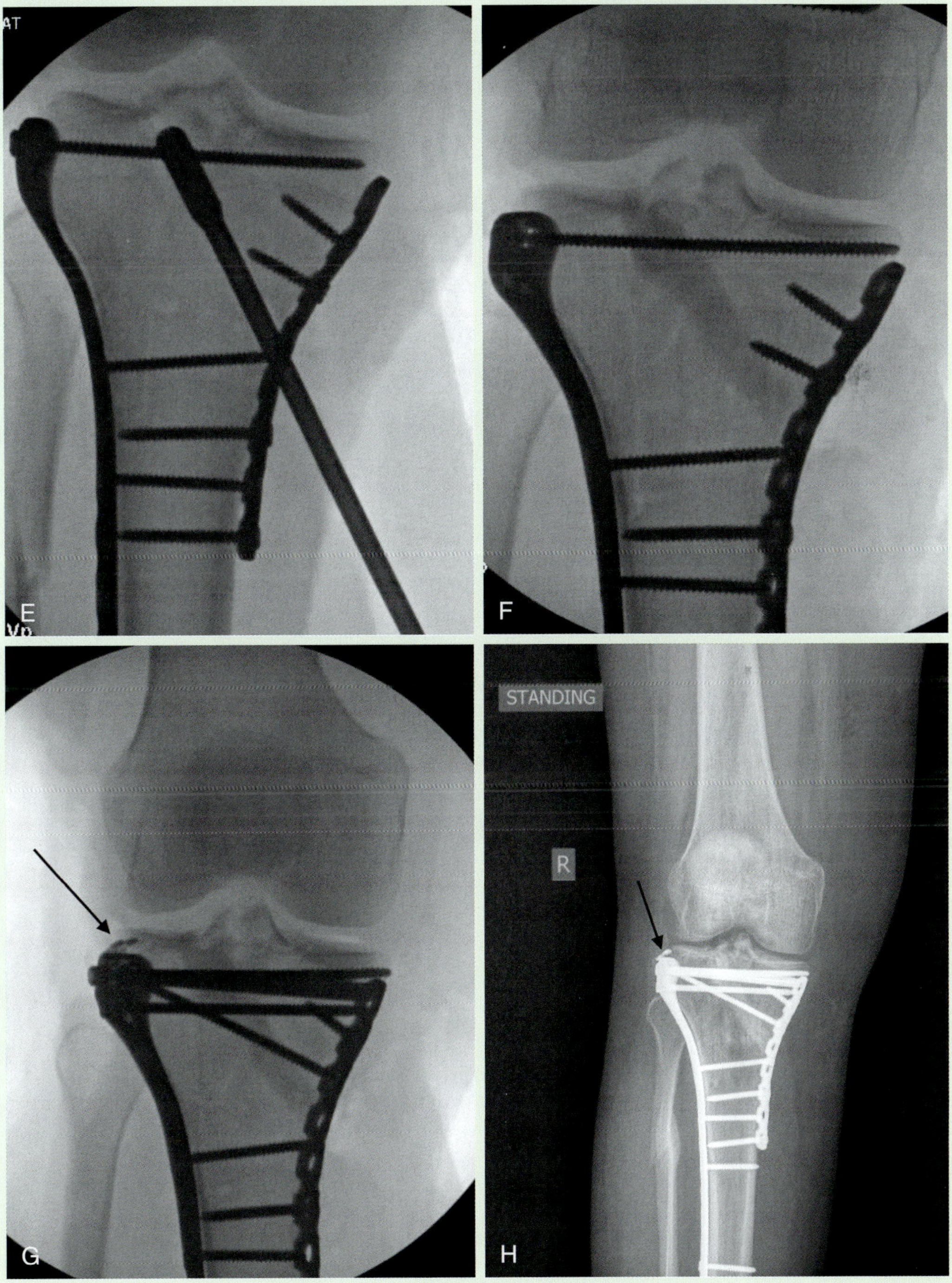

Fig. 6.4 Cont'd

CASE 6.1—CONT'D

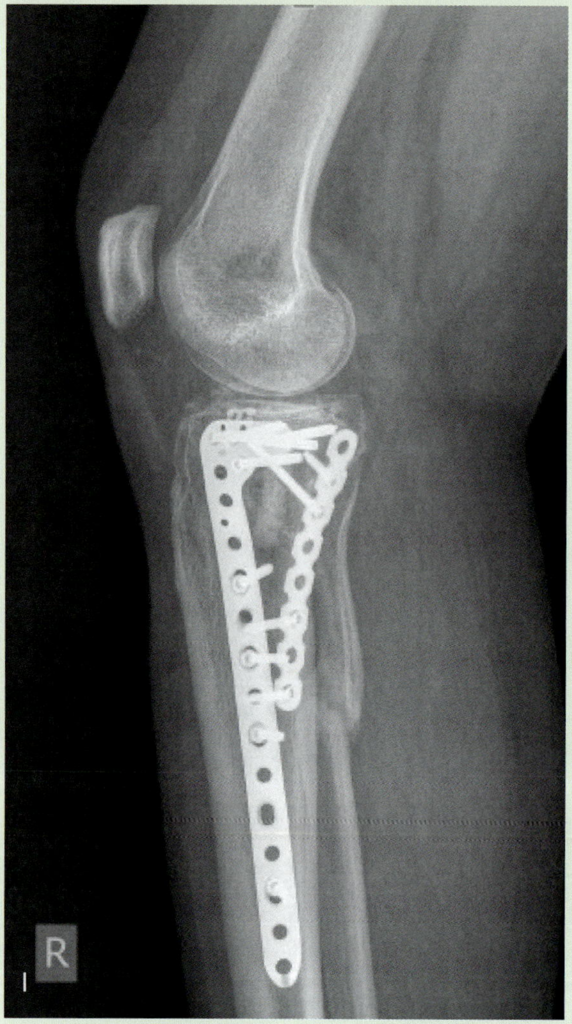

Fig. 6.4 Cont'd

CASE 6.2

A 38-year-old male fell out of a tree while at work, injuring his left knee. Initial radiographs demonstrated a Schatzker type II tibial plateau fracture (Fig. 6.5A). An MRI scan of the left knee showed a comminuted lateral plateau fracture, with multiple articular fragments that were depressed. In addition, a peripheral tear of the lateral meniscus was identified and the MCL seemed to be disrupted off the femur (Fig. 6.5B). The preoperative plan consisted of ORIF of the lateral plateau using a submeniscal arthrotomy and repair of the lateral meniscus. After fixation of the plateau, the MCL would be tested to determine if repair would be warranted.

The tibial plateau was highly comminuted and the depressed fracture fragments had very little subchondral bone. These fragments were stabilized to the lateral plateau using 1.6-mm threaded K-wires. Complicating this further was the fact that the anterior root of the lateral meniscus was attached to one of those fragments. That fragment was also secured with a threaded wire. After stabilizing the free fragments, the lateral plateau underwent reduction and fixation (Fig. 6.5C). Unfortunately, the articular reduction could not be made anatomic, but the condylar widths were restored. After fixation, a valgus stress was applied to evaluate the MCL which showed significant gapping medially (Fig. 6.5D). A medial incision over the femoral epicondyle was made and the MCL was repaired using suture anchors. Stress examination after repair showed good stability to valgus stress (Fig. 6.5E).

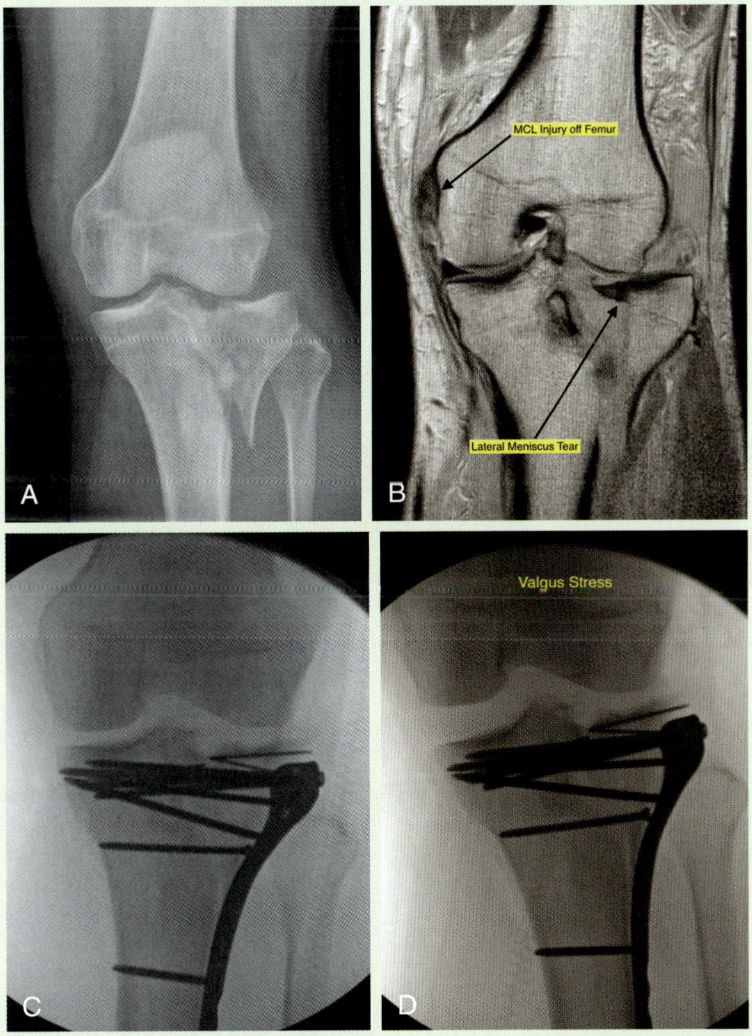

Fig. 6.5 (A) Injury radiographs demonstrating a Schatzker type II tibial plateau fracture. (B) Magnetic resonance imaging showing injury to the femoral attachment of the medial collateral ligament *(MCL)* and a peripheral lateral meniscus tear. (C) Open reduction internal fixation (ORIF) of comminuted lateral tibial plateau fracture. (D) Valgus stress examination after ORIF to assess coronal plane stability. (E) Stress examination after repair of the MCL.

CASE 6.2—CONT'D

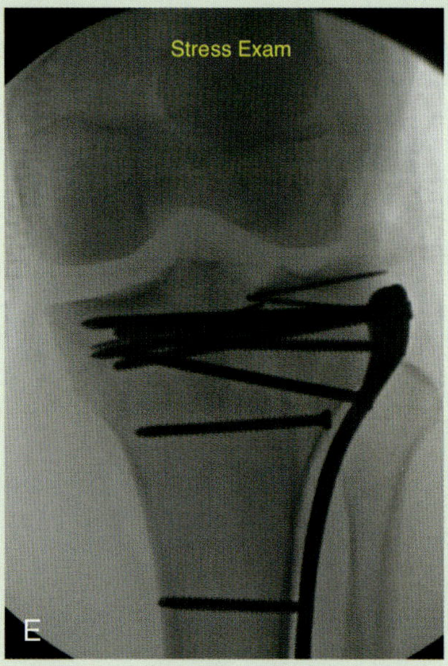

Fig. 6.2 Cont'd

ADAMS' TIPS AND TRICKS

- Consider routine use of MRI for preoperative imaging.
- Routinely use a submeniscal arthrotomy to allow for outside-in repair of lateral meniscal tears.
- Repair collateral ligament avulsions and reconstruct mid-substance tears.
- Stage treatment of cruciate injuries and expect that most will not need reconstruction.
- Always assess coronal plane stability after fixation of plateau. If instability exists, repair or reconstruct as needed.
- Bony stability is the most important part to provide joint stability and maintain alignment. Do not sacrifice reduction or fixation in order to repair or reconstruct soft tissues.

REFERENCES

1. Browner B, Jupiter J, Christian K, Anderson P. *Skeletal Trauma: Basic Science, Management, and Reconstruction*. 6th ed. Philadelphia, PA: Elsevier Inc.; 2019.
2. Stannard JP, Lopez R, Volgas D. Soft tissue injury of the knee after tibial plateau fractures. *J Knee Surg*. 2010;23(4):187–192.
3. Tejwani NC, Achan P. Staged management of high-energy proximal tibia fractures. *Bull Hosp Jt Dis*. 2004;62(1-2):62–66.
4. Watson JT. High-energy fractures of the tibial plateau. *Orthop Clin North Am*. 1994;25(4):723–752.
5. Bennett WF, Browner B. Tibial plateau fractures: a study of associated soft tissue injuries. *J Orthop Trauma*. 1994;8(3):183–188.
6. Wiesel SW, Parvizi J, Rothman RH, et al. *Operative Techniques in Orthopaedic Surgery*. 2nd ed. Lippincott Williams & Wilkins, Philadelphia, PA; 2016.
7. Prat-Fabregat S, Camacho-Carrasco P. Treatment strategy for tibial plateau fractures: an update. *EFORT Open Rev*. 2016;1(5):225–232.
8. Giordano CP, Koval KJ, Zuckerman JD, Desai P. Fracture blisters. *Clin Orthop Relat Res*. 1994;307:214–221.
9. Berkson EM, Virkus WW. High-energy tibial plateau fractures. *J Am Acad Orthop Surg*. 2006;14(1):20–31.
10. Ibrahim DA, Swenson A, Sassoon A, Fernando ND. Classifications in brief: the Tscherne classification of soft

tissue injury. *Clin Orthop Relat Res*. 2017;475(2):560–564.
11. Schatzker J, McBroom R. The tibial plateau fracture. The Toronto experience 1968-1975. *Clin Orthop Relat Res*. 1979;138:94–104.
12. Colletti P, Greenberg H, Terk MR. MR findings in patients with acute tibial plateau fractures. *Comput Med Imaging Graph*. 1996;20(5):389–394.
13. Shepherd L, Abdollahi K, Lee J, Vangsness CT. The prevalence of soft tissue injuries in nonoperative tibial plateau fractures as determined by magnetic resonance imaging. *J Orthop Trauma*. 2002;16(9):628–631.
14. Gardner MJ, Yacoubian S, Geller D, et al. The incidence of soft tissue injury in operative tibial plateau fractures. A magnetic resonance imaging analysis of 103 patients. *J Orthop Trauma*. 2005;19(2):79–84.
15. Moore TM, Harvey JP. Roentgenographic measurement of tibial plateau depression due to fracture. *J Bone Joint Surg*. 1974;56(1):155–160.
16. Delamarter RB, Hohl M, Hopp E. Ligament injuries associated with tibial plateau fractures. *Clin Orthop Relat Res*. 1990;250:226–233.
17. Markhardt BK, Gross JM, Monu JUV. Schatzker classification of tibial plateau fractures: Use of CT and MR imaging improves assessment. *Radiographics*. 2009;29(2):585–597.
18. Tang HC, Chen IJ, Yeh YC, et al. Correlation of parameters on preoperative CT images with intra-articular soft-tissue injuries in acute tibial plateau fractures: a review of 132 patients receiving ARIF. *Injury*. 2017;48(3):745–750.
19. Mui LW, Engelsohn E, Umans H. Comparison of CT and MRI in patients with tibial plateau fracture: Can CT findings predict ligament tear or meniscal injury? *Skeletal Radiol*. 2007;36(2):145–151.
20. Yacoubian SV, Nevins RT, Sallis JG, Potter HG, Lorich DG. Impact of MRI on treatment plan and fracture classification of tibial plateau fractures. *J Orthop Trauma*. 2002;16(9):632–637.
21. Gardner MJ, Yacoubian S, Geller D, et al. Prediction of soft-tissue injuries in Schatzker II tibial plateau fractures based on measurements of plain radiographs. *J Trauma*. 2006;60(2):319–324.
22. Wang J, Wei J, Wang M. The distinct prediction standards for radiological assessments associated with soft tissue injuries in the acute tibial plateau fracture. *Eur J Orthop Surg Traumatol*. 2015;25(5):913–920.
23. Spiro AS, Regier M, de Oliveira AN, et al. The degree of articular depression as a predictor of soft-tissue injuries in tibial plateau fracture. *Knee Surgery, Sport Traumatol Arthrosc*. 2013;21(3):564–570.
24. Chang H, Zheng Z, Shao D, Yu Y, Hou Z, Zhang Y. Incidence and radiological predictors of concomitant meniscal and cruciate ligament injuries in operative tibial plateau fractures: a prospective diagnostic study. *Sci Rep*. 2018;8(1):1–9.
25. Holt MD, Williams LA, Dent CM. MRI in the management of tibial plateau fractures. *Injury*. 1995;26(9):595–599.
26. Lee SY, Jee WH, Jung JY, Koh IJ, In Y, Kim JM. Lateral meniscocapsular separation in patients with tibial plateau fractures: detection with magnetic resonance imaging. *J Comput Assist Tomogr*. 2015;39(2):257–262.
27. Kolb JP, Regier M, Vettorazzi E, et al. Prediction of meniscal and ligamentous injuries in lateral tibial plateau fractures based on measurements of lateral plateau widening on multidetector computed tomography scans. *Biomed Res Int*. 2018;2018.
28. Egol KA, Tejwani NC, Capla EL, Wolinsky PL, Koval KJ. Staged management of high-energy proximal tibia fractures (OTA types 41): the results of a prospective, standardized protocol. *J Orthop Trauma*. 2005;19(7):448–455. discussion 456.
29. Stahl D, Serrano-Riera R, Collin K, Griffing R, Defenbaugh B, Sagi HC. Operatively treated meniscal tears associated with tibial plateau fractures: a report on 661 patients. *J Orthop Trauma*. 2015;29(7):322–324.
30. Tekin AÇ, Çakar M, Esenyel CZ, et al. An evaluation of meniscus tears in lateral tibial plateau fractures and repair results. *J Back Musculoskelet Rehabil*. 2016;29(4):845–851.
31. Westermann RW, Wright RW, Huston LJ, MOON Group, Wolf BR. Meniscal repair with concurrent anterior cruciate ligament reconstruction: operative success and patient outcomes at 6 year follow up. *Am J Sports Med*. 2014;42(9):2184–2192.
32. Laprade RF, Wijdicks CA. Surgical technique: development of an anatomic medial knee reconstruction. *Clin Orthop Relat Res*. 2012;470(3):806–814.
33. LaPrade RF, Ly TV, Wentorf FA, Engebretsen L. The posterolateral attachments of the knee: a qualitative and quantitative morphologic analysis of the fibular collateral ligament, popliteus tendon, popliteofibular ligament, and lateral gastrocnemius tendon. *Am J Sports Med*. 2003;31:854–860.
34. Grimm NL, Levy BJ, Jimenez AE, Bell R, Arciero RA. Open anatomic reconstruction of the posterolateral corner: the Arciero technique. *Arthrosc Tech*. 2020;9(9):e1409–e1414.
35. Warner SJ, Garner MR, Schottel PC, et al. The effect of soft tissue injuries on clinical outcomes after tibial plateau fracture fixation. *J Orthop Trauma*. 2018;32(3):141–147.
36. Stannard JP, Stannard JT, Cook JL. Repair or reconstruction in acute posterolateral instability of the knee: decision making and surgical technique introduction. *J Knee Surg*. 2015;28(6):450–454.

7

Postoperative Care/Rehabilitation

Brendan Shi, MD and Christopher Lee, MD

INTRODUCTION

Postoperative care and rehabilitation for tibial plateau fractures remain areas of surgical management with little standardization. While a significant amount of research has focused on diagnosis, classification, surgical techniques, and operative outcomes of tibial plateau fractures, far less has evaluated appropriate postoperative care. Hence, there are a wide range of postoperative management protocols implemented by orthopedic trauma surgeons worldwide. An ideal postoperative regimen would minimize the risk of losing fracture reduction while also minimizing the risk of wound complications, loss of range of motion, patient deconditioning, and long-term sequelae of these injuries. These at times represent competing interests, with extended immobilization possibly minimizing fracture displacement, while consequently increasing the likelihood of postoperative stiffness in addition to precipitating cartilage loss and subsequent posttraumatic arthritis. The goal of this chapter is to discuss these factors and help guide orthopedic traumatologists to select the appropriate, evidence-based postoperative management protocol.

WOUND CARE

Tibial plateau fractures are high-energy injuries that often present with concomitant soft-tissue sequelae. High-energy plateau fractures often present significant swelling, with rates of compartment syndrome reported to be as high as 28% in bicondylar tibial plateau fractures. Furthermore, surgical site infection rates for tibial plateau fractures treated surgically have been reported as 9.9% in a recent meta-analysis and have been reported to be as high as 13.8%.[1,2] This must be kept in mind when addressing postoperative wound closure and wound care options.

Extensive open injuries with soft-tissue stripping and/or contaminated wounds may require second-look procedures given the high risk of infection. Options for coverage in those scenarios include negative pressure wound therapy (NPWT) followed by secondary closure, skin grafting, and flap coverage, with optimal soft-tissue coverage within 7 days to decrease complications.[3] Details regarding choice of coverage are outside of the scope of this chapter. For a wound to be an optimal candidate for primary closure, it must be free from contamination, contain a viable soft-tissue envelope, and be able to be closed without unnecessary tension. In clean wounds with a viable soft-tissue envelope that have too much tension to be primarily closed after the index surgery, delayed primary closure via gradually tightened subcuticular stitches and the vessel loop shoe-lace method are both options.[4–6]

When amenable to primary closure, wounds should be closed in a layered fashion. For skin closure, vertical mattress and horizontal mattress stitches are preferred for wounds with higher concern for tension as these suture patterns distribute the tension over a greater surface area. A 2008 study by Sagi et al. used a porcine model to explore the effect of suture patterns on cutaneous blood flow, finding that the Allgower-Donati pattern had the least effect on cutaneous blood flow for all levels of tension applied to the repair.[7] More recently, a 2020 study by Shorten and colleagues used laser angiography to measure incisional skin perfusion in patients immediately after ankle fracture surgery.

They found that vertical mattress stitches had equivalent performance to Allgower-Donati stitches and that both allowed for better perfusion than sutures in a horizontal or simple pattern.[8] Finally, a similar study from the Mayo Clinic found vertical mattress stitches to demonstrate superior wound perfusion to staples.[9] However, several trials, systematic reviews, and meta-analysis studies have shown no difference in clinical outcomes between the use of sutures or staples in surgical wound closure. Running subcuticular stitch, the pattern that allows for the most robust wound perfusion in both studies, would not be appropriate for the high-tension wounds seen in tibial plateau fractures. In this author's experience, nylon suture thrown in a vertical mattress fashion provides a secure, strong closure for the vast majority of surgical wounds following fixation of tibial plateau fractures.

After closure, the ideal dressing provides a barrier against potential sources of contamination to prevent infection while also optimizing wound healing. Prior studies have shown that a moist environment helps improve wound healing by preventing tissue dehydration, promoting breakdown of dead tissue and fibrin, and stimulating faster epithelialization than a purely dry dressing.[10,11] A standard three-layer dressing of impregnated gauze (e.g., Xeroform (Covidien, Dublin, Ireland)), standard gauze, and waterproof outer dressing (e.g., Tegaderm (3M, Saint Paul, MN, USA)) provides an ideal healing environment while also wicking away exudate and providing a waterproof barrier on the outside. While research from the arthroplasty literature has suggested that silver-impregnated occlusive dressings are highly effective for wounds with significant drainage and may decrease acute periprosthetic joint infection rates,[12] tibial plateau wounds are far less exudative. Dressings with such high absorptive properties are poorer options for dry wounds.

Initial reports suggested a favorable role for incisional NPWT for major lower extremity trauma to decrease risk of surgical site infection.[13,14] A recent meta-analysis reported a decrease in infections and hospital stays with NPWT use.[14] However, in a recent randomized controlled trial of 1548 adults with lower extremity fractures who underwent primary closure, there was no difference in the deep surgical site infection rate between standard wound dressing and incisional wound vacuum therapy.[15]

BRACING

Postoperative bracing protocol plays a significant role in the recovering patient's functional status after surgery. When considering tibial plateau bracing protocols, the goal is to maximize postoperative range of motion and prevent any loss of knee extension. A combination of locked and unlocked bracing to optimize both has been recommended.

There does appear to be good rationale behind locking the hinged knee brace in extension postoperatively. The expected inflammation and joint swelling after tibial plateau fracture repair cause the knee to rest in a position that maximizes knee joint volume. A position of 15 to 60 degrees of flexion maximizes joint volume and minimizes intraarticular pressure[16]; hence, knee bracing locked in extension is required to prevent the patient from resting in flexion. The elevated levels of inflammatory cytokines in the perioperative period led to arthrofibrosis and subsequent knee stiffness in this flexed position. A loss of even 5 degrees of extension causes a limp and significantly increases energy expenditure. Flexion contractures after tibial plateau fractures are often irreversible: mouse studies have shown that the length of the posterior capsule is permanently shortened even after 1 week of being held in flexion and is not reversible upon remobilization.[17]

Immobilization in extension has its own risks, as the same inflammatory cytokines responsible for flexion contractures can also cause. There are significant benefits to early motion and keeping the knee brace unlocked. Rabbit studies have shown that mobilization of the knee joint postoperatively is associated with a five-fold decrease in proinflammatory interleukin-1 levels, subsequently decreasing release of transforming growth factor beta. Other inflammatory cytokines responsible for fibroblast proliferation.[18] The downstream effects of fibroblast proliferation are significant: a 2015 study from the University of Utah showed that each day of fixed extension after tibial plateau fixation increased the odds of requiring manipulation under anesthesia by 10%.[19] New research also suggests that the downstream effects of mobilization may extend to cartilage health as well. The proinflammatory environment driven by interleukin-1 is associated with chondrocyte death. However, even 8 hours of activity with 16 hours of rest was adequate to block the interleukin-1–mediated proinflammatory gene induction in articular chondrocytes.[20]

In summary, during the immediate postoperative period, the authors recommend a protocol of unlocking the knee brace during the day while locking in −10 degrees of extension at night while the patient sleeps. This protocol yields the antiinflammatory and procartilage benefits of early knee mobilization while also preventing the development of irreversible knee flexion contractures. Patients should be able to maintain full knee extension during the entirety of their recovery period and should achieve 90 degrees of knee flexion by 6 weeks postoperatively. The brace may be discontinued at 6 weeks as there should be sufficient knee motion, especially extension, obtained at this postoperative juncture.

WEIGHT BEARING

The official AO (Arbeitsgemeinschaft für Osteosynthesefragen) recommendation for postoperative weight bearing after tibial plateau repair is restricted weight bearing (nonweight bearing or partial-weight bearing) for roughly 12 weeks. A systematic review of published studies reporting postoperative management of tibial plateau fractures showed that on average surgeons recommend 4 to 6 weeks of nonweight bearing followed by 4 to 6 weeks of partial weight bearing, with increasing Schatzker type being correlated with delayed time to full weight bearing.[21] These restrictions reduce the risk of malreduction by decreasing the amount of force applied to the healing fracture site. Historical studies support these guidelines and have shown that weight bearing in the first 6 weeks postoperatively is associated with increased risk of failure of fixation. Ali and colleagues reported that patients who began partial weight bearing prematurely during the first 6 weeks postoperatively had an 80% rate of loss of reduction compared to 25% of their patients who avoided full weight bearing until after 10 weeks.[22] Other factors that have been associated with loss of reduction include age greater than 60, degree of comminution, and presence of a medial coronal fracture line.[22–24]

It is important to note that there are potential downsides to limiting weight bearing in patients. Restricted weight bearing necessitates increased energy expenditure and changes gait mechanics. Basic scientific studies have shown that joint unloading significantly affects cartilage health and thickness.[25] Historical studies from the 1970s showed that within weeks, knee cartilage thickness was reduced by 50% in dogs with hindlimbs immobilized.[26] Researchers at Kobe University subjected mice to 2, 4, and 8 weeks of hind-limb unloading and found that cartilage thickness was decreased at all time points compared to the control group.[25] Nonweight bearing also contributes to increased muscle atrophy that may contribute to further delays in return to preinjury level of function.[27] Fortunately, these effects are reversible: cartilage can be rebuilt with progressive loading and muscle mass can be recovered with physical therapy.

Recent clinical studies suggest that early weight bearing may not be as detrimental to surgical fixation as previously reported. Haak and colleagues compared immediate weight-bearing protocol to 6 to 8 weeks of initial nonweight bearing in 32 patients with lateral plateau fractures. They found that the immediate weight-bearing group had no increased loss of reduction, fracture displacement, or need for reoperation.[28] A similar study out of the United Kingdom expanded inclusion criteria to include all types of plateau fractures and found that early weight bearing was not associated with joint depression or loss of fixation when compared to 6 weeks of restricted weight bearing.[29] With ever-expanding evidence that postoperative weight bearing may be liberalized past the current guidelines, it may be unsurprising that a recent European survey revealed that many current orthopedic surgeons deviate from official AO guidelines and favor earlier weight bearing.[30]

Despite these recent studies supporting early weight bearing, this author recommends a conservative approach with patients until further conclusive evidence suggests limited risks. Further caution should be used when fractures demonstrate high-risk factors including increased patient age, significant comminution, or presence of a medial coronal fracture line. Overall, randomized clinical trials are required to adequately demonstrate that early weight bearing is not associated with increased risk of fracture malunion or loss of reduction.

EXERCISES AND REHABILITATION

Tibial plateau fractures and the subsequent period of decreased weight bearing and mobilization cause significant weakening of the associated musculature. A study by Gaston et al. in 2005 measured muscle strength in 51 patients who underwent repair of tibial plateau fractures and showed that only 14% returned to baseline quadriceps strength 12 months after surgery.[31] This likely played a large role in their finding that almost one in five patients had sustained flexion contracture of greater than 5 degrees. Aside from helping maintain full extension, quadriceps strengthening also plays a part in knee forces during the gait cycle. As the quadriceps serves to decelerate the leg during the heel strike phase, acting as a shock absorber, weakness in the quadriceps causes an increase in force that ends up being transmitted into the knee and newly repaired tibial plateau.

Hence, the focus of postoperative rehabilitation and exercise should be on maintaining quadriceps and hamstring strength to maximize postoperative range of motion. Unlocking the brace during the day allows the patient to immediately begin active range of motion, delaying quadriceps and hamstring atrophy.

The specific type of exercise used to prevent joint stiffness and strengthen the surrounding muscles depends on stage of weight bearing. During the nonweight bearing stage or the first 4 to 6 weeks, patients and physical therapists should focus on passive and active range of motion, straight leg raises, and stretching. While basic scientific studies have shown decreased arthrofibrosis and improved cartilage healing with continuous passive movement (CPM) machines,[32] these findings have not been replicated in clinical studies. Multiple studies looking at the effect of CPM on total knee replacement patients have found no significant benefit in range of motion or functional outcomes with its use.[33,34] Hence, barring new evidence, we do not see a role for CPM in postoperative rehabilitation. During the partial weight-bearing stage, physical therapists may expand to more intensive strengthening exercises that keep joint reactive forces low such as stationary cycling, aquatic exercises, and rowing. Finally, once the patient has been advanced to full weight bearing, they may progress to closed chain lower body strength exercises such as squats and lunges.

It is crucial for the surgeon to clearly document their weight-bearing recommendations based on the most recent physical examination and radiographs during the rehabilitation process. As each individual has a different fracture pattern and heals at a different rate, communication between the surgeon and physical therapist is crucial to optimize muscle strength while minimizing risk of injury or loss of reduction by progressing with therapy too rapidly.

CASE REPORTS

Here, we present two contrasting cases that emphasize the importance of extension bracing.

CASE 7.1

Patient 1 is a 41-year-old otherwise healthy female, who presented to the emergency department with a closed, bicondylar left tibial plateau fracture after falling off a kick scooter (Fig. 7.1). She was taken to the operating room for open reduction internal fixation with posteromedial and lateral plating (Fig. 7.2A). Significant lateral subchondral depression and tibial spine comminution were noted intraoperatively. There were no surgical complications, and the knee could be brought through full range of motion intraoperatively. Postoperatively, she was made nonweight bearing on the left lower extremity with instructions to lock her hinged knee brace in −10 degrees of extension at night and range as tolerated during the day.

On postoperative day 9, the patient called to clarify the bracing protocol. Despite daily instructions during her inpatient stay by the orthopedic team and her physical therapists, she had been keeping her brace unlocked since discharge. She was reinstructed to keep the hinged knee brace locked in extension at night.

At her 2-week clinic visit, the patient lacked 10 degrees of full extension and was able to flex to 70 degrees. The bracing protocol was reiterated, and she was referred to outpatient physical therapy to work on range of motion.

At her 6-week visit, the patient again lacked 10 degrees of full extension but was able to flex to 100 degrees. The patient reported that she had not been working with physical therapy. She also reported issues with the fit of her hinged knee brace. She was given a Knee Extension System (Dynasplint, Severna Park, MD, USA) for home use and a new physical therapy referral with instructions to go at least five times a week to regain full extension.

Continued

CASE 7.1—CONT'D

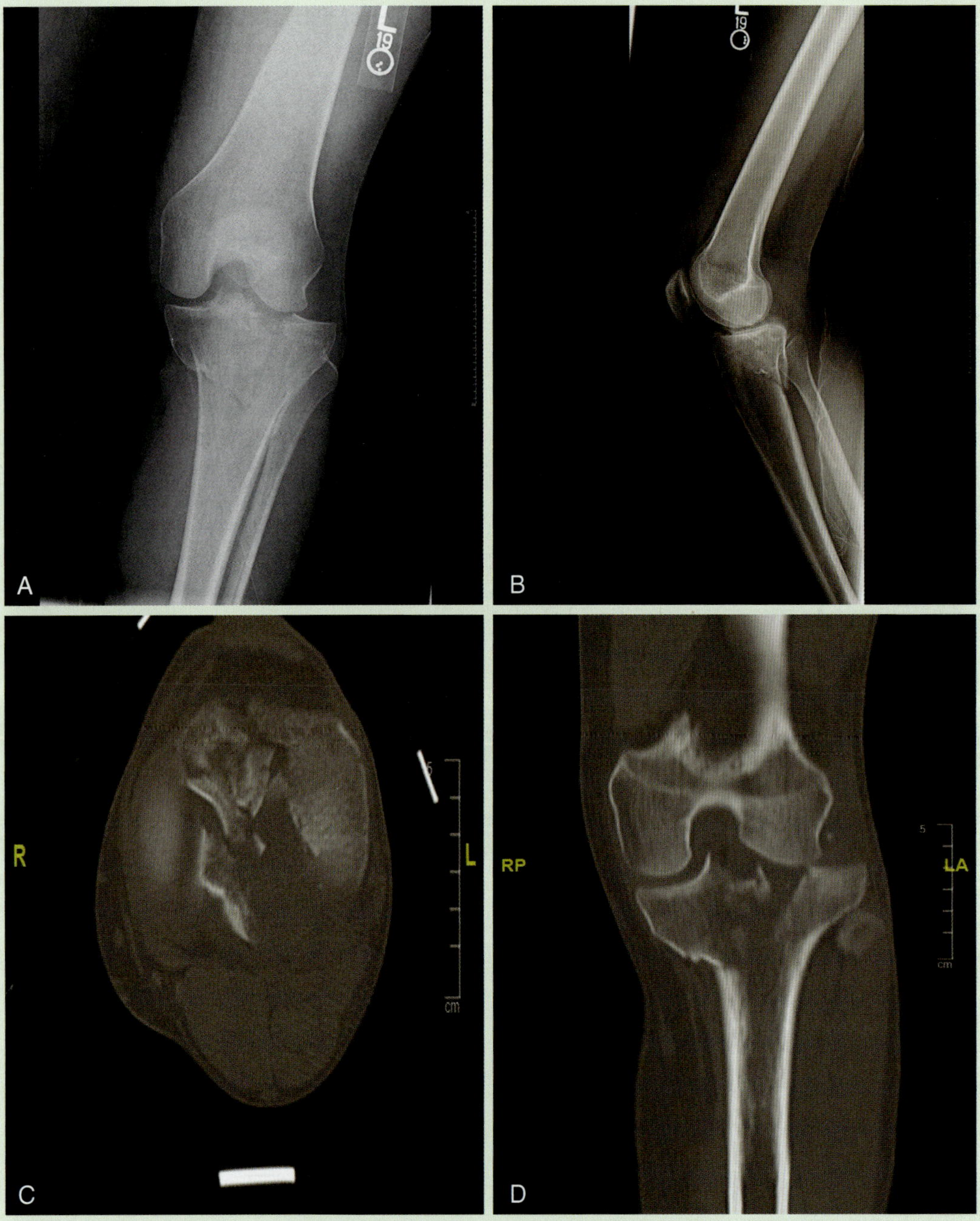

Fig. 7.1 Injury radiographs (A and B) and computed tomography (C and D) images for patient 1 demonstrating left bicondylar plateau fracture with large medial fragment and lateral plateau comminution.

CASE 7.1—CONT'D

By 10 weeks after surgery (Fig. 7.2B), the patient demonstrated interval healing of the fracture and was advanced to full weight bearing of her left lower extremity. With the aggressive physical therapy and Dynasplint use, her knee range of motion was much improved, and she lacked only a few degrees of extension. However, she remained unsatisfied with her range of motion and underwent arthroscopic lysis of adhesions at 3 months, ultimately achieving −1 to 130 degrees of motion.

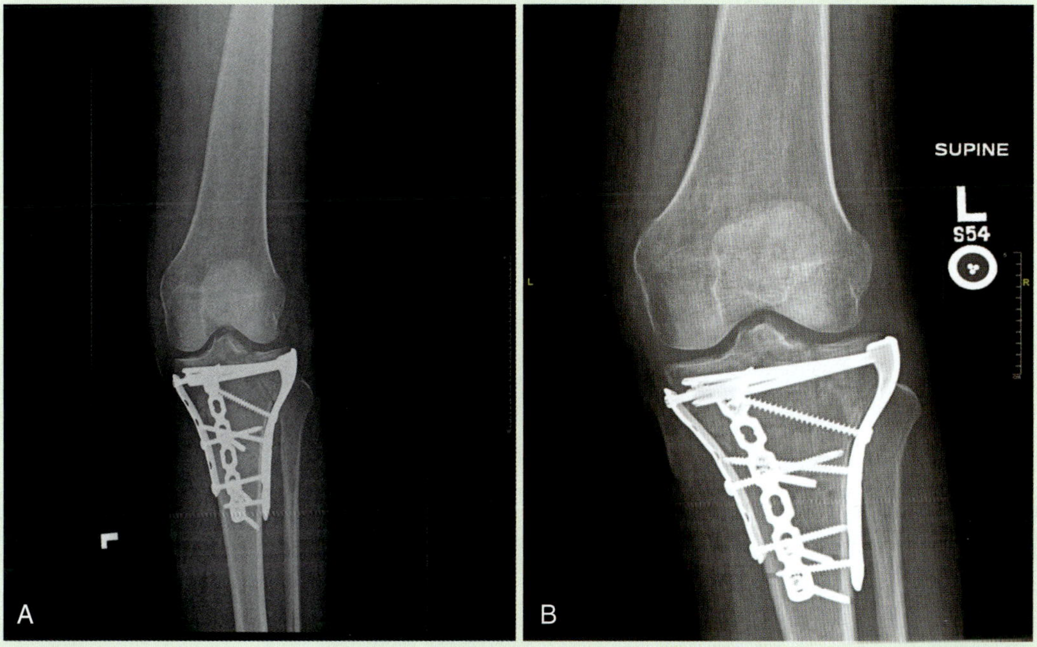

Fig. 7.2 Postoperative radiographs for patient 1 taken (A) in recovery and (B) 10 weeks after surgery.

CASE 7.2

Patient 2 is a 30-year-old otherwise healthy male, who presented with a closed right medial plateau fracture with significant lateral plateau depression after falling from a skateboard (Fig. 7.3). He was taken to the operating room and underwent right medial plateau open reduction internal fixation and placement of right knee spanning external fixator (Fig. 7.4A). Eleven days after index surgery, he underwent a second stage of surgery for external fixator removal and fixation of the lateral plateau. Thirty cubic centimeters of cancellous chips were packed in the large lateral plateau defect prior to plating. After surgery, he was made nonweight bearing on the left lower extremity with hinged knee brace in −10 degrees of extension at night and unlocked during the day. After discharge, he remained compliant with instructions and performed home range of motion exercises during the day.

At his 2-week postoperative visit, he demonstrated full extension and was able to range his knee from 0 to 60 degrees. By 6 weeks, his flexion had improved to 90 degrees. His hinged knee brace was discontinued at this time, and he was instructed to remain nonweight bearing and work on range of motion. By 10 weeks, his knee flexion had improved to 130 degrees. Plain films demonstrated fracture healing (Fig. 7.4B), and he was advanced to full weight bearing. By 5 months postoperatively, he was ambulating normally with full knee range of motion and had advanced to strength training. Radiographs demonstrated intact hardware with no subsidence or failure of fixation.

Continued

CASE 7.2—CONT'D

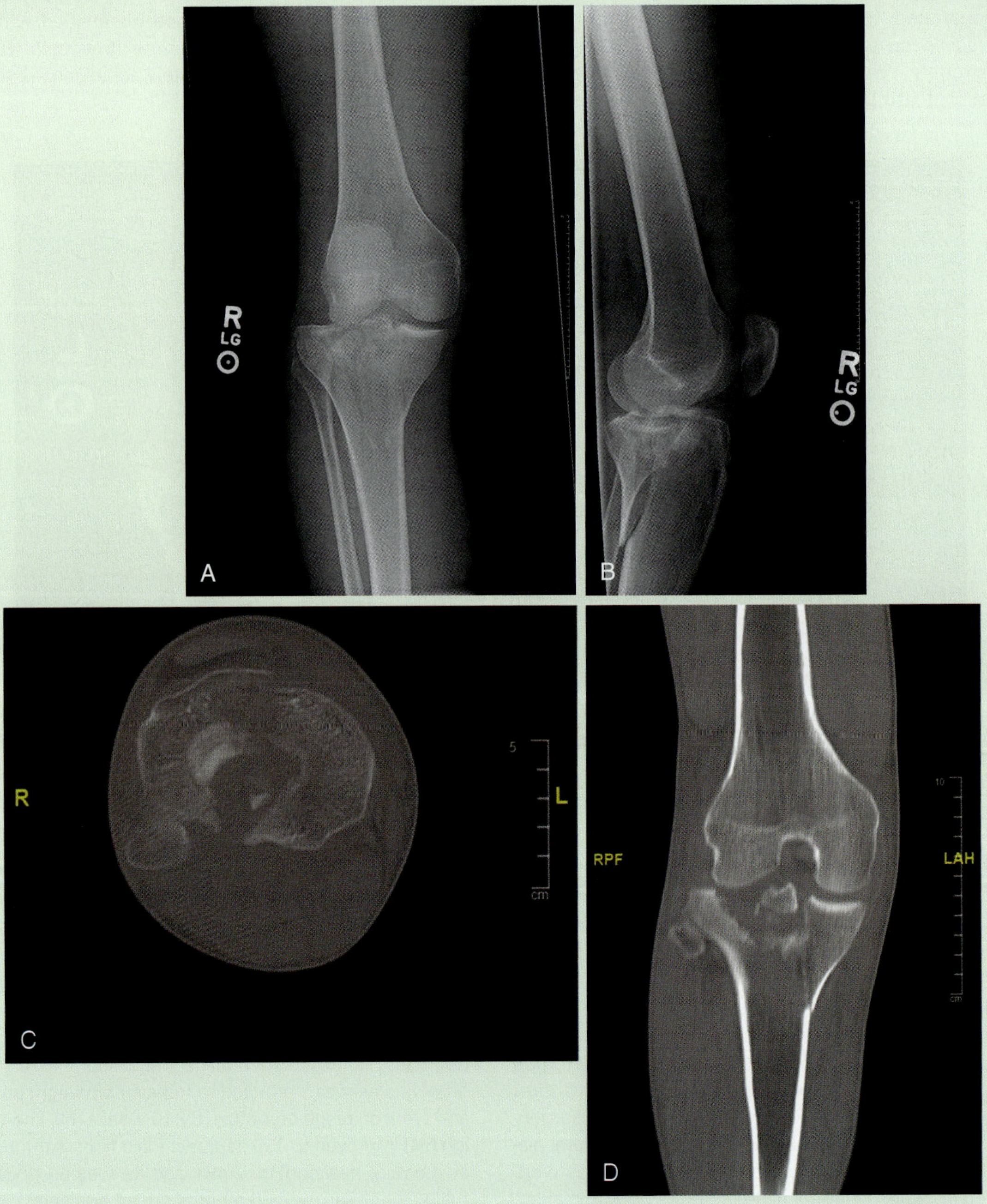

Fig. 7.3 Injury radiographs (A and B) and computed tomography (C and D) images for patient 2 demonstrating right bicondylar plateau fracture with medial fragment and significant lateral joint depression.

CASE 7.2—CONT'D

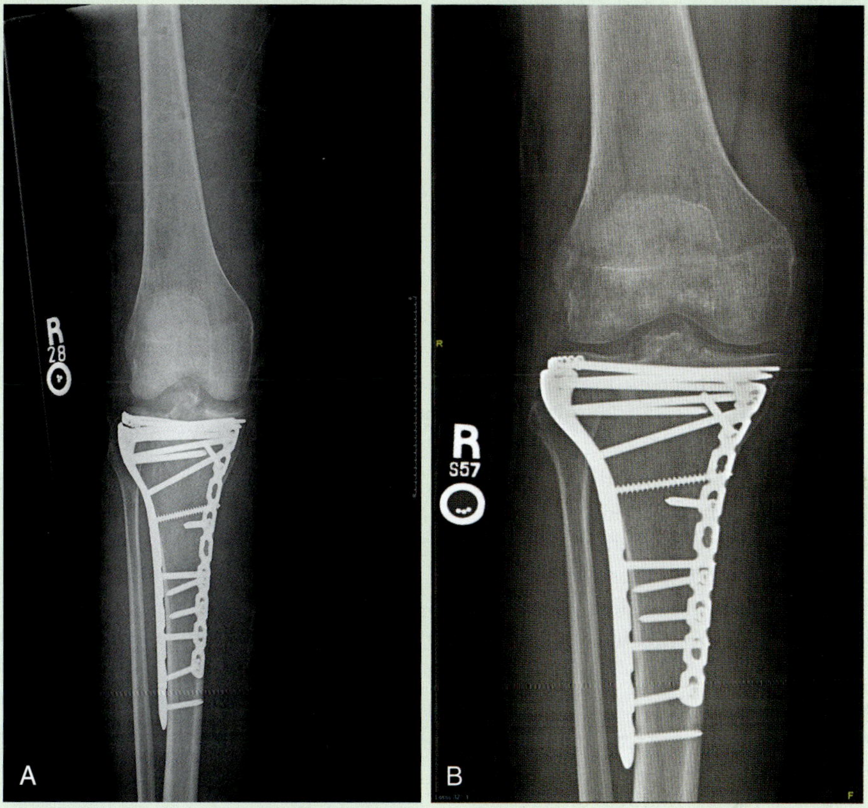

Fig. 7.4 Postoperative radiographs for patient 2 taken (A) in recovery and (B) 10 weeks after surgery.

In this comparison of two young, healthy patients with bicondylar tibial plateau fractures, patient 2 presented with a worse injury requiring a two-stage surgery, but due to compliance with the bracing protocol, he never lost extension and was able to achieve full range of motion by 10 weeks. Patient 1, however, suffered persistent flexion contractures and ultimately elected for arthroscopic lysis of adhesions due to keeping her brace largely unlocked for the first 2 weeks after surgery. These two cases illustrate how quickly knee stiffness can set in during the postoperative period and the relative difficulty of achieving full extension compared to full flexion.

CONCLUSION

Postoperative care remains a challenging endeavor with nonstandardized treatment protocols. The authors recommend very clear communication with the patient and their support team to adhere to and follow rehabilitation protocols. It is oftentimes beneficial to provide clear, written instructions as a patient's recall can vary, especially during the immediate postoperative period. These instructions should include how to care for the wound, how to manage brace use, weight-bearing status, and exercises to be performed while at home.

With regard to wound care, the authors recommend the use of sutures, either in vertical mattress or Allgower-Donati fashion. Occlusive dressings with Xeroform are placed, with the entire leg wrapped. It is not uncommon for dressings to subside and fall with gravity; thus, overwrapping the leg to the thigh can be beneficial.

Postoperative bracing remains challenging, both in terms of patient recall on instructions and in maintaining the brace in the correct position. The authors recommend the brace be locked in −10 degrees of extension at night, as the bulk of the dressings can often induce a slight flexion moment if locked at 0 degrees of extension. With unreliable patients, it can be beneficial to maintain the brace locked in −10 degrees of extension until initial follow-up, as extension is much more difficult to obtain in the future than flexion. Furthermore, the patient and especially support team should be shown how to position the brace, as this will often subside over time, especially as the swelling decreases.

Though evidence as to the optimal time to begin weight bearing remains controversial, the authors recommend a more conservative approach, especially in patients with a high risk for loss of reduction. Optimal patients for early weight bearing may be young and otherwise healthy with isolated lateral plateau fractures.

Finally, physical therapy is often provided on an outpatient basis at initial outpatient follow-up. This, along with beginning open chain exercises, can help facilitate motion and reduce stiffness. A home exercise regimen is also shown to all patients, with the patient encouraged to take an active role in their rehabilitation.

LEE'S TIPS AND TRICKS

- Close skin using techniques that may provide wound edge perfusion such as vertical mattress or Allgower Donati stitches. Dress with Xeroform and gauze, seal dressings, and overwrap leg.
- Loss of extension is harder to regain than loss of flexion: keep hinged knee brace locked in −10 degrees of extension at night and unlock the brace during the day.
- Limit weight bearing for the first 4 to 6 weeks postoperatively and use interval radiographs to determine progression of weight bearing.
- Provide the patient and support team with clear, written instructions describing wound care, bracing, weight-bearing status, and home exercises.

REFERENCES

1. Shao J, Chang H, Zhu Y, et al. Incidence and risk factors for surgical site infection after open reduction and internal fixation of tibial plateau fracture: a systematic review and meta-analysis. *Int J Surg*. 2017;41:176–182.
2. Shah SN, Karunakar MA. Early wound complications after operative treatment of high energy tibial plateau fractures through two incisions. *Bull NYU Hosp Jt Dis*. 2007;65(2):115.
3. Pincus D, Byrne J, Nathens A, et al. Delay in flap coverage past 7 days increases complications for open tibia fractures: a cohort study of 140 North American trauma centers. *J Orthop Trauma*. 2019;33(4):161–168.
4. Friedrich JB, Katolik LI, Hanel DP. Reconstruction of soft-tissue injury associated with lower extremity fracture. *J Am Acad Orthop Surg*. 2011;19(2):81–90.
5. Asgari MM, Spinelli HM. The vessel loop shoelace technique for closure of fasciotomy wounds. *Ann Plast Surg*. 2000;44(2):225–229.
6. Zorrilla P, Marín A, Gómez L, Salido J. Shoelace technique for gradual closure of fasciotomy wounds. *J Trauma*. 2005;59(6):1515–1517.
7. Sagi H, Papp S, DiPasquale T. The effect of suture pattern and tension on cutaneous blood flow as assessed by laser Doppler flowmetry in a pig model. *J Orthop Trauma*. 2008;22(3):171–175.
8. Shorten P, Haimes M, Nesbit R, Bartlett C, Schottel P. Impact of skin suture pattern on incision perfusion using intraoperative laser angiography: a randomized clinical trial of patients with ankle fractures. *J Orthop Trauma*. 2020;34(10):547–552.
9. Wyles CC, Jacobson SR, Houdek MT, et al. The Chitranjan Ranawat Award: running subcuticular closure enables the most robust perfusion after TKA: a randomized clinical trial. *Clin Orthop Relat Res*. 2015;474(1):47–56.
10. Field CK, Kerstein MD. Overview of wound healing in a moist environment. *Am J Surg*. 1994;167(1):S2–S6.
11. Vogt PM, Andree C, Breuing K, et al. Dry, moist, and wet skin wound repair. *Ann Plast Surg*. 1995;34(5):493–500.
12. Grosso MJ, Berg A, LaRussa S, Murtaugh T, Trofa DP, Geller JA. Silver-impregnated occlusive dressing reduces rates of acute periprosthetic joint infection after total joint arthroplasty. *J Arthroplast*. 2017;32(3):929–932.
13. Suh H, Lee A, Park EJ, Hong JP. Negative pressure wound therapy on closed surgical wounds with dead space. *Ann Plast Surg*. 2015;76(6):717–722.
14. Liu S, He C, Cai Y, et al. Evaluation of negative-pressure wound therapy for patients with diabetic foot ulcers: systematic review and meta-analysis. *Ther Clin Risk Manag*. 2017;13:533–544.
15. Costa ML, Achten J, Knight R, et al. Effect of incisional negative pressure wound therapy vs standard wound dressing on deep surgical site infection after surgery for lower limb fractures associated with major trauma: the WHIST randomized clinical trial. *JAMA*. 2020;323(6):519–526.

16. Eyring E, Murray W. The effect of joint position on the pressure of intra-articular effusion. *J Bone Joint Surg Am.* 1964;46(6):1235–1241.
17. Zhou H, Trudel G, Goudreau L, Laneuville O. Knee joint stiffness following immobilization and remobilization: a study in the rat model. *J Biomech.* 2020;99:109471.
18. Ferretti M, Srinivasan A, Deschner J, et al. Anti-inflammatory effects of continuous passive motion on meniscal fibrocartilage. *J Orthop Res.* 2005;23(5):1165–1171.
19. Haller JM, Holt DC, McFadden ML, Higgins TF, Kubiak EN. Arthrofibrosis of the knee following a fracture of the tibial plateau. *Bone Joint J.* 2015;97-B(1):109–114.
20. Madhavan S, Anghelina M, Rath-Deschner B, et al. Biomechanical signals exert sustained attenuation of proinflammatory gene induction in articular chondrocytes. *Osteoarthritis Cartilage.* 2006;14(10):1023–1032.
21. Arnold JB, Tu CG, Phan TM, et al. Characteristics of postoperative weight bearing and management protocols for tibial plateau fractures: findings from a scoping review. *Injury.* 2017;48(12):2634–2642.
22. Ali AM, El-Shafie M, Willett KM. Failure of fixation of tibial plateau fractures. *J Orthop Trauma.* 2002;16(5):323–329.
23. Kim C, Lee C, An K, et al. Predictors of reduction loss in tibial plateau fracture surgery: focusing on posterior coronal fractures. *Injury.* 2016;47(7):1483–1487.
24. Weaver MJ, Harris MB, Strom AC, et al. Fracture pattern and fixation type related to loss of reduction in bicondylar tibial plateau fractures. *Injury.* 2012;43(6):864–869.
25. Nomura M, Sakitani N, Iwasawa H, et al. Thinning of articular cartilage after joint unloading or immobilization. An experimental investigation of the pathogenesis in mice. *Osteoarthritis Cartilage.* 2017;25(5):727–736.
26. Brandt KD. Response of joint structures to inactivity and to reloading after immobilization. *Arthritis Rheum* 2003;49(2):267–271.
27. Yoshiko A, Yamauchi K, Kato T, et al. Effects of post-fracture non-weight-bearing immobilization on muscle atrophy, intramuscular and intermuscular adipose tissues in the thigh and calf. *Skeletal Radiol.* 2018;47(11):1541–1549.
28. Haak KT, Palm H, Holck K, Krasheninnikoff M, Gebuhr P, Troelsen A. Immediate weight-bearing after osteosynthesis of proximal tibial fractures may be allowed. *Dan Med J.* 2012;59(10):A4515.
29. Williamson M, Iliopoulos E, Jain A, Ebied W, Trompeter A. Immediate weight bearing after plate fixation of fractures of the tibial plateau. *Injury.* 2018;49(10):1886–1890.
30. van der Vusse M, Kalmet PHS, Bastiaenen CHG, van Horn YY, Brink PRG, Seelen HAM. Is the AO guideline for postoperative treatment of tibial plateau fractures still decisive? A survey among orthopaedic surgeons and trauma surgeons in the Netherlands. *Arch Orthop Trauma Surg.* 2017;137(8):1071–1075.
31. Gaston P, Will EM, Keating JF. Recovery of knee function following fracture of the tibial plateau. *J Bone Joint Surg Br.* 2005;87(9):1233–1236.
32. Salter RB. The biologic concept of continuous passive motion of synovial joints. The first 18 years of basic research and its clinical application. *Clin Orthop Relat Res.* 1989;(242):12–25.
33. MacDonald SJ, Bourne RB, Rorabeck CH, McCalden RW, Kramer J, Vaz M. Prospective randomized clinical trial of continuous passive motion after total knee arthroplasty. *Clin Orthop Relat Res.* 2000;380(380): 30–35.
34. Yang X, Li G, Wang H, Wang C. Continuous passive motion after total knee arthroplasty: a systematic review and meta-analysis of associated effects on clinical outcomes. *Arch Phys Med Rehabil.* 2019;100(9):1763–1778.

8

Complications

Brandi Hartley, MD, Travis Parkulo, MD, and James Gainer, MD

INTRODUCTION

Tibial plateau fractures occur when a varus or valgus stress is applied to the knee in conjunction with axial loading. Younger individuals sustain this fracture through high-energy mechanisms such as motor vehicle accidents, pedestrian strikes, or falls from heights.[1] In older individuals, it typically occurs due to their poor bone quality and a low-energy fall.[1,2] This section will focus on the sequelae and complications involved in the treatment of these fractures. Complications/sequelae include but are not limited to wound healing problems, deep infection, compartment syndrome, neurovascular injury, posttraumatic osteoarthritis (PTOA) of the ipsilateral knee and ankle, knee instability, arthrofibrosis, loss of muscle function/strength around the knee, ankle, and foot, malunion, nonunion, and loss of limb. For the sake of clarity, we will focus here on four of the most common and devastating problems: compartment syndrome, wound healing issues, arthrofibrosis, and PTOA. Complications can be minimized through proper history and physical examination (bearing in mind the mechanism of injury and overall amount of energy imparted to cause fracture), consideration of the soft-tissue health and whether staged treatment is necessary, and excellent surgical technique with a focus on anatomic reduction using limited incisions and meticulous soft-tissue handling.[3,4]

COMPARTMENT SYNDROME

Acute compartment syndrome (ACS) most often occurs following a fracture or crush injury to a limb.[5] Following an injury, accumulation of blood and other tissue fluids results in significant swelling within the myofascial compartment. This accumulation of fluid results in venous hypertension and transudation of further fluid into the compartment.[6] The progressive increase in compartment fluid causes an increase in pressure, which may result in tissue ischemia and necrosis without prompt intervention.[7] Treatment for ACS involves urgent fasciotomy with the release of skin and muscle fascia to allow a reduction in compartment pressure.

Diagnosis

Fractures about the tibia and specifically bicondylar tibial plateau fractures have an increased incidence of severe soft-tissue injury and are associated with ACS.[8,9] Patients who are male and younger have been found to be at increased risk of ACS following tibial plateau fracture.[10] Clinical signs of compartment syndrome that are generally well accepted are pain that is out of proportion to what should be expected, pain with passive stretch of the involved muscle, and paresthesias in the distribution of sensory nerves within the compartment. However, when used as a screening test, these clinical signs and symptoms have been shown to have low sensitivity when diagnosing ACS.[11] If the clinical signs are at all in question regarding a diagnosis of ACS, then intramuscular pressures should be obtained. Numerous studies advocate for the use of routine intramuscular pressures in the general diagnosis of compartment syndrome.[12,13] Others advocate for the use of serial intramuscular pressures that provide more information regarding absolute changes in compartment pressures and changes in perfusion pressures. McQueen et al. found a sensitivity of 94% and a specificity of 98% when using continuous anterior compartment measurements, and a diagnosis of ACS was made when patients' differential pressure remained less than 30 mmHg for more than 2 hours.[13]

At the author's institution, clinical signs and symptoms are typically used for diagnosis of ACS. If physical examination and patient symptoms are in question, then intramuscular pressures are taken at the anterior and posterior compartments with fasciotomies performed when a 30-mmHg threshold for absolute compartment pressures and a perfusion pressure of less than 30 mmHg result.

Treatment

Our bias is to have more false positives and err on the side of surgical release rather than watchful waiting. A delayed diagnosis/treatment of ACS can result in significant morbidity for the patient,[14] not to mention legal repercussions for the treating team. A two-incision technique to release all four compartments is utilized to allow for evaluation of muscle viability and adequate debridement as necessary in all four compartments of the lower leg (Fig. 8.1). A knee spanning external fixator is routinely placed at the time of fasciotomies to allow for fracture stabilization and allows the patient to mobilize if other injuries are not present. Vessel loops, rubber bands, or prolene sutures can be utilized at the fasciotomy sites in a "roman sandal" configuration to allow for skin tension but also permit swelling and expansion of wound as needed (Fig. 8.2). Multiple second look evaluations may be required, and definitive closure with fracture fixation must not occur until the soft-tissue envelope permits, with all necrotic tissue removed and wounds able to undergo either delayed closure or split-thickness skin grafting.

Conclusion

ACS is a dangerous complication that can occur with tibial plateau fractures. Early diagnosis is critical to prevent significant morbidity for the patient. Surgeons must be aware of patients who are at increased risk, specifically those who are involved in high-energy accidents sustaining bicondylar tibial plateau fractures with significant displacement and obvious soft-tissue injury. Specific attention must be paid to the soft-tissue envelope at the initial evaluation. Additionally, heightened awareness is necessary regarding pain that is out of proportion to what should be expected, pain with passive stretch of the involved compartment, and paresthesias in the distribution of sensory nerves within the compartment. Surgeons must remain vigilant in diagnosis and perform compartment release when indicated.

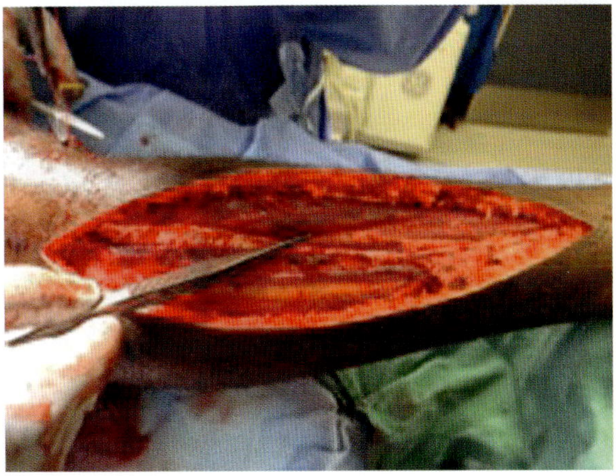

Fig. 8.1 Compartment release identifying a small portion of anterior compartment damage.

WOUND HEALING ISSUES

Complications from wound healing and their associated infections continue to be a significant source of morbidity in orthopedic trauma surgery.[15] In the case of tibial plateau fractures, where the mechanism tends to be associated with significant soft-tissue damage in the form of inflammation and swelling, there is a relatively high incidence of wound complications that can have a drastic impact on acute and long-term surgical outcomes.[16]

Wound healing is a multifactorial process whose variants include the wound bed itself, the surrounding tissue, as well as the biology of the host individual. Wounds heal through either primary intention, usually by means of suture or adhesives allowing for scar formation, and its resultant maturation. In some instances, primary intention as a means of closure either fails or is not achievable, either due to the character of the wound or its contamination from the mechanism of injury. In these instances, when primary closure and healing is not realistic, closure by secondary intention is necessary. Wound healing through secondary intention is achieved through the formation of granulation tissue over a vascular soft-tissue bed.[15] In certain injuries, where the individual is at higher risk for dehiscence or infection in the setting of primary closure, the secondary intention is the superior method of wound healing as it may avoid surgical complications.[17] Secondary wound healing presents a challenge as it relates to fracture care due to retained hardware and bacterial biofilm formation.

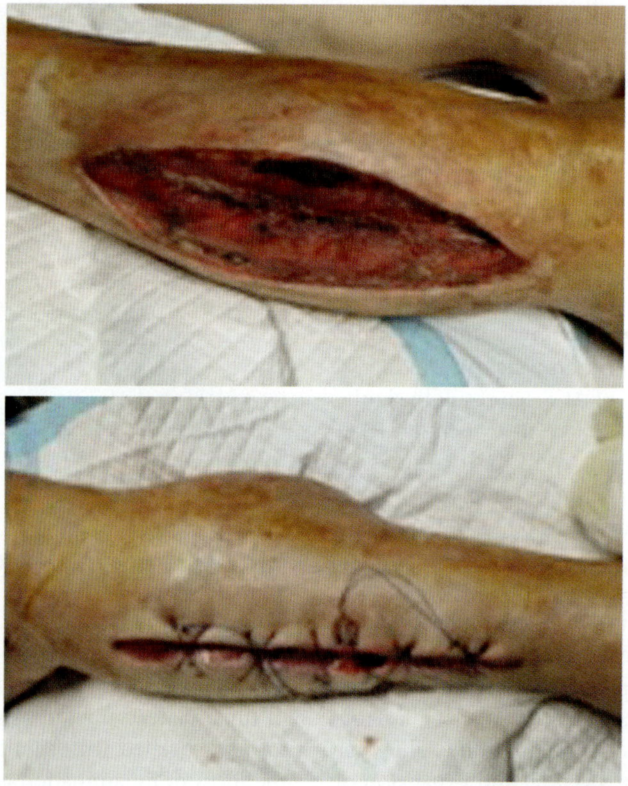

Fig. 8.2 Lateral compartment release (A). Temporary closure option for a fasciotomy wound (B).

An issue that can add to the complexity of management with tibial plateau fractures is the development of fracture blisters in high-energy injuries. These blisters are sentinels of soft-tissue damage beneath them and are concerning due to increased risk of infection and as a possible hindrance to surgical approach for definitive fracture management, as well as increased time to operation.[18] These blisters are either clear filled or blood filled and are theorized to form due to the separation of the dermis and epidermis at the time of injury. This skin separation leads to edema, venous stasis/thrombosis, development of epidermal necrosis, and the eventual formation of blisters. A histological study of these blisters has demonstrated that the contents of the clear-filled blisters are sterile transudate and those of the blood-filled blisters are hemorrhagic.[18]

Despite a lack of extensive investigation into management or clinical outcomes of fracture blisters, there are multiple management options. Some surgeons elect to allow them to rupture on their own. The obvious limitation to this being in the event that the blister overlies the desired incision site, there could be a delay in surgical fixation of the underlying fracture. On histological examination of blisters that have healed without issue and those that have developed wound complications, the main factor leading to wound complications was the lack of re-epithelialization or false epithelialization of the blister bed.[19] Tolpinrud et al. demonstrated that simple unroofing of these blisters leads to almost immediate colonization of the blister transudate and blister bed by skin flora, including *Staphylococcus epidermidis* and *S. aureus* shortly after unroofing.[19] In addition, Tolpinrud et al. demonstrated that unroofing the blister to the edge of healthy tissue and applying Silvadene twice a day with associated dry dressing changes resulted in 90% of their patient cohort healing without wound issues.[19] Most recently, there was investigation into utilization of negative pressure wound therapy with sterile saline instillation (NPWT-id) in the management of both ankle and tibial plateau fractures. Hasegawa et al. theorized that the mechanism of the NWPT allows for faster re-epithelization, reduction of soft-tissue swelling, and

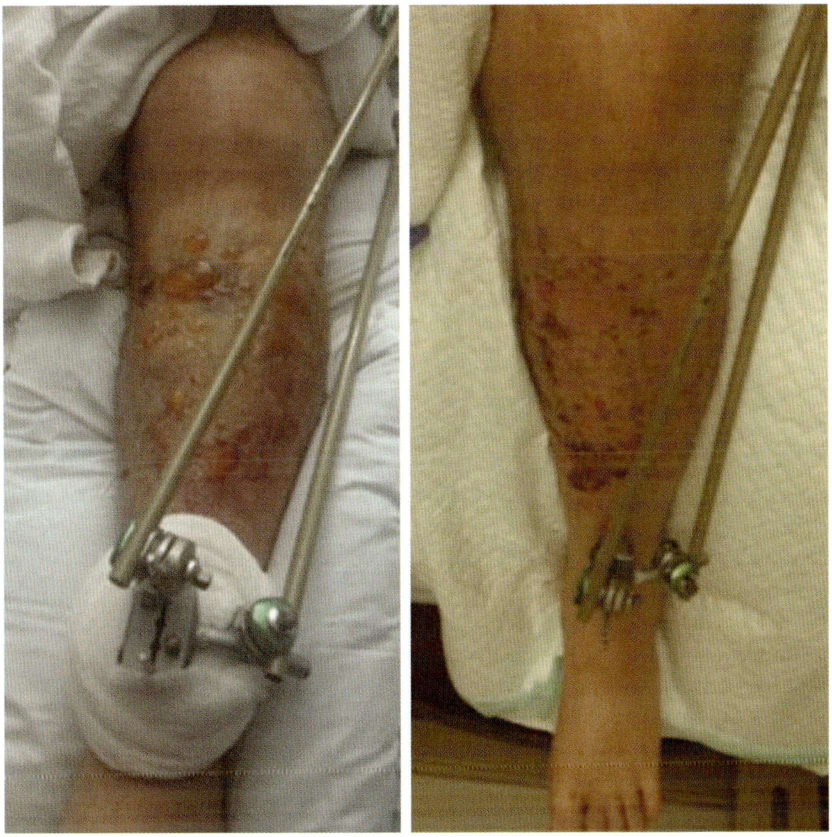

Fig. 8.3 Fracture blisters from a bicondylar tibial plateau following a fall from height (A). Resolution of the blisters with time (B).

faster time to surgery. In their limited case study, there was no incidence of complications related to wound healing.[20]

In the case of tibial plateau fractures, frequently there is a period of immobilization preceding surgery to decrease soft-tissue swelling due to increased complications with acute fixation. This period of immobilization and allowing swelling to subside prior to surgery can absolutely be used to the surgeon's advantage with concomitant management of the fracture blisters (Fig. 8.3). Ultimately, the management of fracture blisters is a surgeon's preference as no best management strategy has been proven.

The prevalence of surgical site infections (SSIs) and wound dehiscence in tibial plateau fractures have historically ranged anywhere from 5% to 80% with a mean of 27% after open reduction and fixation[16] and most recently, reports of an 18% deep infection rate after open reduction and fixation of high-energy tibial plateau fractures.[16] Due to a high incidence of complications from these injuries, there has been significant investigation and research in the realm of how to manage the wounds from the initial insult and surgical fixation. In many cases, these injuries are approached with staged management to optimize surgical outcomes.[21] While the management of these surgical complications is far from algorithmic, there are emerging techniques, technology, and materials that can be a great aid in these potentially debilitating injuries and complications.

One of these emerging methods is NPWT. In cases of primary intention, NPWT reduces edema, increases perfusion, and augments the apposition of wound edges.[17] NPWT aids secondary intention by increasing the speed at which these wounds heal and by allowing stability of the wounds margins.[22] NPWT promotes granulation tissue formation, lessens the bacterial concentration, and increases the expression of intracellular signaling molecules that promote angiogenesis and healing, such as vascular endothelial growth factor and platelet-derived growth factor.[22] The net effect being positively augmented healing with the use of NPWT at macroscopic and microscopic levels.

Recently, there have been numerous studies comparing NPWT to traditional dressings in closed incisions in orthopedic trauma. These cases were primarily of the lower extremity. These studies found that utilization of NPWT decreased the incidence of superficial SSI, deep SSI, and wound dehiscence. It was also found that the use of NPWT can decrease the overall risk of infection of open fractures and increase the rate of healing in these traumatic injuries.[17,22] One reason for this could be due to the fact that when using NPWT, there is a decreased need for dressing changes, which is a significant opportunity for contamination of the wound by healthcare workers. While there have been acceptable results in the study of NPWT as a modality for management of surgical wounds in the trauma setting, there are many instances where traditional dressings and NPWT fail to meet the needs of the wound, and in these instances, various tissue grafts and/or flap coverage remains a mainstay of management.[22,23]

In conclusion, management of wounds in the setting of tibial plateau fractures can be a difficult surgical issue, and there is not always a clear cut way to address the problem. While there have been significant advances in the field of wound management in the setting of tibial plateau fractures, each case must be addressed in light of the wound itself, the mechanism by which the injury was inflicted, and the patients' underlying medical comorbidities. Current management indicates not only staged fixation of the bony insult but also the soft-tissue insult using the vast array of recent medical advances to achieve the best surgical outcome for the patient.

ARTHROFIBROSIS

Inflammation about the knee joint secondary to injury, surgery, or infection can result in excessive collagen production and adhesions that cause decreased joint motion and pain.[24] Approximately 3% to 18% of patients develop a stiff knee following tibial plateau fracture fixation.[25] Decreased knee motion can cause difficulty with activities of daily living as these typically occur in the flexion-extension range of 10 to 120 degrees (raising from a chair, climbing stairs, descending stairs).[26] Kugelman et al. found nonwhite ethnicity, older age, higher body mass index (BMI), and polytrauma to be independent predictors for decreased range of motion following operative treatment of tibial plateau fracture 6 months post surgery.[25] Others have found that increased time in a temporizing external fixator or bilateral tibial plateau fractures can lead to decreased knee range of motion requiring treatment.[27,28]

Nonoperative management begins with aggressive physical therapy; however, if the patient is failing to progress with physical therapy and flexion remains less than 90 degrees, then manipulation under anesthesia is warranted. Haller et al. demonstrated that earlier time to manipulation (mean 2.9 months) leads to greater return in knee motion versus later manipulation (mean 4.86 months).[28] Continuous passive motion (CPM) has been employed to prevent arthrofibrosis postoperatively. Hill et al. found that 48 hours post surgery, there was increased range of motion when using CPM; however, long-term outcomes showed no difference in motion.[29] In contrast, Haller et al. found that the use of CPM to be associated with decreased development of arthrofibrosis with the mean follow-up of 6 months.[28]

Surgical options for treatment of arthrofibrosis include arthroscopic lysis of adhesions or an open debridement with or without a Judet quadricepsplasty. According to Middleton et al., arthroscopic lysis of adhesions correlated with significantly improved overall range of motion at 12 weeks, improved flexion at 12 weeks, as well as improved extension at 12 weeks.[30] Additionally, patients who had previously undergone external fixation had significantly improved motion at 12 weeks following lysis of adhesions.[30] The Judet quadricepsplasty procedure can be used as a last line of treatment for complex knee stiffness.[31] This involves sequential release of restricting adhesions until desired motion is achieved. Release includes resection of intra-articular adhesions (through a medial arthrotomy or arthroscopically) and a lateral incision used to free up lateral retinaculum, release of pin site adhesions, and extraperiosteal release of adhesions to vastus lateralis, vastus intermedius, and rectus femoris. Fractional lengthening of fascia lata, debulking of fibrotic vastus intermedius, and overabundant fracture callus may be necessary as well. The procedure has been found to have a high complication rate (extensor lag, wound dehiscence, deep infection) cited as high as 23%.[32] In a retrospective case series of 11 patients, Bidolegui et al. were able to increase knee flexion from a preoperative mean of 36 degrees to a mean of 98 degrees following a modified Judet quadricepsplasty combined with physical therapy.[33]

POSTTRAUMATIC ARTHRITIS

Does a tibial plateau fracture doom the patient to advanced PTOA and need for an arthroplasty? This clinical debate continues, with the literature clearly acknowledging the radiographic development of arthrosis; however, the clinical outcomes are more varied. Ostrum stated that many lateral tibial plateau fractures do not progress to severe PTOA and do not require total knee arthroplasty (TKA).[34] Ostrum stated that the "literature does not support the belief that an intra-articular tibial plateau fracture will progress to arthritis."[34] Scott et al. reported a 3.3% conversion rate to TKA following periarticular knee fractures with risk factors, including female sex, tibial plateau fractures (versus distal femur), and obesity.[35] Snoeker et al. utilized a young adult cohort study to demonstrate a sixfold increase in arthrosis following any injury to the knee, including meniscal pathology, anterior cruciate ligament tears, and fractures.[36] What are the factors that contribute to clinical outcomes, PTOA, and the need for TKA after intraarticular tibial plateau fracture?

Articular Step-off

Dirschl et al. stated that articular incongruity was well tolerated after tibial plateau fractures.[37] They noted that there is "little support in the literature for the assertion that accurate reduction of tibial plateau fractures, particularly to tolerances <2 mm, is critical for a good clinical outcome."[37] Baumlein et al. reported increased rates of radiographic osteoarthritis in the entire cohort of skiers examined in all compartments of the knee; however, at a mean follow-up of 10.3 years, the Hospital for Special Surgery (HSS) knee score was 96.5 (range 74–100), suggesting satisfactory functional outcomes.[38] Giannoudis et al. noted that articular incongruities were well tolerated for tibial plateau fractures.[39] These authors noted that other factors (features only partially related to articular reduction, e.g., joint stability, retention of the meniscus, and coronal plane alignment) were more important in determining the outcome than articular step-off alone.[39] Of the 11 studies reviewed, five showed no effect on the outcome comparing articular step-off and no step-off.[40–43] Of the other six studies, one showed acceptable results with a step-off of less than 10 mm,[44] and another study showed inferior results with a step-off of more than 10 mm.[45] Wilde stated that preserving the normal alignment of the knee was critical to the end result of the treatment of tibial plateau fractures.[46] He further noted, "Joint depression, per se, if not associated with malalignment, does not necessarily cause poor results."[46] In terms of the effect of joint stability, he noted that joint depression in a stable knee was not necessarily associated with a poor result, but a depression of more than 4 mm did have an effect on outcome.[46] Ehlinger et al. reviewed 13 patients who were surgically treated for a Schatzker type IV-VI tibial plateau fracture after a mean follow-up of 39.1 months.[47] The average Lysholm score was 94.1, the mean HSS score was 93.6, and all patients previously employed returned to work after 4.5 months. Five patients were noted to have an articular step-off of more than 2 mm, yet all 13 patients demonstrated no radiographic evidence of osteoarthritis at final evaluation.[47]

The current literature suggests that articular step-off following intraarticular fractures of the tibial plateau is less of a determinant of outcome when the step-offs are small (4 mm or less), and the fracture involves mainly the lateral tibial plateau.

Variables Other Than Articular Step-off

Dirschl et al. noted that the tibial plateau has thicker articular cartilage than many other joints and that the effect of factors other than articular reduction, such as knee instability, malalignment, and meniscectomy, was more important to the outcome.[37] Ostrum also noted that certain plateau fractures (e.g., medial tibial plateau fractures and those having had an excision of the meniscus) have a much poorer prognosis.[34] Rademakers et al. reported a 31% incidence of radiographic arthritis after operatively treated tibial plateau fractures at 14 years, but most were asymptomatic.[48] However, results were much worse with malalignment of more than 5 degrees. Twenty-seven percent of patients reported moderate to severe symptoms.[48] A study of 73 patients following tibial plateau fracture with a mean follow-up of 54 months demonstrated a correlation with valgus malalignment of more than 5 degrees and advanced osteoarthritis along with a depression of more than 2 mm.[36] Interestingly, the valgus malalignment or articular depression had no effect on outcome scores.[49]

Multiple studies demonstrate poorer clinical, radiographic, and functional outcome scores with increasing fracture classification number using the Schatzker classification.[50–53] Prasad et al. reviewed 40 Schatzker type V and VI tibial plateau fractures treated with dual plating with 4-year follow-up and showed good clinical outcomes in association with good radiographic outcomes.[54] All patients had a final radiographic articular step-off of less than 2 mm, good coronal and sagittal plane alignment, and mean condylar width of less than 5 mm. Final clinical outcome was assessed by the Oxford Knee Score. Thirty-two of 40 had a final score of more than 30 (excellent), and only 8 patients had a score between 20 and 29 (good).[54]

Clearly, there is an association between arthrosis and articular fracture/injury. Wasserstein et al. utilized a cohort analysis to determine a significant increase in TKA risk with an overall hazard ratio of 5.29. Higher rates of TKA were associated with increasing age, bicondylar fracture, and greater comorbidities.[55] A Denmark study by Elsoe et al. noted that 5.7% of 7950 patients who suffered a tibial plateau fracture were managed with a TKA within 13.9 years, a 3.5 times higher hazard ratio than a match cohort without articular fracture.[56] According to van Dreumel, 40.6% (39/71) of proximal tibia fractures developed radiographic arthrosis at 1 year, noting an increase in those with bicondylar fractures (57.5%); yet, there was no correlation to functional outcome measures obtained.[57] Mattiassich et al. evaluated 31 patients at 3 years and 22 years following a tibial plateau fracture documenting deterioration in functional outcomes over time; however, 10 patients (32%) developed no radiographic evidence of arthritis, and at the long-term follow–up, 10 patients had the best scores possible on a clinical examination scale.[58] Some patients developed severe symptoms, while others remained the same or even improved at long-term follow-up.[58] The study did not comment or examine the etiology of their findings as the vast variety of outcome scores are likely multifactorial. However, it appears that malalignment and articular step-off of more than 2 to 4 mm may contribute significantly to the development of posttraumatic arthritis and poorer clinical outcomes after tibial plateau fracture. Because articular step-offs in the tibial plateau are well tolerated, nonarticular step-off factors (malalignment, ligamentous stability) seem to be more important factors in determining outcome for the fractured tibial plateau and the knee joint as a whole. The literature continues to demonstrate that end-stage osteoarthritis following a tibial plateau fracture remains relatively rare. More information on posttraumatic arthritis after tibial plateau fracture can be found in Chapter 9.

CASE 8.1

A 40-year-old helmeted male firefighter presented in the early morning with isolated right leg pain following a motorcycle accident with no palpable or dopplerable pulses, no motor or sensory function, and a transverse laceration over the knee measuring 14 cm × 6 cm with exposed tendon. There were no significant medical history and no history of surgery. He lives 2 hours from the trauma center, is married, and has two young sons. Imaging demonstrated a bicondylar tibial plateau fracture dislocation (Fig. 8.4). Computed tomography angiogram demonstrated a popliteal artery injury requiring emergent surgical intervention (Fig. 8.5). The patient underwent a saphenous vein graft bypass with lower leg fasciotomies (performed by vascular surgery), aggressive debridement with single-layer wound closure, along with reduction and external fixation (performed by orthopedics) (Fig. 8.6).

Postoperative day 1 examination, the patient remained insensate below midtibia and with motor function distal to injury; however, pulses were dopplerable at bedside. The patient complained of significant thigh pain with tense compartments. The trauma surgery team urgently took the patient for thigh fasciotomies, noting increased pressure with minimal nonviable musculature. Upper and lower leg fasciotomies managed with negative pressure dressings per the trauma team. Postoperative day 5, patient was taken to the operating room (OR) with orthopedics for closure of right thigh fasciotomy that had notable extension to the suprapatellar knee wound; however, muscle was viable, and wound was clean. The thigh fasciotomy was closed in a layered fashion, while leaving the fascia open. Lower leg lateral fasciotomy was also clean with minimal debridement

CASE 8.1—CONT'D

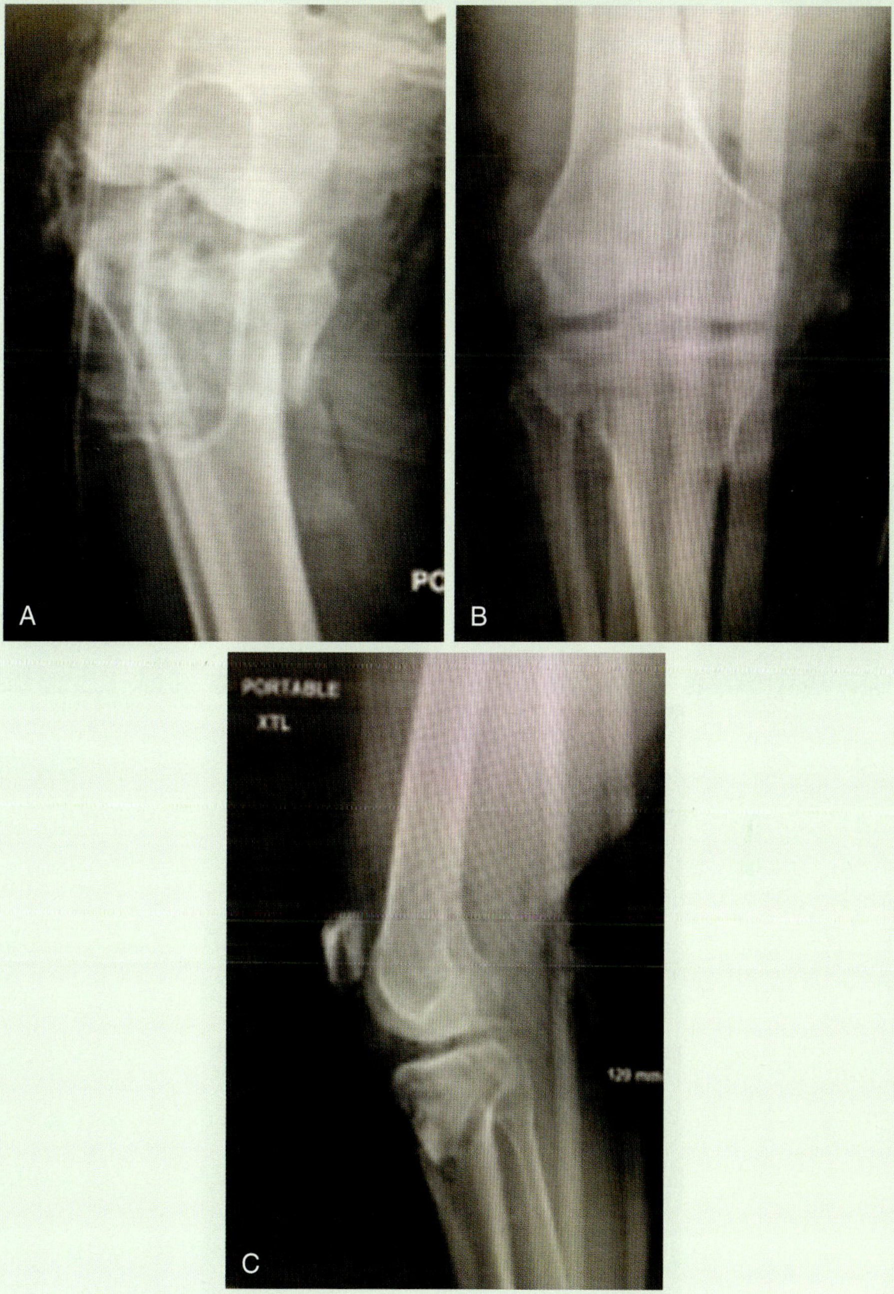

Fig. 8.4 (A) Initial film. (B and C) Postreduction films in a knee immobilizer.

Continued

CASE 8.1—CONT'D

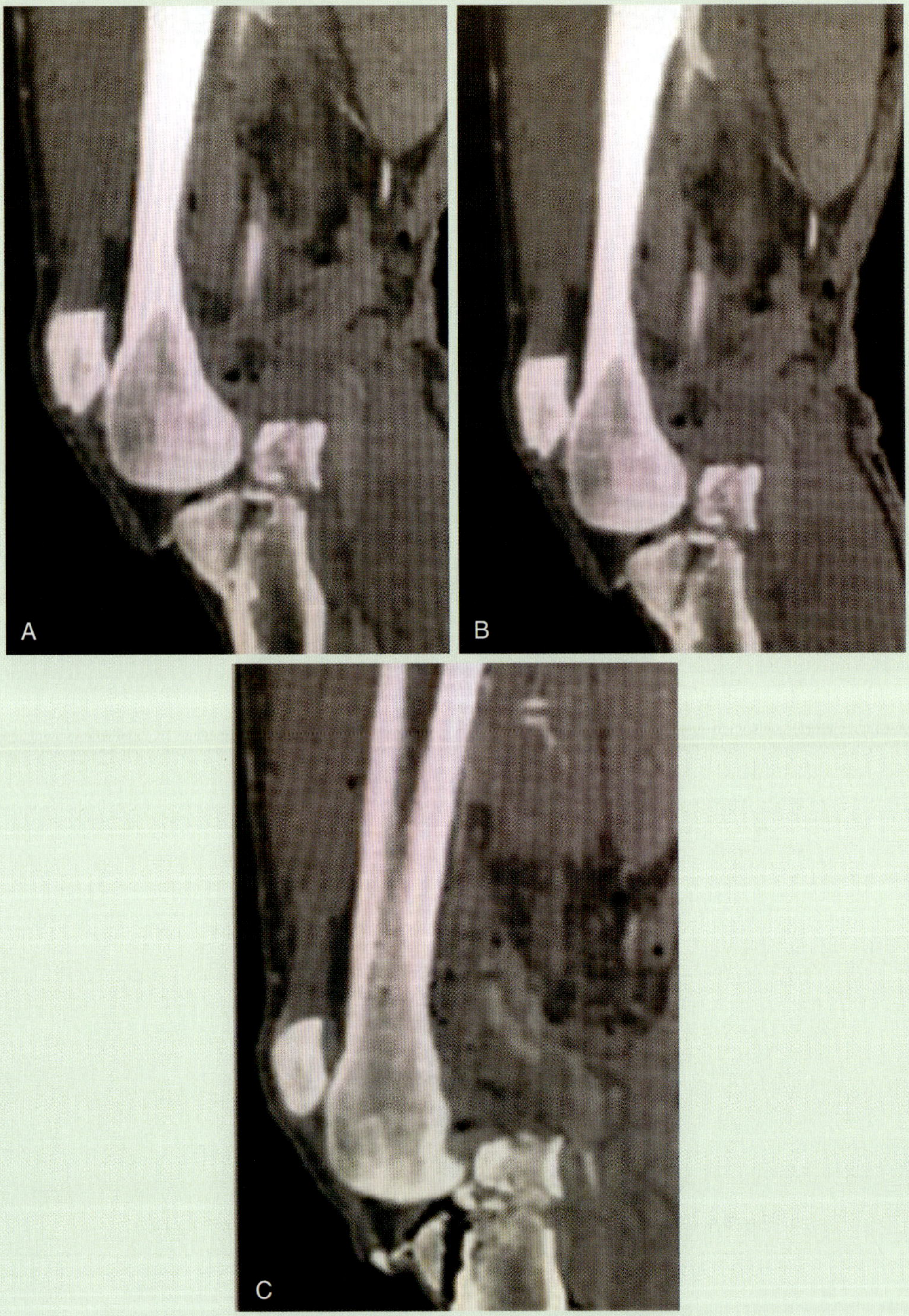

Fig. 8.5 Sequential images of a sagittal computed tomography angiogram demonstrating attenuation of the popliteal artery (A–C).

CASE 8.1—CONT'D

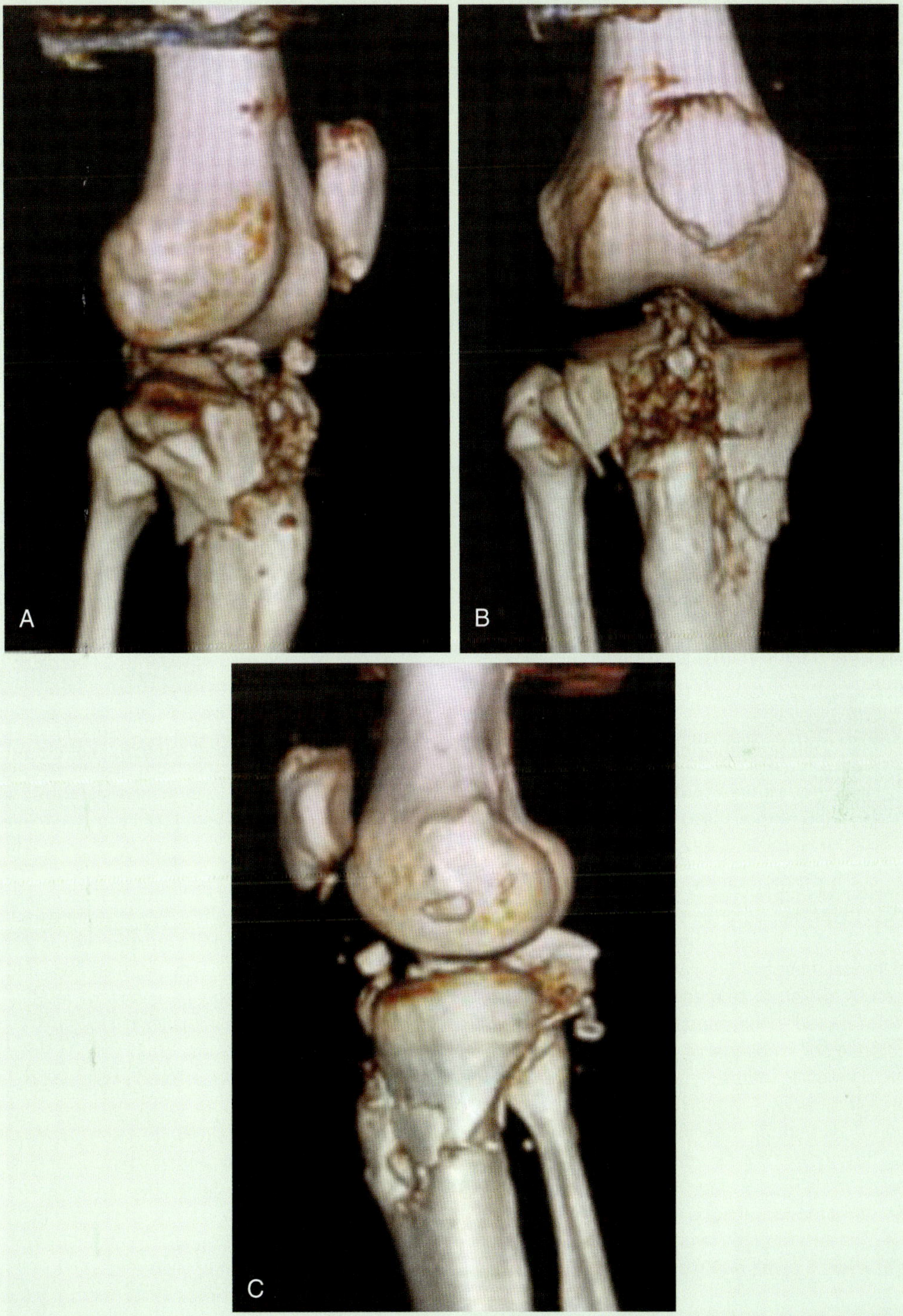

Fig. 8.6 (A–C) 3D CT reconstruction demonstrates the comminution and complexity of the fracture following external fixation.

Continued

CASE 8.1—CONT'D

necessary, negative pressure dressing applied. Unfortunately, extensive medial and deep compartment necrosis was identified and aggressively debrided. Negative pressure dressing was applied to the lower leg. Two more debridements and vacuum-assisted closure (VAC) changes were performed in the OR prior to definitive fixation on postinjury day 9. Definitive fixation of the tibial plateau (Fig. 8.7) was performed in conjunction with repair of the patella tendon avulsion, split-thickness skin grafting of the lateral lower leg fasciotomy, and repeat debridement of the medial fasciotomy with VAC dressing application, along with external fixator removal. The knee was placed in a hinged knee brace locked in extension postoperatively.

Two days following bony fixation, a repeat debridement of the medial fasciotomy noted some concerning deep fluid sent for culture with even further debridement performed. At this time, near-complete resection of the medial gastrocnemius and soleus has been performed with complete exposure of the medial tibia periosteum. Cultures were ultimately positive for a polymicrobial infection (*Escherichia coli*, *Serratia marcescens*, *Enterococcus faecalis*). Infectious disease was consulted, and broad-spectrum antibiotics were started. Three more debridements were performed with continued purulence and necrosis encountered. Multiple discussions with patient and family ensued throughout his hospitalization regarding goals of care and treatment options. Ultimately on postinjury day 26, a right above-knee amputation was performed. The patient was discharged home 3 days following his amputation with intravenous antibiotics for 6 weeks. Outpatient follow-up continued with proper incisional healing and, ultimately, a temporary prosthetic leg within 2 months of his amputation. Primary prosthesis was obtained at 4 months. Ultimately, the patient returned to firefighting at 9 months from his injury. He has since returned to all prior activities, including hunting/fishing, hiking, running, water skiing, and even rock climbing (Fig. 8.8). He also has become an amputee mentor for others around the country.

Key Case Points

1. Wait, wait, wait. Allow the soft tissues to fully demarcate prior to definitive fixation.
2. Always suspect an infection with cultures obtained at subsequent debridements.
3. Keep an open line of communication with the patient *and family*. Provide resources for grief and loss when able (psychiatry, prosthetics consultation, and amputee mentorship).

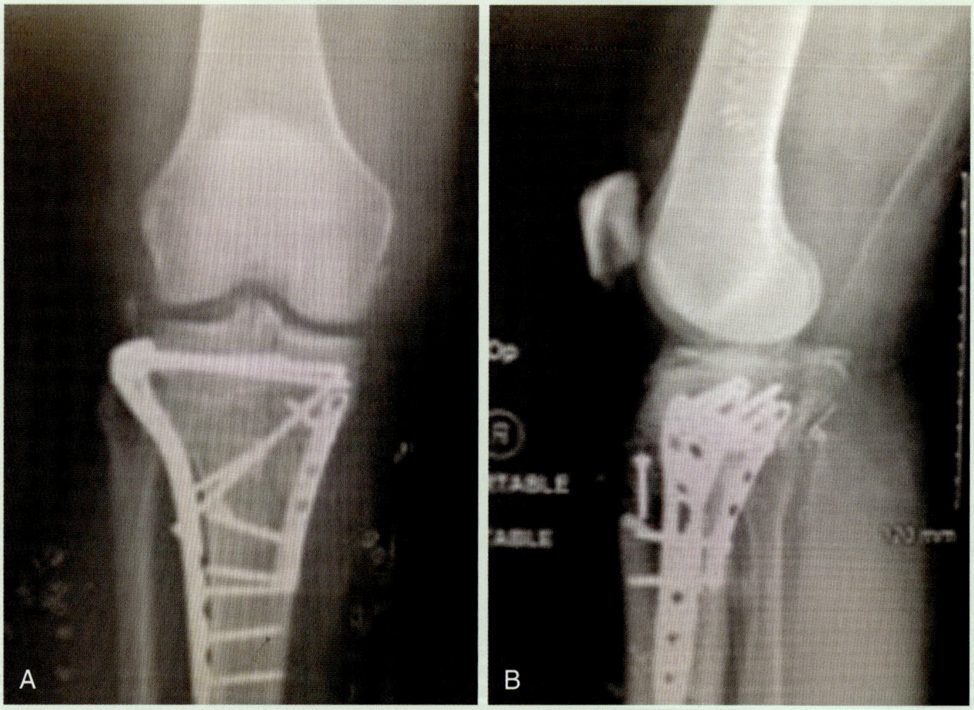

Fig. 8.7 Postoperative anteroposterior (A) and lateral (B) images of the knee.

CASE 8.1—CONT'D

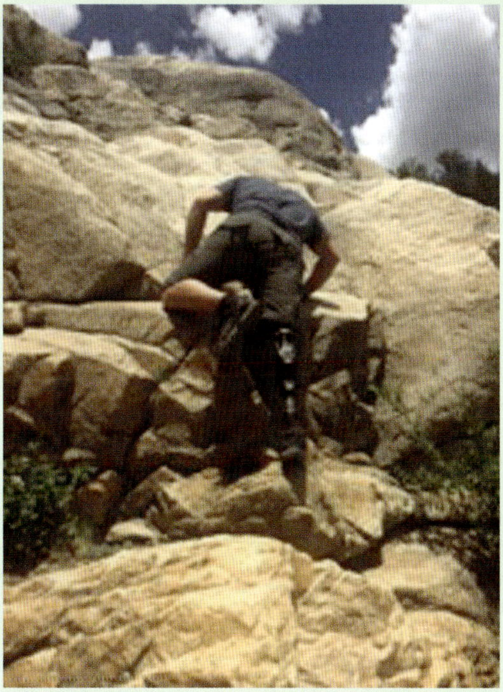

Fig. 8.8 The patient in Case 8.1 rock climbing following above-knee amputation less than 2 years from his injury.

HARTLEY'S TIPS AND TRICKS

- Maintain a high index of suspicion for compartment syndrome, and when diagnosed, perform fasciotomies promptly.
- Negative pressure wound therapy is an effective treatment in wounds where healing by primary or secondary intention is the goal.
- Arthrofibrosis can be treated by manipulation under anesthesia alone if addressed early in the postoperative course, whereas later may require quadricepsplasty and/or intraarticular lysis of adhesions.
- Lateral submeniscal arthrotomy can be performed for nearly all lateral tibial plateau fractures. This improves visualization and allows for reduction confirmation.
- Obtain internal and external rotation intraoperative images to properly view the medial and lateral articular surfaces. Also, obtain images perpendicular to the joint line in the anteroposterior (AP); correct the C-arm as necessary if limb on a triangle, bump, foam, etc.
- Accept that anatomic reduction is occasionally not possible. The cure cannot be worse than the disease. Recall the important aspects of fixation: alignment, ligamentous stability, and medial > lateral articular reduction.

REFERENCES

1. Kugelman D, Qatu A, Haglin J, Leucht P, Konda S, Egol KA. Complications and unplanned outcomes following operative treatment of tibial plateau fractures. *Injury*. 2017;48(10):2221–2229.
2. Egol KA, Koval KJ, Zuckerman JD. *Handbook of Fractures*. 4th ed. Philadelphia, PA: Lippincott Williams & Wilkins; 2010.
3. Papagelopoulos PJ, Partsinevelos AA, Themistocleous GS, Mavrogenis AF, Korres DS, Soucacos PN. Complications after tibia plateau fracture surgery. *Injury*. 2006;37(6):475–484.
4. Colman M, Wright A, Gruen G, Siska P, Pape HC, Tarkin I. Prolonged operative time increases infection rate in tibial plateau fractures. *Injury*. 2013;44(2):249–252.

5. McQueen MM, Gaston P, Court-Brown CM. Acute compartment syndrome. Who is at risk? *J Bone Joint Surg Br*. 2000;82:200–203.
6. Matsen FA. Compartment syndrome. A unified concept. *Clin Orthop Rel Res*. 1975;113:8–14.
7. Schmidt AH. Acute compartment syndrome. *Injury*. 2017;48:S22–S25.
8. Berkson EM, Virkus WW. High-energy tibial plateau fractures. *J Am Acad Orthop Surg*. 2006;14(1):20–31.
9. Weinlein J, Schmidt A. Acute compartment syndrome in tibial plateau fractures—beware!. *J Knee Surg*. 2010;23(1):9–16.
10. Marchand LS, Working ZM, Rane AA, Elliott IS, Gilbertson E, Rothberg DL. Compartment syndrome in tibial plateau fractures: do previously established predictors have external validity? *J Orthop Trauma*. 2020;34(5):238–243.
11. Ulmer T. The clinical diagnosis of compartment syndrome of the lower leg: are clinical findings predictive of the disorder? *J Orthop Trauma*. 2002;16(8):572–577.
12. Finkelstein JA, Hunter GA, Hu RW. Lower limb compartment syndrome: course after delayed fasciotomy. *J Trauma Acute Care Surg*. 1996;40(3):342–344.
13. Hope MJ, McQueen MM. Acute compartment syndrome in the absence of fracture. *J Orthop Trauma*. 2004;18(4):220–224.
14. Sheridan GW, Matsen 3rd FA. Fasciotomy in the treatment of the acute compartment syndrome. *J Bone Joint Surg Am*. 1976;58(1):112–115.
15. Kim PJ, Attinger CE, Steinberg JS, Evans KK. Negative pressure wound therapy with instillation: past, present, and future. *Surg Technol Int*. 2015;26:51–56.
16. Liu X, Zhang H, Cen S, Huang F. Negative pressure wound therapy versus conventional wound dressings in treatment of open fractures: a systematic review and meta-analysis. *Int J Surg*. 2018;53:72–79.
17. Kunze KN, Hamid KS, Lee S, Halvorson JJ, Earhart JS, Bohl DD. Negative-pressure wound therapy in foot and ankle surgery. *Foot Ankle Int*. 2020;41(3):364–372.
18. Strauss EJ, Petrucelli G, Bong M, Koval KJ, Egol KA. Blisters associated with lower-extremity fracture: results of a prospective treatment protocol. *J Orthop Trauma*. 2006;20(9):618–622.
19. Tolpinrud WL, Rebolledo BJ, Lorich DG, Grossman ME. A case of extensive fracture bullae: a multidisciplinary approach for acute management. *JAAD Case Rep*. 2015;1(3):132–135.
20. Hasegawa IG, Livingstone JP, Murray P. A novel method for fracture blister management using circumferential negative pressure wound therapy with instillation and dwell. *Cureus*. 2018;10(10):e3509.
21. Wang C, Zhang Y, Qu H. Negative pressure wound therapy for closed incisions in orthopedic trauma surgery: a meta-analysis. *J Orthop Surg Res*. 2019;14(1):427.
22. Semsarzadeh NN, Tadisina KK, Maddox J, Chopra K, Singh DP. Closed incision negative-pressure therapy is associated with decreased surgical site infections: a meta-analysis. *Plast Reconstr Surg*. 2015;136:592–602.
23. Dingemans SA, Birnie MFN, Backes M, et al. Prophylactic negative pressure wound therapy after lower extremity fracture surgery: a pilot study. *Int Orthop*. 2018;42(4):747–753.
24. Usher KM, Zhu S, Mavropalias G, Carrino JA, Zhao J, Xu J. Pathological mechanisms and therapeutic outlooks for arthrofibrosis. *Bone Res*. 2019;7(1):1–24.
25. Kugelman DN, Qatu AM, Strauss EJ, Konda SR, Egol KA. Knee stiffness after tibial plateau fractures: predictors and outcomes. *J Orthop Trauma*. 2018;32(11):e421–e427.
26. Magit D, Wolff A, Sutton K, Medvecky MJ. Arthrofibrosis of the knee. *J Am Acad Orthop Surg*. 2007;15(11):682–694.
27. Reahl GB, Marinos D, O'Hara NN, et al. Risk factors for knee stiffness surgery after tibial plateau fracture fixation. *J Orthop Trauma*. 2018;32(9):e339–e343.
28. Haller JM, Holt DC, McFadden ML, Higgins TF, Kubiak EN. Arthrofibrosis of the knee following a fracture of the tibial plateau. *Bone Jt J*. 2015;97(1):109–114.
29. Hill AD, Palmer MJ, Tanner SL, Snider RG, Broderick JS, Jeray KJ. Use of continuous passive motion in the postoperative treatment of intra-articular knee fractures. *J Bone Joint Surg Am*. 2014;96(14):e118.
30. Middleton AH, Perlewitz MA, Edelstein AI, Vetter CS. Knee arthrofibrosis following tibial plateau fracture treated with arthroscopic lysis of adhesions with manipulation [published online ahead of print October 27, 2020]. J Knee Surg. doi: 10.1055/s-0040-1718679.
31. Judet R, Judet J, Lagrange I. Technic of liberation of the extensor apparatus in knee stiffness [Une technique de liberation de l'apparielextenseur dans les raiduers du genou]. *Mem Acad Chir (Paris)*. 1956;82:944–947 (in French).
32. Masse A, Biasibetti A, Demangos J, Dutto E, Pazzano S, Gallinaro. The Judet quadricepsplasty: long-term outcome of 21 cases. *J Trauma*. 2006;61(2):358–362.
33. Bidolegui F, Sebastian PP, Robinson EP. Safety and efficacy of the modified Judet quadricepsplasty in patients with post-traumatic knee stiffness. *Eur J Orthop Surg Tramatol*. 2021;31(3):549–555.
34. Ostrum RF. Orthopaedic trauma mythbusters: intra-articular fractures. *Instr Course Lect*. 2013;62:29–33.
35. Scott BL, Lee CS, Strelzow JA. Five-year risk of conversion to total knee arthroplasty after operatively treated periarticular knee fractures in patients over 40 years of age. *J Arthroplasty*. 2020;35:2084–2089.
36. Snoeker B, Turkiewicz T, Magnusson K, et al. Risk of knee osteoarthritis after different types of knee injuries in young adults: a population-based cohort study. *Br J Sports Med*. 2020;54:725–730.

37. Dirschl DR, Marsh JL, Buckwalter JA, et al. Articular fractures. *J Am Acad Orthop Surg*. 2004;12(6):416–423.
38. Baumlein M, Hanke A, Gueorguiev B, et al. Long-term outcome after surgical treatment of intra-articular tibial plateau fractures in skiers. *Arch Orthop Trauma Surg*. 2019;139:951–959.
39. Giannoudis PV, Tzioupis C, Papathanassopoulos A, Obakponovwe O, Roberts C. Articular step-off and risk of post-traumatic osteoarthritis. *Evidence today. Injury*. 2010;41:986–995.
40. Brown TD, Anderson DD, Nepola JV, Singerman RJ, Pedersen DR, Brand RA. Contact stress aberrations following imprecise reduction of simple tibial plateau fractures. *J Orthop Res*. 1988;6:851–862.
41. Honkonen SE. Indications for surgical treatment of tibial condyle fractures. *Clin Orthop Relat Res*. 1994;302:199–205.
42. Koval KJ, Sanders R, Borrelli J, Helfet D, DiPasquale T, Mast JW. Indirect reduction and percutaneous screw fixation of displaced tibial plateau fractures. *J Orthop Trauma*. 1992;6:340–346.
43. Weigel DP, Marsh JL. High-energy fractures of the tibial plateau. Knee function after longer follow-up. *J Bone Joint Surg Am*. 2002;84-A:1541–1551.
44. Lucht U, Pilgaard S. Fractures of the tibial condyles. *Acta Orthop Scand*. 1971;42:366–376.
45. Lansinger O, Bergman B, Korner L, Andersson GB. Tibial condylar fractures. A twenty-year follow-up. *J Bone Joint Surg Am*. 1986;68:13–19.
46. Wilde GP. The knee. In: Foy M, Fagg P, eds. *Medicolegal Reporting in Orthopaedic Trauma*. 4th ed. London, UK: Churchill Livingstone; 2010:273–286.
47. Ehlinger M, Rahme M, Moor B-K, et al. Reliability of locked plating in tibial plateau fractures with a medial component. *Orthop Traumatol Surg Res*. 2012;98:173–179.
48. Rademakers MV, Kerkhoffs GM, Sierevelt IN, Raaymaker EL, Marti RK. Operative treatment of 109 tibial plateau fractures: five- to 27-year follow-up results. *J Orthop Trauma*. 2007;21(1):5–10.
49. Parkkinen M, Madanat R, Mustonen A, Koskinen SK, Paavola M, Lindahl J. Factors predicting the development of early osteoarthritis following lateral tibial plateau fractures: mid-term clinical and radiographic outcomes of 73 operatively treated patients. *Scand J Surg*. 2014;103:256–262.
50. Dall'Oca C, Maluta T, Lavini F, Bondi M, Micheloni GM, Bartolozzi P. Tibial plateau fractures: compared outcomes between ARIF and ORIF. *Strategies Trauma Limb Reconstr*. 2012;7:163–175.
51. Jagdev SS, Pathak S, Kanani H, Salunke A. Functional outcome and incidence of osteoarthritis in operated tibial plateau fractures. *Arch Bone Jt Surg*. 2018;6(6):508–516.
52. Kraus TM, Martetschlager F, Muller D, et al. Return to sports activity after tibial plateau fractures. 89 cases with minimum 24-month follow-up. *Am J Sports Med*. 2012;40(12):2845–2852.
53. Malakasi A, Lallos SN, Chronopoulos E, Korres DS, Efstathopoulos NE. Comparative study of internal and hybrid external fixation in tibial condylar fractures. *Eur J Orthop Surg Traumatol*. 2013;23:97–103.
54. Prasad GT, Kumar TS, Kumar RK, Murthy GK, Sundaram N. Functional outcomes of Schatzker type V and VI tibial plateau fractures treated with dual plates. *Indian J Orthop*. 2013;47(2):188–194.
55. Wasserstein D, Henry P, Paterson JM, Kreder HJ, Jenkinson R. Risk of total knee arthroplasty after operatively treated tibial plateau fracture. A matched-population-based cohort study. *J Bone Joint Surg Am*. 2014;96:144–150.
56. Elsoe R, Johansen MB, Larsen P. Tibial plateau fractures are associated with a long-lasting increased risk of total knee arthroplasty a matched cohort study of 7,950 tibial plateau fractures. *Osteoarthr Cartil*. 2019;27:805–809.
57. van Dreumel RLM, van Wunnik BPW, Janssen L, Simons PCG, Janzing HMJ. Mid- to long-term functional outcome after open reduction and internal fixation of tibial plateau fractures. *Injury*. 2015;46:1608–1612.
58. Mattiassich G, Foltin E, Scheurecker G, Schneiderbauer A, Kropfl A, Fischmeister M. Radiographic and clinical results after surgically treated tibial plateau fractures at three and twenty two years postsurgery. *Int Orthop*. 2014;38:587–594.

9

Posttraumatic Reconstruction

Daniel O. Johansen, MD and Adam A. Sassoon, MD, MS

INTRODUCTION

As discussed in Chapter 5, the surgical management of tibial plateau fractures relies primarily on open reduction and internal fixation (ORIF) using various fracture fixation principles. Reconstruction, however, does serve an important role in select cases in the acute fracture setting. Additionally, arthroplasty is the primary surgical treatment for addressing posttraumatic end-stage arthrosis after tibial plateau fractures. Unicompartmental and total knee arthroplasty (TKA) for treatment after tibial plateau fractures are not without challenges and postoperative complications. Preoperative and intraoperative planning are crucial for successful outcomes when addressing these challenging surgical cases.

PRIMARY TOTAL KNEE ARTHROPLASTY

Rationale for Primary TKA

ORIF of the tibial plateau is the mainstay of treatment in most operative cases of tibial plateau fractures.[1] The goal of periarticular fracture fixation is to restore joint congruity and limb alignment using a stable fixation construct. Unfortunately, not all patients are ideal candidates for ORIF due to the presence of a complex fracture pattern and compromised healing related to their soft tissue and bone biology. Olderly patients with osteoporotic bone who suffer tibial plateau fractures can be considered potential candidates for an acute primary TKA as a definitive form of treatment for their injury.[2]

Complications after ORIF of tibial plateau fractures have been shown to be higher in patients older than 60 years old.[2–4] When considering ORIF in this patient population, the surgeon should be aware of the most common complications, including fixation failure, posttraumatic arthritis, nonunion, malunion, and medical complications related to a prolonged period of immobilization.[5] In this patient population, the higher complication rate is believed to be due to more significant metaphyseal comminution, poor bone quality, and compromised soft-tissue envelope around the knee.[2] In one retrospective study, a 79% fixation failure rate was documented in patients older than 60 compared with only 7% in younger patients.[3] Additionally, the elderly have been shown to have a more difficult time adhering to weight-bearing precautions, which are crucial for success in the early weeks following ORIF.[6] Poor compliance with weight-bearing restrictions has been shown to be an independent risk factor for fixation failure.[3]

Indications and Benefits of Performing a Primary TKA

Primary TKA for a tibial plateau fracture has few indications and should only be undertaken in a specific patient population. Considering the complications associated with ORIF in this population, the elderly patient with preexisting knee osteoarthritis who is found to have a complex periarticular tibial plateau fracture in the setting of osteoporotic bone could be a candidate for definitive treatment with a primary TKA. Reconstruction with a TKA in this patient population treats both the fracture and concomitant knee osteoarthritis. The clinical finding of preexisting and symptomatic knee osteoarthritis is important in these patients as the absence of arthritis would favor a trial of nonoperative management versus ORIF. If the patient subsequently developed knee osteoarthritis, a TKA could then be considered at a later date.

Elderly patients with these fractures can often have medical comorbidities that would likely be exacerbated by prolonged immobilization after ORIF or can lead to the development of decubitus complications (e.g., pneumonia, deep vein thrombosis, decubitus ulcers).[7] A clear benefit of performing a primary TKA is the ability to allow for immediate full weight bearing and knee range of motion without bracing. Similarly, select elderly polytrauma patients with other injuries that would preclude them from early mobilization (e.g., a contralateral lower limb fracture or an upper extremity fracture making use of assistive devices difficult) can also be considered for primary TKA.

Postoperative Outcomes Following Primary TKA

Postoperative outcomes after primary TKA for tibial plateau fractures are favorable in regard to functional scores. A recent systematic review of all studies performing primary TKA for tibial plateau fractures revealed excellent Knee Society Knee Scores and fair Knee Society Function Scores.[8,9] On average, in this systematic review, postoperative knee range of motion at midterm follow-up was found to be 108 ± 10 degrees.[8] To date, there are no studies that directly compare outcomes of primary TKA versus ORIF for the treatment of tibial plateau fractures. Malviya et al.[2] reported patient satisfaction of 90% and noted that 81% of patients returned to their premorbid functional status after primary TKA in their retrospective series of elderly patients. On average, these patients returned to ambulation without use of assistive devices by postoperative day 24.[2]

In the literature, the complication rate averages 15% (range 0%–50%) in these primarily small and retrospective studies.[8] In the largest case series in the literature (n = 30), a reoperation rate of 23% was described.[10] Complications requiring reoperation included: wound complications, periprosthetic fracture, deep infection, removal of loose cement, and revision for aseptic loosening.[10] At midterm follow-up, mortality rates averaged 4.8%.[8]

These results suggest that primary TKA is a valid option for a select group of elderly patients with tibial plateau fractures. Patient selection is important, given the potential complications that this surgery holds. Additionally, it is recommended that a surgeon comfortable with revision arthroplasty techniques performs the reconstruction, given the complexity of the case, which is more similar to revision arthroplasty than a standard TKA for atraumatic osteoarthritis.

Surgical Approach and Decision-Making

As with any complex surgery, preoperative workup and planning are essential for a successful outcome. Examination of the affected extremity should be evaluated for skin and soft-tissue compromise, particularly in an elderly population that is more likely to have a friable soft-tissue envelope following acute trauma. Surgical timing depends on the soft-tissue envelope, but a significant delay is not required. In one study, TKA was performed within an average of 4 days from injury; only one postoperative wound complication was noted.[2] A thorough preoperative medical evaluation must be undertaken to ensure that the patient is optimized to undergo a complex arthroplasty procedure.

Preoperative imaging should include plain radiographs and computed tomography (CT) of the injured knee for fracture pattern identification. Plain radiographs of the ipsilateral tibia and femur should be obtained to rule out any extraarticular deformity, as well as any proximal or distal hardware as the final arthroplasty components often require long stems. Consider obtaining plain radiographs of the contralateral knee to assist with preoperative templating.

Implant choice should be carefully considered well in advance of the operation. Generally, an implant system that creates a balanced knee restores the joint line, and provides knee stability with the least constraint possible should be selected, given concern for earlier aseptic failures with a higher level of constraint.[11] Given that ligamentous injury has been reported to be as high as 71% after tibial plateau fractures, implants with various levels of constraint ought to be made available in the event of compromised collateral ligaments.[12] Similarly, bone loss in these osteoporotic patients can create instability requiring a higher level of constraint such as a condylar constrained implant or even a rotating hinge implant for more significant bony defects. Restoration of bone defects with the use of cement, bone graft, tibial sleeves, or cones must be anticipated. A modular system with stemmed implants should be available as fractures that extend from the plateau into the metaphysis or diaphysis should be bypassed by at least two cortical diameters.[13] Stems also offer the advantage of dispersed stress across the fractured tibia and should be considered with the use of more constrained implants.[14] Additionally, fracture fragment trays, locking plates, and cerclage wires should be available to recreate a stable bony platform prior to the placement of arthroplasty components.

A standard midline incision is recommended. A medial parapatellar arthrotomy is generally sufficient for visualization; however, extensile exposures may be required. Hsu et al. recommend the following systematic approach when performing primary TKA for treatment of periarticular fractures around the knee.[13] First, they recommend preventing fracture propagation using cerclage wires around any fractures that extend into the metadiaphyseal region. Cerclage wires will facilitate the use of intramedullary guides to minimize the risk of fracture propagation or displacement. Next, any fractures of the medial and lateral plateaus are reduced and temporarily fixed with K-wires. Standard fracture fixation principles are followed with the use of plates and/or screws to reconstruct the normal plateau anatomy or to unite any metadiaphyseal fracture fragments.

Following fracture stabilization, attention is turned to reconstruction of the tibial platform.[13] Intramedullary guides are used to make a bone preserving proximal tibia cut. Any bone defects are noted and fill of contained or uncontained defects can be planned with the above-mentioned techniques. If a tibial stem is required, intramedullary preparation is performed. Attention can then be turned to femoral preparation. According to standard knee arthroplasty principles, care must be taken to recreate the joint line and posterior condylar offset in order to optimize knee kinematics.[15]

At this point, the level of implant constraint is selected based on the integrity of the collateral ligaments and the bony architecture. Our most commonly employed implant in this patient population is a semi-constrained knee with stems that bypass the fracture site. However, there is no consensus in the literature regarding the level of constraint required for these cases; these case series with favorable outcomes range from the use of posterior stabilized implants up to rotating hinge systems.[16] Following the placement of trial components, knee kinematics are assessed, and joint stability is verified prior to final component placement. Standard cement techniques are used for implant placement. With a stable construct and well-stabilized knee, the patient is allowed to bear weight as tolerated and fully range the knee without use of a brace.

POSTTRAUMATIC TOTAL KNEE ARTHROPLASTY

Indications for Posttraumatic TKA

Posttraumatic arthritis is a debilitating complication that can develop after tibial plateau fractures. As discussed in Chapter 8, this complication occurs and appears to be related to the severity of the trauma, articular malalignment, and older patient age.[17] Treatment for posttraumatic arthritis begins with nonoperative management. Once the patient has failed conservative treatment, reconstruction should be considered. A TKA is indicated in patients with symptomatic tricompartmental arthritis and can also be considered in cases of end-stage arthritis involving one or two compartments of the knee (Fig. 9.1).[16] Although there are no strict age cut-offs, this procedure is generally reserved for adult patients older than 50, given that patients younger than 50 undergoing TKA are at higher risk for revision.[18] However, any adult patient in whom nonoperative management has failed and who shows signs of end-stage arthritis can be considered for knee arthroplasty. In the literature, the average age at the time of TKA due to posttraumatic arthritis after tibial plateau fractures ranged from 56 to 65 years old.[19–23]

Another potential indication for TKA after tibial plateau fractures is in cases of nonunion. Although rare, nonunion after tibial plateau fractures can occur and does so more frequently in elderly patients or in cases of ORIF complicated by infection.[4] In cases of tibial plateau nonunion, treatment strategies include revision ORIF with bone grafting versus reconstruction with bulk allograft.[24] For elderly patients, especially in the setting of preexisting osteoarthritis, TKA for treatment of the nonunion should be considered.[24,25]

Outcomes of TKA for Posttraumatic Arthritis

The prevalence of posttraumatic arthritis varies between 21% and 44% after tibial plateau fractures.[26] The rate of patients undergoing TKA for management of posttraumatic arthritis, however, is much lower and ranges between 3% and 7.3% in the literature.[16] As expected, with increasing time from injury, the rates of TKA conversion increase.[16] When compared to age-matched controls without a history of plateau fracture, at 2, 5, and 10 years after ORIF, the percentage of patients undergoing TKA are 0.32% versus 0.29%, 5.3% versus 0.82%, and 7.3% versus 1.8%, respectively.[27] Overall, patients with a

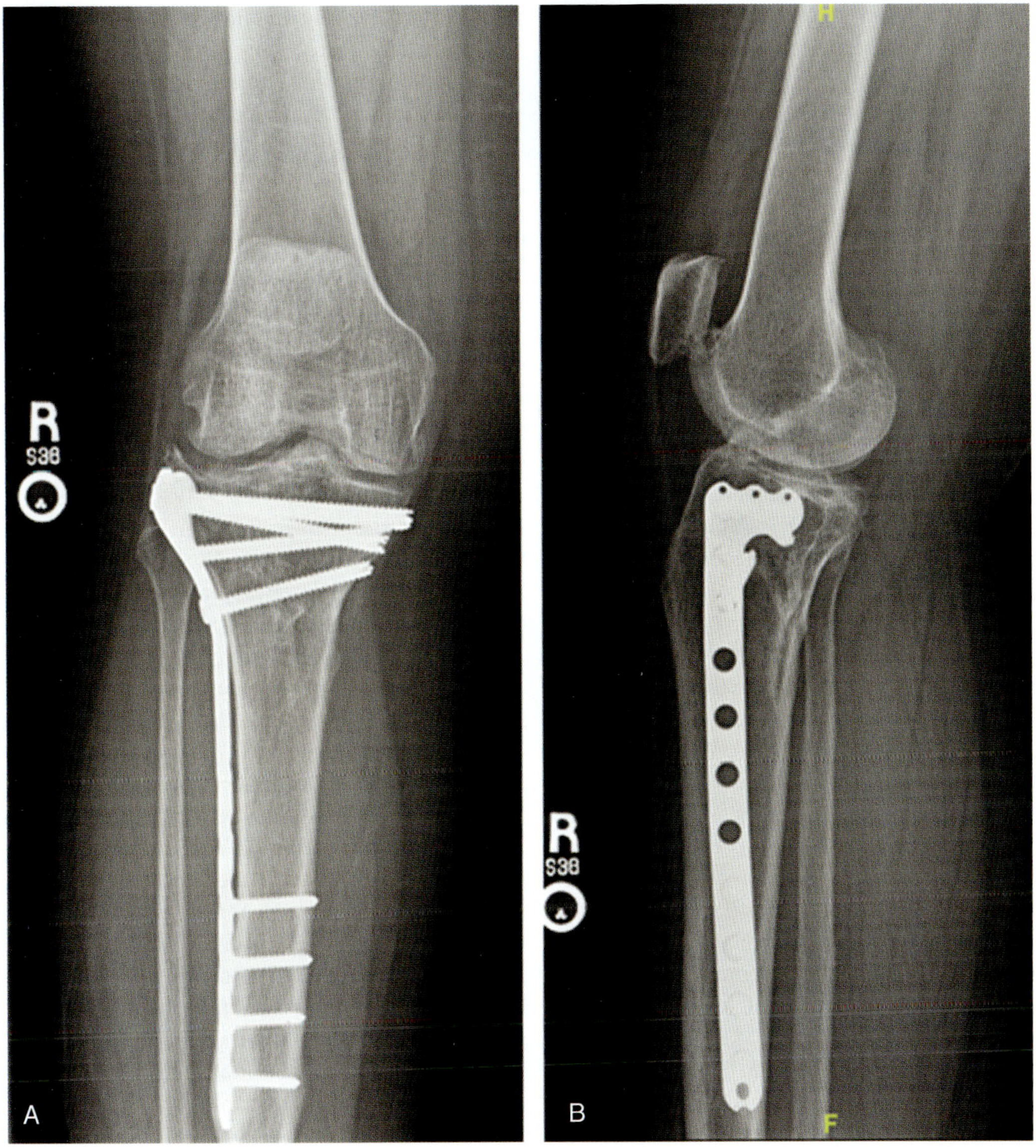

Fig. 9.1 Anteroposterior (A) and lateral (B) knee radiographs of a patient with posttraumatic tricompartmental arthritis after undergoing tibial plateau open reduction internal fixation for a lateral plateau fracture. (Images courtesy Dr. Erik Zeegen.)

history of tibial plateau ORIF are 5.3 times more likely to undergo TKA than age-matched patients without a history of tibial plateau fracture.[27] Factors that influence the risk of needing a TKA are patient age, female sex, presence of medical comorbidities, and bicondylar plateau fractures.[27]

Earlier studies showed that TKA for posttraumatic arthritis resulted in lower functional scores when compared to TKA for primary knee osteoarthritis.[28] However, more recent studies have shown that postoperative knee function scores and patient-reported outcomes are comparable to patients undergoing TKA for primary osteoarthritis.[21,26] TKA after tibial plateau fractures has been shown to significantly improve knee function and decrease knee pain.[19–23,26] Posttraumatic knee stiffness can be a debilitating complication for patients after sustaining tibial plateau fractures. Following TKA, knee range of motion has been shown to increase 4 to 18 degrees compared to preoperative range of motion.[19,20,23,29] At midterm follow-up, most patients are satisfied after undergoing TKA for posttraumatic arthritis; there was no significant difference in patient satisfaction compared to an age-matched cohort of patients undergoing TKA for primary osteoarthritis.[21]

Implant survivability following TKA for posttraumatic arthritis has also shown to be favorable at mid- and long-term follow-up.[21,23,26] Complications are not insignificant in this patient population, but revisions for mechanical complications are not significantly different when compared to a control group undergoing TKA for primary osteoarthritis.[21,26] Implant survival free of revision due to aseptic loosening is as high as 96% at 15-year follow-up, a number comparable to revision rates of TKA for primary osteoarthritis.[23]

Surgical Challenges and Complications

Although TKA for posttraumatic arthritis after tibial plateau fracture is a useful surgical option, it is not without its challenges and complications. When compared with TKA for primary osteoarthritis, TKA after tibial plateau fractures is associated with significantly higher rates of intraoperative and postoperative complications.[19,21,23,26] The higher rate of intra- and postoperative complications is likely related to posttraumatic stiffness, previous incisions that may have compromised the soft-tissue envelope, malalignment, ligamentous instability, presence of retained hardware, possible occult infection, and bony defects.

Intraoperative complications can include fractures, damage to the extensor mechanism, and collateral ligament injury.[19,21,23,26] These intraoperative complications are likely higher as a result of difficulty with obtaining adequate visualization. Posttraumatic changes after fracture and/or ORIF can make the knee very stiff, which can impede intraoperative visualization similar to that of a revision TKA procedure. In certain cases, one may require the use of a more extensile exposure such as the quadriceps snip, VY turndown, or a tibial tubercle osteotomy. Additionally, extensive soft-tissue releases off the femoral condyles can substantially improve visualization and help protect the extensor mechanism. If such releases are anticipated or planned, a constrained or hinged implant option should be available.

Postoperative complications occur at higher rates compared with TKA for primary osteoarthritis, particularly within the first 2 years after surgery.[21,23] At 15-year follow-up, one recent study showed that complications occurred at a rate as high as 34%, with 90% of these complications occurring within the first 2 years after TKA.[23] One of the most common postoperative complications has been shown to be early wound complications, likely due to compromised soft-tissue envelope in the setting of previous surgical incisions, retained hardware, and posttraumatic changes after a fracture.[21,23,26] Other notable complications can include arthrofibrosis, infection, extensor mechanism injury, aseptic loosening, patellar subluxation, and periprosthetic fracture.[20–23,26]

Preoperative Workup and Planning

In order to optimize the patient's outcome intraoperatively and postoperatively, a thorough preoperative examination and surgical plan are required. The surgeon should approach the preoperative workup in a manner similar to that of a complex revision arthroplasty case. Starting with the physical examination, the skin and soft tissues must be inspected. As mentioned, the wound complication rates after TKA for posttraumatic arthritis are much higher than in primary TKA cases.[21,23,26] The surgical scars and the location of any prior grafts or flaps should be noted and documented to plan out the surgical approach. For the patient with multiple revisions, skin may be thin and significantly adherent to the proximal tibia, patella, or femur. A plastic surgery consultation should be considered if there is concern about postoperative wound closure that may require skin grafting or flap coverage.

Knee range of motion should be assessed preoperatively. It is well documented that knee stiffness is a common complication after tibial plateau fractures following operative or nonoperative treatment.[3,4,16] One-third of patients treated with ORIF for their tibial plateau fractures underwent conversion to TKA due to pain and stiffness.[21] Identification of knee contractures is useful to help plan for necessary releases intraoperatively. Although TKA for posttraumatic arthritis has been shown to increase knee range of motion by 4 to 18 degrees, expectations of postoperative knee range of motion should be discussed with the patient as it has been shown that preoperative knee range of motion is one of the biggest determinants of postoperative knee range of motion.[19,20,23,29]

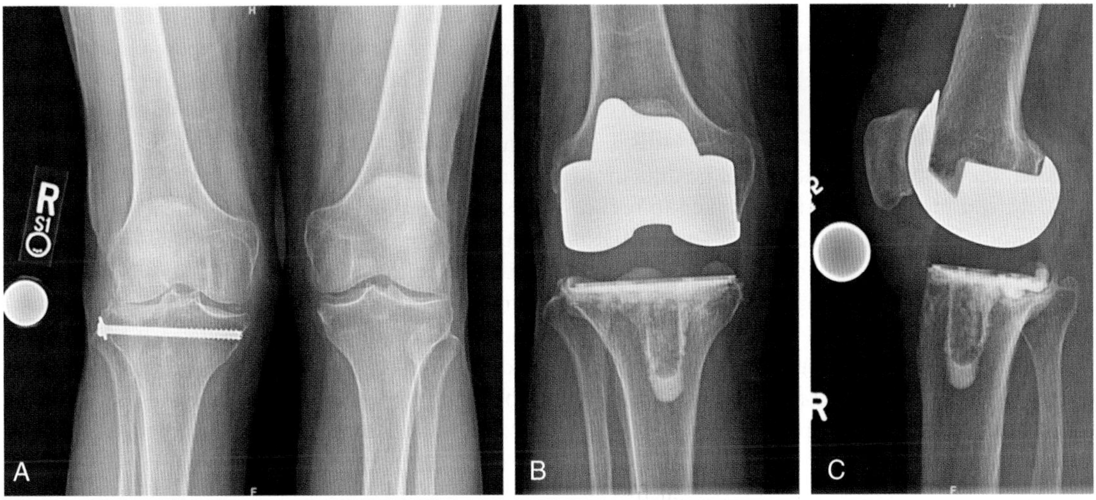

Fig. 9.2 Anteroposterior standing knee radiograph (A) of a patient who had previously undergone screw fixation for treatment of a lateral tibial plateau fracture. The patient has posttraumatic arthritis, most significant within the lateral compartment. Anteroposterior (B) and lateral (C) postoperative radiographs show that a total knee arthroplasty was performed using posterior stabilized implants.

A thorough ligamentous examination should be performed, given the high rate of ligamentous injury following tibial plateau fractures.[12] Identification of incompetent collateral ligaments will help guide decision-making regarding the level of implant constraint. We recommend the use of an implant system that creates a balanced knee, restores the joint line, and provides knee stability with the least constraint possible (Fig. 9.2). Even in patients without evidence of preoperative ligament insufficiency or significant bone loss on imaging, revision TKA implant systems need to be available on the day of surgery in anticipation of potential intraoperative complications such as collateral ligament injury or bone defects.

Preoperative imaging should include plain radiographs of the knee and weight-bearing hip-to-ankle radiographs to assess leg alignment and presence of hardware and to evaluate for extraarticular deformity, which could complicate component positioning or the use of long-stemmed implants. The use of intraoperative computer navigation can be helpful in cases with hardware or extraarticular deformity of the tibia or femur.[30] CT of the knee is not required but can be useful to rule out nonunion or osseous defects that are not readily appreciated on plain radiographs.

Infection is a significant complication in this patient population and has occurred at a rate of 3.2% to 20% in the literature, which is higher than that of TKA for treatment of primary osteoarthritis.[20–23,26] For this reason, a thorough preoperative history and workup should be undertaken. Red flags include any history of wound complication, failure of fixation, nonunion, multiple surgeries, or a history of an open tibial plateau fracture. In addition to complete blood count, consider obtaining a C-reactive protein (CRP) and erythrocyte sedimentation rate (ESR) prior to surgery. Aspiration and synovial fluid analysis with culture should be performed in patients who have had a history of previous wound healing problems, tibial nonunion, or elevated inflammatory markers.

The presence of hardware around the joint may complicate the surgical approach and will most often require hardware removal. Preoperative planning should include the decision to perform either a one- or two-stage conversion from ORIF to TKA. In most cases in the literature, conversion to TKA was performed in a single-stage fashion.[20–23,31] There is some evidence that the history of ORIF around the knee and the presence of retained hardware following TKA may increase the risk of infection postoperatively.[32] More recent studies have shown a trend toward higher infection rates for one- or two-stage procedures and a trend toward more mechanical complications for cases where previous hardware is fully or partially retained after TKA, but these results did not reach statistical significance.[31,33] The decision to remove the hardware in a staged fashion should be made, in part, based on any history of past infection, signs or symptoms of current infection, and with the patient's skin and soft-tissue envelope in mind.

Surgical Approach and Decision-Making

As discussed, the posttraumatic knee can be difficult to expose safely, and precautions must be taken to reduce the risk of wound complications. For patients without previous knee surgery, a standard midline incision is recommended. If previous incisions have been made, the most recent incision should be used as long as it can be modified to provide adequate exposure.[16] Using the most lateral incision is recommended as this will avoid interrupting the blood supply to the lateral flap that obtains its most robust dermal blood supply from the medial aspect of the knee.[16,34] If transverse scars are present, they can be most safely crossed at a 90-degree angle.[16] Caution should be taken when raising flaps in order to preserve the blood supply as best as possible.

A medial parapatellar arthrotomy is our standard approach to the joint. Cultures of the synovial fluid can be taken, especially in patients treated with previous tibial plateau ORIF. Extensive release of scar within the gutters, suprapatellar pouch, and the peritendinous tissues may be required to sublux the patella for adequate visualization. The use of more extensile exposures such as the quadriceps snip, femoral epicondylar peel, or a tibial tubercle osteotomy may be required in order to prevent iatrogenic injury to the extensor mechanism.

Following adequate releases to obtain sufficient visualization, the knee can be prepared for arthroplasty components. As in primary TKA, the goal in this setting is to provide a stable knee that restores neutral mechanical alignment and sagittal and coronal balance, preserves the joint line and posterior tibial slope, and obtains normal patellar tracking.[35] Posttraumatic malunion, nonunion, bone defects, extraarticular deformity, and ligament deficiency will make this a challenge.

A subperiosteal release of the proximal tibia soft tissue is performed to expose the medial plateau. Any bony defects and the extent of articular malalignment are assessed. We utilize intramedullary guides for tibial preparation, but extramedullary guides or navigation may be required in cases with intramedullary hardware or significant extraarticular deformity. Preoperative templating can assist with planned bone cuts to restore mechanical alignment. If proximal tibial hardware is located within the planned cut, the hardware will need to be fully or partially removed. Ideally, this should be done as minimally invasive as possible and is incorporated into the incision. If needed, the proximal aspect of the plate can be cut with a diamond-tipped burr a and the remainder of screws and distal plate can be retained; metal debris must be thoroughly removed (Fig. 9.3).

Collateral ligament integrity is then assessed and will guide the level of implant constraint. We have found that semi-constrained or hinged implants are often required in these cases due to previous ligament injury, as a result of intentional releases of the collaterals for the purpose of adequate visualization, or as a result of ligament injury following large tibial or femoral bone cuts due to intraarticular malalignment. Other indications for more constrained implants are for obese patients or patients with neuropathic arthropathy (Fig. 9.4). Following bone cuts, the tibia is prepared, and bone defects are addressed using bone grafting, cement fill, metal sleeves, or cones (Fig. 9.5). We recommend the use of diaphyseal engaging stems, particularly in cases where bone loss is present, a higher constrained implant is used, or when the stress riser needs to be bypassed. The stem disperses stress across the proximal tibia, which is important in a case with defects due to a previous fracture.[36] Modular offset stem couplers can be used to avoid stem and component malposition and maximize the metaphyseal coverage in cases of deformity of the tibia. The stem and tibial components are cemented using either a total cementation technique or a hybrid fixation technique with a cementless diaphyseal engaging stem and cemented fixation of the metaphyseal components.[36] This decision is typically based on surgeon preference, but the quality of the diaphyseal bone may play a role in technique selection.

Following the placement of final implants, a final verification of knee kinematics and stability is performed. Due to significantly higher rates of postoperative infection following TKA for treatment of tibial plateau fractures,[20–23,26] we routinely use calcium sulfate beads containing vancomycin and tobramycin for infection prophylaxis. A layered closure of the wound is performed taking great care to respect the soft-tissue envelope during wound closure. Intraarticular drains and a negative pressure wound dressing are recommended. Postoperatively, the patient is allowed to be weight-bearing as tolerated with full range of motion. If necessary, full flexion may be restricted for a short period of time in certain patients with tenuous skin in order to prevent wound dehiscence.

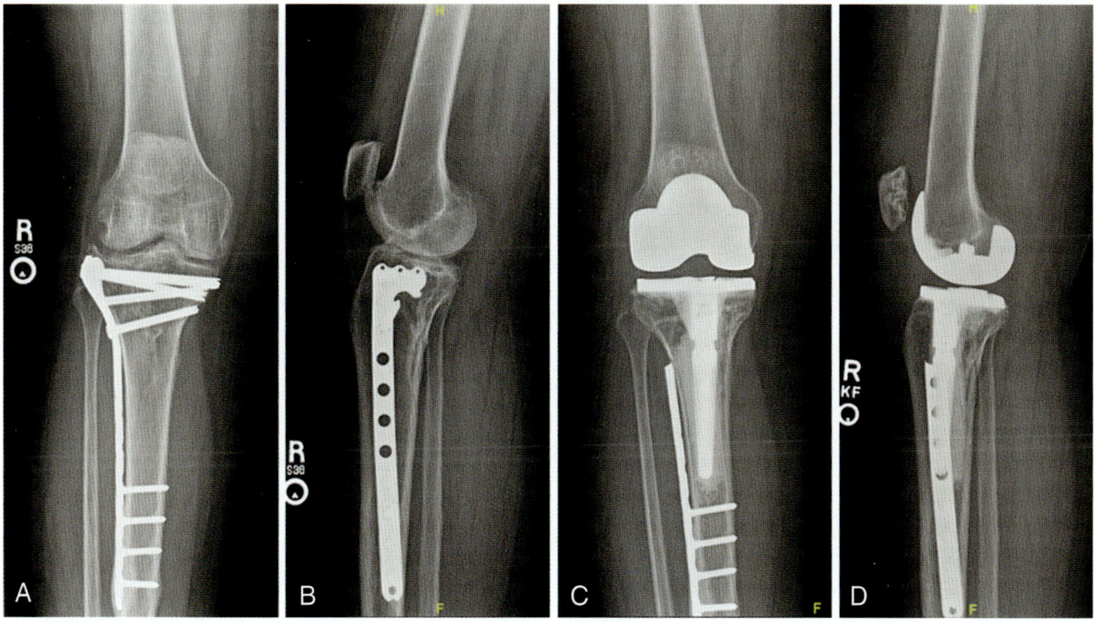

Fig. 9.3 Anteroposterior (A) and lateral (B) radiographs of a patient with posttraumatic knee arthritis after undergoing open reduction internal fixation for a lateral plateau fracture. Postoperative anteroposterior (C) and lateral (D) radiographs demonstrate the use of posterior stabilized knee implants. Intraoperatively, the plate was found to interfere with tibial component position. A diamond-tipped burr was used to cut and remove the proximal portion of the plate in order to avoid a more extensive approach that would have been required for entire plate removal. (Images courtesy Dr. Erik Zeegen.)

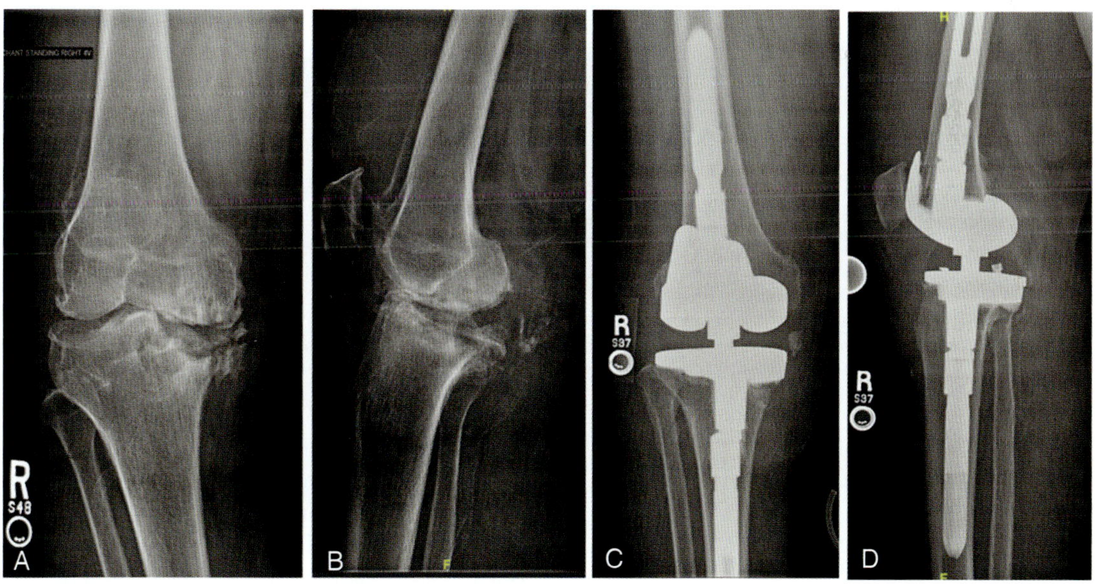

Fig. 9.4 Anteroposterior (A) and latera (B) radiographs of a patient with diabetes and Charcot arthropathy of the right knee. Due to the presence of neuropathic arthropathy, a hinged total knee arthroplasty system was utilized in order to prevent postoperative instability that can be seen in this patient population when lower levels of constraint are used. An augment was used for the medial tibial base plate in order to address medial sided bone loss. Postoperative anteroposterior (C) and lateral (D) radiographs are shown.

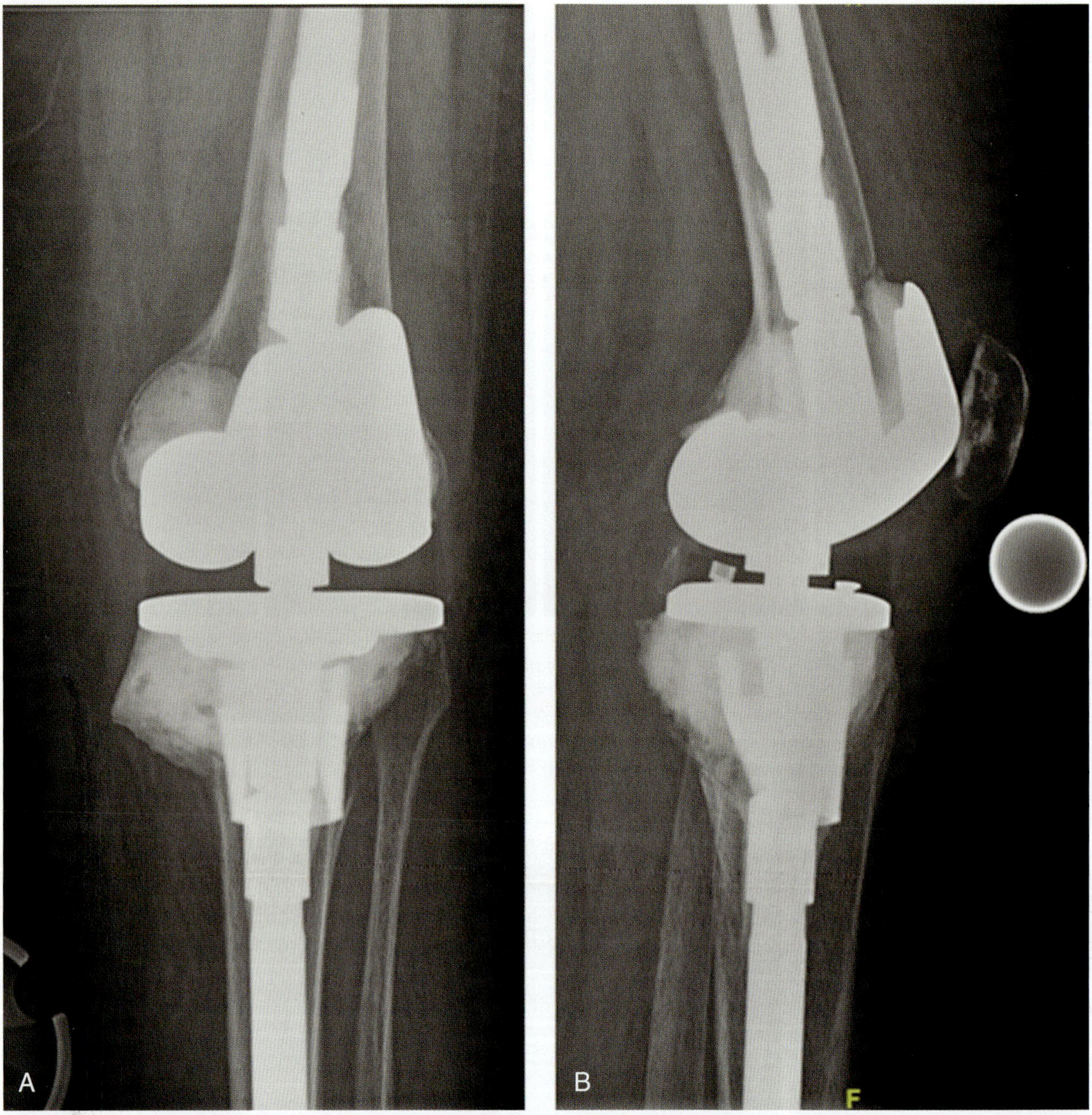

Fig. 9.5 Anteroposterior (A) and lateral (B) radiographs of a knee with use of hinged total knee arthroplasty implants. Intraoperatively, the patient was noted to have severe bone loss on the femoral and tibial side. The defects were addressed with use of a tibial metaphyseal cone as well as cement fill at the periphery.

UNICOMPARTMENTAL KNEE ARTHROPLASTY

Indications for Unicompartmental Knee Arthroplasty

Tibial plateau fractures involving the medial or lateral plateau in isolation can result in knee arthritis due to the intraarticular injury and posttraumatic degeneration resulting from unequal forces across a malunited joint.[37] In cases of symptomatic unicompartmental femorotibial arthritis, a unicompartmental knee arthroplasty (UKA) is a surgical treatment that can be considered in select patients. Considerations for patient selection for UKA in the posttraumatic setting include age, activity level, grade of arthritis, ligament stability, and amount of knee malalignment.[38]

Patients with radiographic findings of moderate or severe single-compartment posttraumatic arthritis are considered as cases of mild osteoarthritis can be treated nonoperatively or with a corrective osteotomy.[38] Patient age and activity level are considered when deciding between a UKA or an alternative treatment option for posttraumatic arthritis. Although it has been suggested that younger (i.e., less than 50 years old) and more active patients are at higher risk of revision, more recent studies have questioned this, showing lower revision rates than previously reported.[39,40] In a study of patients undergoing lateral compartment UKA for posttraumatic arthritis after tibial plateau fracture, the average patient age was 50 with a range from 25 to 67 years.[41]

Additional factors that are considered are the degree of the malalignment of the knee. Knees with more than 15 degrees of varus or valgus malalignment are generally contraindicated, but the main factor in decision making should be whether or not the knee deformity is correctable on examination. When it is not correctable on examination, this would require soft-tissue release, which could result in instability.[42] Anterior cruciate ligament (ACL) integrity is also a requirement for UKA as ACL-deficient knees have been shown to have higher rates of femoral rollback and altered kinematics, which can result in higher failure rates or liner wear.[38,39,42]

Outcomes of UKA for Posttraumatic Arthritis

There are limited studies specifically addressing outcomes following UKA for posttraumatic arthritis after tibial plateau fractures.[41,43,44] These studies included patients who underwent lateral UKA, which is consistent with the fact that tibial plateau fractures most commonly involve the lateral tibial plateau.[41,43,44] Functional outcomes were improved as postoperative knee scores increased compared to preoperative scores.[41,43,44] The postoperative range of motion was noted to be, on average, equal to the arc of motion that was present prior to surgery, which is consistent with the postoperative range of motion following TKA for posttraumatic arthritis.[19,20,23,41] Valgus malalignment at final follow-up was significantly improved compared to preoperative measurements.[43] In one study, prosthesis survivorship was shown to be 100% at 5- and 10-year follow-up and 80% at 15-year follow-up.[41]

In a comparative study of lateral UKAs for primary knee osteoarthritis versus posttraumatic knee osteoarthritis, postoperative functional outcomes were significantly better in the primary osteoarthritis group.[44] However, in a more recent study, there was no significant difference in postoperative knee scores or in 9-year prosthesis survival rates (92% in both groups).[43]

The sparse data on this topic show that the indication for UKA after posttraumatic arthritis due to tibial plateau fractures is rare overall. However, when patients are selected appropriately, these studies show that UKA for posttraumatic arthritis after tibial plateau fracture is an effective treatment for improving knee function and alignment with a low overall revision rate. Further studies are required to better elucidate any differences in outcomes compared to UKA for primary osteoarthritis.

Preoperative Planning and Surgical Approach

The preoperative workup and plan are similar to that of preparing for a TKA for the treatment of posttraumatic knee arthritis. A physical examination is required to assess for previous scars or incisions as this can influence the surgical approach. Performing a ligamentous examination is important in these patients as ACL insufficiency is considered a contraindication for UKA. An assessment of the knee alignment should be performed with emphasis on determining if the varus/valgus alignment is correctable to neutral. As mentioned, if the knee deformity cannot be corrected, a larger release is likely required, which could destabilize the UKA.

Preoperative imaging includes weight-bearing radiographs of the knee to classify the level of arthritis and rule out multicompartment arthritis. A standing hip-to-ankle radiograph is also useful to calculate the degree of malalignment and to identify any extraarticular deformity or additional hardware above or below the knee. Additionally, a stress radiograph can be performed to objectively assess if the knee deformity is correctable. CT can be considered if there is concern of nonunion or significant bone loss. A magnetic resonance imaging (MRI) can also be considered if the ACL or collateral ligament integrity is in question; however, the presence of hardware from an ORIF may result in a significant artifact.

Implant selection is based upon the surgeon's preference in regard to fixed- versus mobile-bearing implants. The current studies of lateral UKA for posttraumatic arthritis have primarily utilized a fixed-bearing design. We routinely use fixed-bearing designs for our UKAs to avoid the risk of mobile-bearing dislocation. As with any arthroplasty procedure, backup equipment and implants should be made available. A TKA implant system should be on hand in the event that a conversion to TKA is required.

The incision for a UKA depends on the surgeon's preference and on which femorotibial compartment is being replaced. A standard midline incision can be used, or the incision can be translated laterally or medially. A medial parapatellar arthrotomy or midvastus approach is typically utilized for a medial UKA. A medial or lateral parapatellar arthrotomy has been described for access to the lateral compartment when performing a lateral UKA.[42,44] After entering the joint, the contralateral femorotibial and patellofemoral compartments are assessed for the extent of arthritis to determine whether to proceed with UKA or TKA.

The decision to remove any hardware is made based on whether or not it would interfere with the tibial bone cuts. Hardware removal should be undertaken in a soft-tissue friendly manner in order to avoid wound complications postoperatively. The tibia is then assessed for the extent of bony defects. Bony defects should be relatively minimal; otherwise, a TKA should be considered. Bone defects can be filled with autograft from the femoral bone cuts. In cases of comminution or depression of the plateau, the use of bone graft with reinforcing screws to support the subchondral bone has been described.[41] Once a stable plateau is recreated, trial components can be placed. Knee stability and kinematics are then tested prior to cementing the final components into place. Postoperatively, these patients are allowed to weight-bear with full range of motion as tolerated.

CASE STUDY 9.1

History of Present Illness

The patient was a 53-year-old female who presented to the clinic for consultation regarding her right knee. The patient had a fall from a ladder 8 months prior and suffered a closed Schatzker type VI tibial plateau fracture. She was treated at an outside hospital with external fixation followed by definitive fixation approximately 4 weeks later. She denied any revision surgeries or infections. She was able to weight bear with a cane but complained of instability and significant knee pain. Her x-rays in the clinic showed a significantly comminuted plateau fracture treated with medial and lateral plate fixation (Fig. 9.6 A, B). On physical examination, she had well-healed incisions over the medial and lateral proximal tibia. There was a notable prominence of the tibial tuberosity with a thin soft-tissue envelope. The passive knee range of motion was limited to 10 to 85 degrees. She had 4 out of 5 quadriceps motor strength with a 15-degree extension lag. There was significant laxity with no endpoint when varus and valgus stress were applied to the knee.

Preoperative Planning

When planning for TKA in cases such as these, with significant comminution, joint line disruption, pain, instability, and a compromised soft-tissue envelope, a staged approach is recommended. Prior to hardware removal, a CT scan was done to confirm fracture healing. Hardware removal was performed as minimally invasive as possible using the previous incisions (Fig. 9.6C, D). Cultures performed during the procedure were negative for bacterial growth. The patient was doing well until about 6 weeks after hardware removal when she presented to an outside hospital with swelling and pain. The outside facility believed that she had osteomyelitis based on MRI findings and began treating her with intravenous antibiotics. She re-presented to our facility and was found to have elevated ESR and CRP with persistent pain and swelling. An aspiration of the joint was negative for bacteria, and synovial white blood cell count was within normal limits. An ultrasound was negative for deep vein thrombosis. Due to concern for likely infection, the decision was then made to proceed with a two-stage TKA with placement of an antibiotic spacer prior to undergoing final component placement.

Antibiotic Spacer Placement

Prior to surgery, preoperative templating was done to estimate the size of our proposed implants. Based on imaging and physical examination findings, we anticipated that she would ultimately require a hinged TKA. Rather than using the medial or lateral incisions, a midline incision was utilized in anticipation of the future TKA procedure. A medial parapatellar arthrotomy was performed. Synovial fluid was sent for culture. An extensive synovectomy was performed, given the possibility of infection. Tissue samples were also sent for culture. We elected to perform an articulating antibiotic spacer in order to preserve as much knee range of motion as possible. The femur and tibia were prepared using the revision system cutting guides. The patella was also cut in preparation of future resurfacing. A thorough irrigation was performed using dilute betadine followed by a pulse irrigator. Sizing of each component was done and

CASE STUDY 9.1—CONT'D

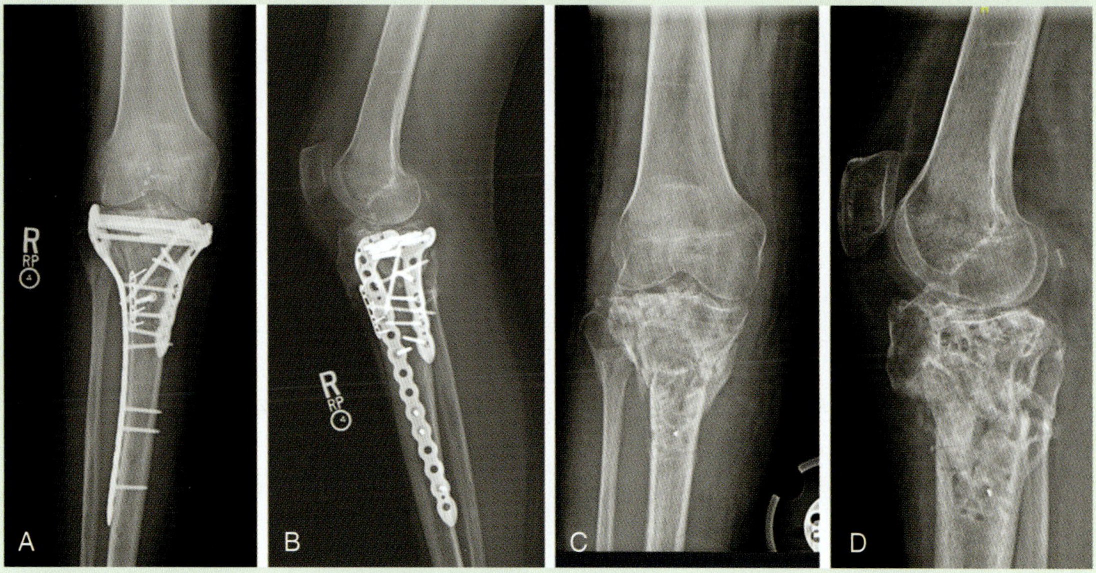

Fig. 9.6 Anteroposterior (A) and lateral (B) radiographs of a patient who had undergone internal fixation for treatment of a Schatzker type VI tibial plateau fracture. There is severe posttraumatic arthrosis of the medial and lateral compartments of the knee. Hardware removal was performed for a planned staged reconstruction. Anteroposterior (C) and lateral (D) radiographs of the knee reveal posttraumatic arthritis and malunion.

was consistent with our preoperative template. Disposable spacer molds using cement mixed with vancomycin and tobramycin were utilized to create the femoral and tibial components (Fig. 9.7). Care was taken to avoid oversizing the spacer to prevent undue tension on the wound closure. Calcium sulfate beads mixed with vancomycin and tobramycin were placed within the joint. A thorough, layered wound closure was performed. A negative pressure wound dressing was applied. Postoperatively, the patient was made touch-toe weight bearing with use of a walker. Postoperative cultures grew out *Cutibacterium acnes*. Infectious disease consultants recommended a 6-week course of intravenous antibiotics.

TKA Procedure

Prior to implantation of the TKA implants, the knee was aspirated after a 2-week antibiotic holiday. Cultures from this aspiration were negative. Three months after the cement spacer placement, the incisions were healed. Knee range of motion was restricted to 45 degrees of flexion, and her extensor mechanism remained intact. One additional aspiration of the knee was performed prior to the surgical date, again verifying no evidence of intraarticular infection. Inflammatory markers had normalized.

The previous midline incision and medial parapatellar arthrotomy were utilized. The knee was noted to be extremely stiff, and visualization was impaired due to difficulty subluxing the patella. Given that we had planned for a hinged prosthesis, we extensively released the soft-tissue attachments from the medial and lateral epicondyles in order to gain visualization of the joint without injuring the extensor mechanism. A tibial tubercle osteotomy was not required. The antibiotic spacer was removed using an osteotome. An osseous debridement was performed on all cut bony surfaces using a burr. The intramedullary canals were reamed with flexible reamers. The intramedullary canals and joints were irrigated with dilute betadine followed by a copious amount of saline irrigation. We then brought in new drapes and performed a glove and gown change prior to bringing in our clean set-up trays for reconstruction.

The tibial diaphysis was prepared for a diaphyseal fitting press-fit stem in order to bypass the previous fracture site and most distal screw holes. An additional 2 mm of proximal tibia was cut to freshen the surface for the planned implant. A fibrous union was noted at the proximal tibial metaphysis, resulting in a malaligned position of the metaphysis relative to the diaphysis. A stem offset

Continued

CASE STUDY 9.1—CONT'D

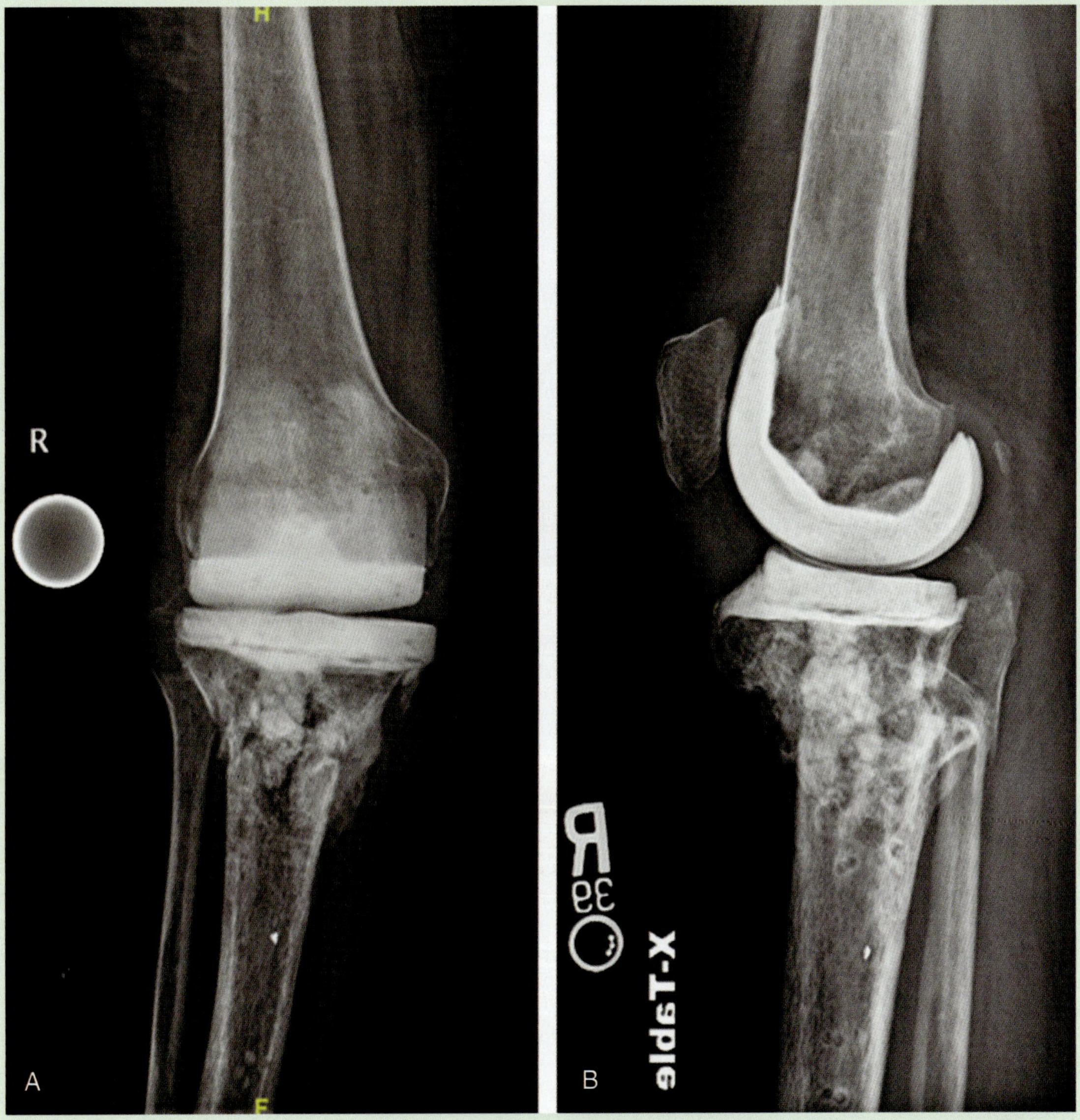

Fig. 9.7 Anteroposterior (A) and lateral (B) radiographs of a patient who has undergone antibiotic cement spacer placement for planned two-stage implant reconstruction in the setting of infection. Disposable spacer molds were utilized to create this articulating antibiotic cement spacer.

CASE STUDY 9.1—CONT'D

coupler was required in order to appropriately place the tibial component. Tibial augments were required both medially and laterally to preserve the joint line. Attention was then turned to femoral preparation. Femoral cuts were revisited to freshen the cut surfaces. Given the constraint of the hinged implant, a long stem was prepared. Following all cuts for the femoral component, trials were placed and insert thickness was selected based on soft-tissue tensioning. The patella was cut and prepared based on a measured cut. The knee was found to achieve full extension and 105 degrees of flexion with normal patellar tracking.

Trial components were removed. A tourniquet was inflated prior to cement preparation. A hybrid cement fixation technique was used for the tibial component. The stem was press-fit, and cement was used from the level of the offset coupler to the tibial tray. The femoral and patellar components were then cemented into place. Once the cement had cured, the hinge mechanism was constructed using the appropriate insert size. The knee was noted to be stable, and range of motion was recreated. A final irrigation was performed. Calcium sulfate beads containing vancomycin and tobramycin were placed into the joint prior to wound closure (Fig. 9.8). A negative pressure wound dressing was applied. Postoperatively, the patient was allowed to fully weight-bear, and full range of motion was encouraged.

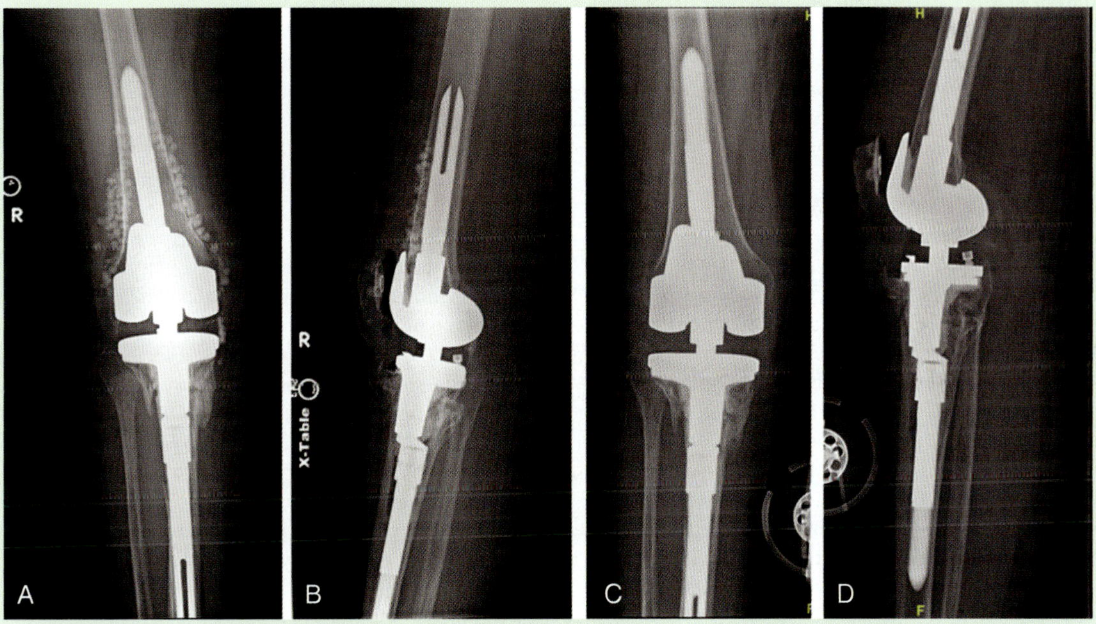

Fig. 9.8 Anteroposterior (A) and lateral (B) postoperative radiographs after spacer removal and hinged total knee implant reconstruction. Hybrid implant fixation was performed. Calcium sulfate beads containing vancomycin and tobramycin were placed prior to wound closure for infection prophylaxis, given the history of infection. At 3 months postoperatively, the anteroposterior (C) and lateral (D) knee radiographs show a well-fixed and well-aligned total knee arthroplasty. The calcium sulfate beads have resorbed and are no longer visible on imaging.

SASSOON'S TIPS AND TRICKS

- Prepare plans A, B, and C during these difficult cases. Implants with varying levels of constraint need to be available in the operating room.
- Exposure is key to preventing injury to the extensor mechanism. If you are unable to obtain adequate visualization, a tibial tubercle osteotomy should be considered.
- When the collateral ligaments are incompetent from past injury, the soft-tissue attachments around the femur and tibia can be released as the knee will require a hinged component. These releases may be enough to provide exposure without having to perform a tibial tubercle osteotomy.

REFERENCES

1. Wang Y, Luo C, Zhu Y, et al. Updated three-column concept in surgical treatment for tibial plateau fractures - a prospective cohort study of 287 patients. *Injury*. 2016;47(7):1488–1496.
2. Malviya A, Reed MR, Partington PF. Acute primary total knee arthroplasty for peri-articular knee fractures in patients over 65 years of age. *Injury*. 2011;42(11):1368–1371.
3. Ali AM, El-Shafie M, Willett KM. Failure of fixation of tibial plateau fractures. *J Orthop Trauma*. 2002;16(5):323–329.
4. Rozell JC, Vemulapalli KC, Gary JL, Donegan DJ. Tibial plateau fractures in elderly patients. *Geriatr Orthop Surg Rehabil*. 2016;7(3):126–134.
5. Bohm ER, Tufescu TV, Marsh JP. The operative management of osteoporotic fractures of the knee: to fix or replace? *J Bone Joint Surg Br*. 2012;94(9):1160–1169.
6. Seo H, Lee GJ, Shon HC, et al. Factors affecting compliance with weight-bearing restriction and the amount of weight-bearing in the elderly with femur or pelvic fractures. *Ann Rehabil Med*. 2020;44(2):109–116.
7. Parratte S, Ollivier M, Argenson JN. Primary total knee arthroplasty for acute fracture around the knee. *Orthop Traumatol Surg Res*. 2018;104(1S):S71–S80.
8. Wong MT, Bourget-Murray J, Johnston K, Desy NM. Understanding the role of total knee arthroplasty for primary treatment of tibial plateau fracture: a systematic review of the literature. *J Orthop Traumatol*. 2020;21(1):7.
9. Scuderi GR, Bourne RB, Noble PC, Benjamin JB, Lonner JH, Scott WN. The new Knee Society Knee Scoring System. *Clin Orthop Relat Res*. 2012;470(1):3–19.
10. Haufe T, Förch S, Müller P, Plath J, Mayr E. The role of a primary arthroplasty in the treatment of proximal tibia fractures in orthogeriatric patients. *Biomed Res Int*. 2016;2016:6047876.
11. Pitta M, Esposito CI, Li Z, Lee YY, Wright TM, Padgett DE. Failure after modern total knee arthroplasty: a prospective study of 18,065 knees. *J Arthroplasty*. 2018;33(2):407–414.
12. Stannard JP, Lopez R, Volgas D. Soft tissue injury of the knee after tibial plateau fractures. *J Knee Surg*. 2010;23(4):187–192.
13. Hsu J, Pappas N, Lee GC. A systematic approach to simultaneous periarticular fracture fixation and primary non-hinged knee replacement in patients with comminuted periarticular fractures about the knee. *Curr Orthop Pract*. 2011;22(6):567 572.
14. Anderson JA, Sculco TP. Implant selection in revision total knee replacement. *Techn Orthop*. 2011;26(2):94–98.
15. Samson AJ, Hamilton DF, Loh B, MacPherson G, Burnett R. Optimizing posterior condylar offset and joint line restoration in revision total knee arthroplasty using a contemporary implant system. *Techn Orthop*. 2019;34(2):e5–e8.
16. Stevenson I, McMillan TE, Baliga S, Schemitsch EH. Primary and secondary total knee arthroplasty for tibial plateau fractures. *J Am Acad Orthop Surg*. 2018;26(11):386–395.
17. Pinter Z, Jha AJ, McGee A, et al. Outcomes of knee replacement in patients with posttraumatic arthritis due to previous tibial plateau fracture. *Eur J Orthop Surg Traumatol*. 2020;30(2):323–328.
18. Dy CJ, Marx RG, Bozic KJ, Pan TJ, Padgett DE, Lyman S. Risk factors for revision within 10 years of total knee arthroplasty. *Clin Orthop Relat Res*. 2014;472(4):1198–1207.

19. Saleh KJ, Sherman P, Katkin P, et al. Total knee arthroplasty after open reduction and internal fixation of fractures of the tibial plateau: a minimum five-year follow-up study. *J Bone Joint Surg Am.* 2001;83(8):1144–1148.
20. Parratte S, Boyer P, Piriou P, et al. Total knee replacement following intra-articular malunion. *Orthop Traumatol Surg Res.* 2011;97(suppl 6):S118–S123.
21. Scott CE, Davidson E, MacDonald DJ, White TO, Keating JF. Total knee arthroplasty following tibial plateau fracture: a matched cohort study. *Bone Joint J.* 2015;97-B(4):532–538.
22. Shearer DW, Chow V, Bozic KJ, Liu J, Ries MD. The predictors of outcome in total knee arthroplasty for post-traumatic arthritis. *Knee.* 2013;20(6): 432–436.
23. Abdel MP, von Roth P, Cross WW, Berry DJ, Trousdale RT, Lewallen DG. Total knee arthroplasty in patients with a prior tibial plateau fracture: a long-term report at 15 Years. *J Arthroplasty.* 2015;30(12): 2170–2172.
24. Chan DB, Jeffcoat DM, Lorich DG, Helfet DL. Nonunions around the knee joint. *Int Orthop.* 2010;34(2):271–281.
25. Kress KJ, Scuderi GR, Windsor RE, Insall JN. Treatment of nonunions about the knee utilizing custom total knee arthroplasty with press-fit intramedullary stems. *J Arthroplasty.* 1993;8(1):49–55.
26. Lizaur-Utrilla A, Collados-Maestre I, Miralles-Muñoz FA, Lopez-Prats FA. Total knee arthroplasty for osteoarthritis secondary to fracture of the tibial plateau. A prospective matched cohort study. *J Arthroplasty.* 2015;30(8):1328–1332.
27. Wasserstein D, Henry P, Paterson JM, Kreder HJ, Jenkinson R. Risk of total knee arthroplasty after operatively treated tibial plateau fracture: a matched-population-based cohort study. *J Bone Joint Surg Am.* 2014;96(2):144–150.
28. Roffi RP, Merritt PO. Total knee replacement after fractures about the knee. *Orthop Rev.* 1990;19(7): 614–620.
29. Marczak D, Synder M, Sibiński M, Okoń T, Kowalczewski J. One-stage total knee arthroplasty with pre-existing fracture deformity: post-fracture total knee arthroplasty. *J Arthroplasty.* 2014;29(11): 2104–2108.
30. Tigani D, Masetti G, Sabbioni G, Ben Ayad R, Filanti M, Fosco M. Computer-assisted surgery as indication of choice: total knee arthroplasty in case of retained hardware or extra-articular deformity. *Int Orthop.* 2012;36(7):1379–1385.
31. Pinter Z, Jha AJ, McGee A, et al. Outcomes of knee replacement in patients with posttraumatic arthritis due to previous tibial plateau fracture. *Eur J Orthop Surg Traumatol.* 2020;30(2):323–328.
32. Suzuki G, Saito S, Ishii T, Motojima S, Tokuhashi Y, Ryu J. Previous fracture surgery is a major risk factor of infection after total knee arthroplasty. *Knee Surg Sports Traumatol Arthrosc.* 2011;19(12): 2040–2044.
33. Manrique J, Rasouli MR, Restrepo C, et al. Total knee arthroplasty in patients with retention of prior hardware material: what is the outcome? *Arch Bone Jt Surg.* 2018;6(1):23–26.
34. Osei DA, Rebehn KA, Boyer MI. Soft-tissue defects after total knee arthroplasty: management and reconstruction. *J Am Acad Orthop Surg.* 2016;24(11):769–779.
35. Tanzer M, Makhdom AM. Preoperative planning in primary total knee arthroplasty. *J Am Acad Orthop Surg.* 2016;24(4):220–230.
36. Kang SG, Park CH, Song SJ. Stem fixation in revision total knee arthroplasty: indications, stem dimensions, and fixation methods. *Knee Surg Relat Res.* 2018;30(3): 187–192.
37. Phen HM, Schenker ML. Minimizing posttraumatic osteoarthritis after high-energy intra-articular fracture. *Orthop Clin North Am.* 2019;50(4):433–443.
38. Deschamps G, Chol C. Fixed-bearing unicompartmental knee arthroplasty. Patients' selection and operative technique. *Orthop Traumatol Surg Res.* 2011;97(6). 648–661.
39. Kuipers BM, Kollen BJ, Bots PC, et al. Factors associated with reduced early survival in the Oxford phase III medial unicompartment knee replacement. *Knee.* 2010;17(1):48–52.
40. Greco NJ, Lombardi Jr AV, Price AJ, Berend ME, Berend KR. Medial mobile-bearing unicompartmental knee arthroplasty in young patients aged less than or equal to 50 years. *J Arthroplasty.* 2018;33(8):2435–2439.
41. Lustig S, Parratte S, Magnussen RA, Argenson JN, Neyret P. Lateral unicompartmental knee arthroplasty relieves pain and improves function in posttraumatic osteoarthritis. *Clin Orthop Relat Res.* 2012;470(1):69–76.
42. Ollivier M, Abdel MP, Parratte S, Argenson JN. Lateral unicondylar knee arthroplasty (UKA): contemporary indications, surgical technique, and results. *Int Orthop.* 2014;38(2):449–455.

43. Romagnoli S, Vitale JA, Marullo M. Outcomes of lateral unicompartmental knee arthroplasty in post-traumatic osteoarthritis, a retrospective comparative study. *Int Orthop*. 2020;44(11):2321–2328.

44. Sah AP, Scott RD. Lateral unicompartmental knee arthroplasty through a medial approach. Surgical technique. *J Bone Joint Surg Am*. 2008;90(suppl 2, pt 2):195–205.

INDEX

Page numbers followed by '*f*' indicate figures, those followed by '*t*' indicate tables, and '*b*' indicate boxes.